Pediatric Palliative Care

Pediatric Palliative Care

Special Issue Editor

Stefan J. Friedrichsdorf

MDPI • Basel • Beijing • Wuhan • Barcelona • Belgrade

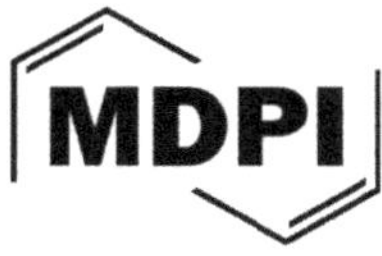

Special Issue Editor
Stefan J. Friedrichsdorf, MD, FAAP
Department of Pain Medicine, Palliative Care & Integrative Medicine,
Children's Hospitals and Clinics of Minnesota
Minneapolis, Minnesota, USA

Editorial Office
MDPI
St. Alban-Anlage 66
4052 Basel, Switzerland

This is a reprint of articles from the Special Issue published online in the open access journal *Children* (ISSN 2227-9067) from 2017 to 2018 (available at: https://www.mdpi.com/journal/children/special_issues/palliative_care)

For citation purposes, cite each article independently as indicated on the article page online and as indicated below:

LastName, A.A.; LastName, B.B.; LastName, C.C. Article Title. *Journal Name* **Year**, *Article Number*, Page Range.

ISBN 978-3-03897-350-8 (Pbk)
ISBN 978-3-03897-351-5 (PDF)

Cover image courtesy of a boy with serious illness: *"PAIN. Once I felt as if an I.V. was exploding in my arm!"*
The child then described the excruciating pain he had felt when someone tripped over his IV pole that then came crashing down. The boldly colored, nightmarish image with foreboding slashes of black conveys the extreme pain and the associated anxiety. and vulnerability. At the bottom of the picture—totally overwhelmed by the chaos—is his arm, the site of the pain.

Contents

About the Special Issue Editor

Stefan J. Friedrichsdorf, MD, FAAP is an Asssociate Professor of Pediatrics at the University of Minnesota and the medical director of the Department of Pain Medicine, Palliative Care and Integrative Medicine at Children's Hospitals and Clinics in Minnesota, Minneapolis/St. Paul (USA) —one of the largest and most comprehensive programs of its kind in the country. He is the president-elect of the Special Interest Group on Pain in Childhood of the International Association for the Study of Pain (IASP). The interdisciplinary pain program is devoted to prevent and treat acute, procedural, neuropathic, psycho-social-spiritual, visceral, and persistent pain for all pediatric patients in close collaboration with all subspecialties at Children's Minnesota. The palliative care team provides holistic care for pediatric patients with life-limiting diseases and adds an extra layer of support to the care of children with serious illness and their families. Integrative Medicine provides and teaches integrative, non-pharmacological therapies (such as massage, acupuncture/acupressure, biofeedback, aromatherapy, self-hypnosis) to provide care that promotes optimal health and supports the highest level of functioning in all individual child's activities. Dr. Friedrichsdorf sees pediatric patients as inpatients, in the interdisciplinary pain clinic, or in the palliative care clinic. He is the sponsor of the system-wide lean value stream "The Comfort Promise: We do everything possible to prevent and treat pain" at Children's Minnesota to minimize and prevent pain caused by needles for all in- and outpatients, reaching more than 200,000 children annually. In 2015 the department opened an award winning, unique 10,000 square feet "Healing Environment" Pain, Palliative and Integrative Medicine Clinic. Dr. Friedrichsdorf received the 2016 "Elizabeth Narcessian Award for Outstanding Educational Achievements in the Field of Pain" by the American Pain Society and the 2011 "Hastings Center Cunniff-Dixon Physician Award". The department received the "Circle of Life Award" by the American Hospital Association in 2008, was selected as a Palliative Care Leadership Center for the Center to Advance Palliative Care (CAPC) 2008-2015, and the 2013 recipient of the "Clinical Centers of Excellence in Pain Management Award" by the American Pain Society. In 2016 Children's Minnesota received the prestigious ChildKind International pain relief certification. He is associate editor of the Journal of Pain and Symptom Management, the principal investigator of a 2010–2017 National Institutes of Health (NIH) / National Cancer Institute (NCI) multisite study on the creation, implementation and evaluation of a Pediatric Palliative Care Curriculum (EPEC-Pediatrics) and he founded and continues to direct the annual Pediatric Pain Master Class, a week-long intensive interdisciplinary course for health professionals. Dr. Friedrichsdorf has presented more than 650 lectures about pediatric pain medicine and palliative care in 28 countries on all six continents and has a track record of research and publications in the field, including contributions to more than 20 books on the subject. Dr. Friedrichsdorf received his MD degree from the Medical University of L übeck, Germany, completed his pediatric residency at the University of Witten/Herdecke, Germany (Children's Hospital in Datteln), and undertook his fellowship in Pediatric Pain & Palliative Care at the University of Sydney, Australia (Children's Hospital at Westmead). He is board certified in Pediatrics, a Fellow of the American Academy of Pediatrics and trained in hypnosis.

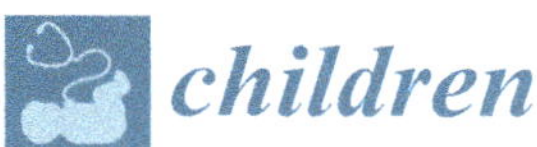

MDPI

Editorial

Delivering Pediatric Palliative Care: From Denial, Palliphobia, Pallilalia to Palliactive

Stefan J. Friedrichsdorf [1,2,*] and Eduardo Bruera [3]

1 Children's Hospitals and Clinics of Minnesota, 2525 Chicago Ave S, Minneapolis, MN 55403, USA
2 University of Minnesota Medical School, 420 Delaware Street SE, Minneapolis, MN 55455, USA
3 Department of Palliative Care and Rehabilitation Medicine, The University of Texas, MD Anderson Cancer Center, 1515 Holcombe Blvd., Houston, TX 77030, USA; ebruera@mdanderson.org
* Correspondence: stefan.friedrichsdorf@childrensMN.org; Tel.: +1-612-813-7888; Fax: +1-612-813-7199

Received: 23 August 2018; Accepted: 28 August 2018; Published: 31 August 2018

Abstract: Among the over 21 million children with life-limiting conditions worldwide that would benefit annually from a pediatric palliative care (PPC) approach, more than eight million would need specialized PPC services. In the United States alone, more than 42,000 children die every year, half of them infants younger than one year. Advanced interdisciplinary pediatric palliative care for children with serious illnesses is now an expected standard of pediatric medicine. Unfortunately, in many institutions there remain significant barriers to achieving optimal care related to lack of formal education, reimbursement issues, the emotional impact of caring for a dying child, and most importantly, the lack of interdisciplinary PPC teams with sufficient staffing and funding. Data reveals the majority of distressing symptoms in children with serious illness (such as pain, dyspnea and nausea/vomiting) were not addressed during their end-of-life period, and when treated, therapy was commonly ineffective. Whenever possible, treatment should focus on continued efforts to control the underlying illness. At the same time, children and their families should have access to interdisciplinary care aimed at promoting optimal physical, psychological and spiritual wellbeing. Persistent myths and misconceptions have led to inadequate symptom control in children with life-limiting diseases. Pediatric Palliative Care advocates the provision of comfort care, pain, and symptom management concurrently with disease-directed treatments. Families no longer have to opt for one over the other. They can pursue both, and include integrative care to maximize the child's quality of life. Since most of the sickest children with serious illness are being taken care of in a hospital, every children's hospital is now expected to offer an interdisciplinary palliative care service as the standard of care. This article addresses common myths and misconceptions which may pose clinical obstacles to effective PPC delivery and discusses the four typical stages of pediatric palliative care program implementation.

Keywords: pediatric palliative care; program development; barriers; hospice; myths; program implementation

---

1. Introduction

The special edition "Pediatric Palliative Care" in *Children* (http://www.mdpi.com/journal/children/special_issues/palliative_care) has collated 20 outstanding articles from many of the leading pediatric palliative care researchers and clinicians worldwide allowing us to present an overview of advances, research, and challenges in pediatric palliative care (PPC). As the guest editor, I thank the authors for their strong contributions to this edition, in assisting children with serious illness and their families, as well as to moving our field further along.

Over 21 million children 0–19 years would benefit annually from a palliative care approach worldwide, more than eight million needing specialized PPC [1,2]. In the United States alone, more than

42,000 children died in 2013, fifty-five percent of them infants younger than one year [3]. The leading causes of pediatric deaths include accidents (7645 children), suicide (2143), and homicide (2021). Leading life-limiting conditions include congenital malformations and chromosomal abnormalities (5740) followed by malignancies (1850). Minorities, such as Latinos, appear to have higher barriers to accessing PPC [4].

PPC is about matching treatment to patient goals and is considered specialized medical care for children with serious illness. It is focused on relieving pain, distressing symptoms, and stress of a serious illness and appropriate at any age and at any stage, together with curative treatment. The primary goal is to improve quality of life for both the child and his or her family. In the words of an ill child: "Palliative care no longer means helping children die well, it means helping children and their families to live well, and then, when the time is certain, to help them die gently." (Mattie Stepanek, 1990–2007). Sadly, advances in the control of symptoms in children dying of diseases such as cancer have not kept pace with treatment directed at curing the underlying disease. The majority of distressing symptoms in children with advanced cancer (such as pain, dyspnea and nausea/vomiting) were not treated, and when treated, therapy was commonly ineffective [5–9].

In this editorial we will address the four steps of PPC program implementation [10], followed by an evaluation of common assumptions, myths and barriers, which may hinder the implementation of PPC into the care of a child or teenager with serious illnesses [11,12].

2. Implementing Institutional Change: The Four Stages of PPC Program Implementation

Although the majority of children's hospitals in the United States do have a pediatric palliative care program, most of them appear to be understaffed and underfunded. A survey by Feudtner et al. in 2013 among 226 US children's hospitals (of which 162 responded) showed that 112 (69% of respondents; at least 49.6% of all children's hospitals) have PPC program [13]. However, most programs offer only inpatient services, and most only during the work week.

A universal reality is that, overwhelmingly, in places where palliative care has not existed before, will require major cultural adaptation [10]. We have adapted the following four stages, initially described by Bruera in 2004 [10], to pediatric palliative care program implementation.

2.1. Stage 1: Denial

Clinical leaders suggesting the implementation of a new PPC program in a pediatric institution are very likely to face significant denial by clinical colleagues and hospital executives, who may not be aware of the need for a PPC program. Often, there are limited or no measurement of the amount of physical and emotional distress suffered by children and their families with serious illness. The limited documentation on the need of PPC is complicated by perceptions (which are unfortunately not based on reality) such as "Our patients here usually have very good symptom control" or "We here at ... " (insert the name of any pediatric primary service or subspecialty here) " ... already got it and we cover everything and don't need an extra palliative care service."

An important approach to expect and address denial, would be to carefully and rapidly document the level of unmet need in patients and families in the pediatric institution, including in the patients under care by individuals, who are in denial. Simple surveys of uncontrolled symptoms or emotional distress might be extremely useful. Parents' testaments, in writing or in a short movie clip, might be particularly helpful to overcome denial during a presentation to colleagues and leadership.

2.2. Stage 2: Palliphobia

The second stage of PPC program implementation in a pediatric institution can be best described as the recognition that there is a problem, but usually this meets consistent fear about consequences of the problem and the possible solutions it entails. Although this might represent fear of the unknown, it is not unheard of that sometimes people react with great anger towards it. In fact, many individuals can react in negative way to developing a PPC team. Physicians, nurse practitioners and other health professionals may feel their professional competence is being questioned or even threatened by the new PPC team. In fact, they may be afraid of referring patients to the PPC service because of concerns over criticism of their symptom control, communication or overall treatment strategies they have used for many years. Hospitals executives may be afraid of being found lacking in compassion and holistic care among all the competing priorities in a shifting landscape of pediatric healthcare and scarce funding.

Common phrases PPC teams may hear include "The parents are not ready", "We asked them and they said no" (although surprisingly few parents are asked for permission to include other services, such as infectious disease services),"She is not dying now", "There is always something else we can try", "It is too early", "Hospice? That's wonderful, but that is for other people", "You talking to the family means destroying hope", "We are still fighting".

Unfortunately, further exacerbation of Palliphobia can be expected, if the PPC team tries too hard and/or is too fast in making changes in patient care. After a major confrontation with the neonatologist, oncologist etc. (a.k.a. the bull-in-the-china-shop-strategy—"move aside, the palliative care doctor has arrived ... "), the PPC usually succeeds in changing and improving analgesia, communication strategies or changing discharge planning, but likely will not receive further consults/referrals from this team or unit, resulting in a negative reputation among colleagues in the institution.

A useful technique is to approach a limited number of possible referring clinicians and ask them to become supporters and mentors of the program. Once a significant number of patients have been treated, it is then safe to make a presentation in Grand rounds or Medical staff meetings showing the results, ideally with the presence of the referring clinicians. In absence of data, all opinions (including palliphobic ones) are good, but the presence of data on positive outcomes and testimonials from the initial team of referring clinicians can be very reassuring to those who are still uncommitted to refer patients.

"Palliphobia" is more difficult to overcome than "Denial", and requires disciplined planning and rapid conflict resolution: Useful strategies to overcome this stage may include making great efforts at reassuring the existing clinical pediatric team that the PPC of course will work in an integrated fashion collaboratively with them. Importantly, members of the PPC team will not disqualify their patient care plan, but rather enhance them by focusing on aspects not addressed so far. "How can I help?" is commonly a useful question posed to the primary clinician, followed by a detailed discussion of who does what ("Would you like me to prescribe the methadone, or do you prefer me simply giving recommendations and you take care of it?").

2.3. Stage 3: Pallilalia

A large number of PPC programs worldwide appear to be stuck in the 3rd stage "Pallilalia". Usually about two to four years after implementing a PPC program, repetitive absurdities are spoken about palliative care in general and the PPC program specifically, without anything being done to advance its development. This is in fact the most dangerous stage, as it has a high risk resulting in burnout among PPC professionals.

Hospital leadership and executives describe PPC as "very important" or "a major priority", but actually there's no significant allocation of personnel, space, money, curriculum time etc. Colleagues within the pediatric institution frequently talk about how useful they feel PPC is, and how happy they are with the PPC team, but as a matter of fact refer only small minority of their patients—usually the ones with terrible psycho-social-medical and/or mental health problems. With this attitude, a PPC program is simply financially and administratively not viable.

Children's hospitals at this stage frequently "appoint a committee to discuss PPC", or propose "a major study whether PPC works in our institution" or, suggest the PPC lead applies for external grants, so "funds can be obtained for a pilot program in a year or two". There have also been cases, where hospital leadership decided that the 6-figure donation to the PPC program were used to offset general losses in other departments instead.

Most understaffed PPC programs (commonly lead by a 0.2 FTE physician, who was on-call 24/7 and during his/her vacations), have disappeared at this stage. Clinical colleagues and institutions became used to the beneficial presence of the PPC team, while having made no major commitment to support it.

A useful technique to overcome Pallilalia is to use benchmarks for clinical and time burden that might allow for fair comparisons. While some of the referring teams may see a mix of more and less time demanding encounters, palliative care teams always see time demanding patients and they frequently allow the referring teams to shorten their own encounter with the patients they refer. Therefore, clinical time may be a better measure than number of encounters. Since this is not always easy to measure, one palliative care team compared data from parking records to determine the additional burden on the palliative care team.

It is important to anticipate this developmental stage by gathering data of provided clinical services, number of patients seen, details of teaching conducted, research studies, etc. The PPC team should aim mostly at leaders of hospital and medical schools, rather than just immediate supervisors or peers, when providing documentation of work. They should request, that information be compared to output and resources of other programs within the institution and on a national level. PPC teams may ask for external review by national or international PPC leaders in the field. Sadly, not infrequently, only through resignation of the PPC leader, institutions come to realize that PPC has been badly under-resourced, and start corrective measures during the process of recruiting a successor.

2.4. Stage 4: Palliactive

A PPC program has reached the final level of development, when recognized by robust appointment and funding of professional interdisciplinary team PPC members. It is recommended to seek a designation of an administrative structure equal to oncology or infectious disease programs (department or division). Other important components of this stage include allocation of space, formal curriculum space and medical training program rotations.

PPC is truly recognized when colleagues actively refer patients to PPC and encourage other colleagues to do the same. Unfortunately, regression can happen at any time—frequently due to changes in administrative leadership within the institution. Also, in large children's hospitals on certain units is not unlikely that a robust established PPC team may encounter all four stages on the very same day, depending on which physician they encounter.

3. Common Myths and Misconceptions in Pediatric Palliative Care (PPC)

3.1. Myth 1: PPC Is Primarily for Children with a Malignancy

The majority of children dying of serious illness do not have cancer [14]. In 2013 a total of 42,328 children 0–19 years died in the United States, more than 55% (23,440) of them infants younger than one year [3]. The leading causes of pediatric deaths include accidents (7645 children), suicide (2143), and homicide (2021). In 2015 a total of 11,933 children, adolescents and young adults 0–24 years died due to a life-limiting disease: Leading conditions include congenital malformations and chromosomal abnormalities (5965), followed by malignancies (2688), and heart disease (1354) [15]. Although the prognosis for children with cancer has improved considerably over the last decades, malignancies now remains the leading cause of non-accidental death in childhood only in children older than one year of age. In pediatric cancer units, the presence of "trigger diagnoses" (triggering automatic referral to PPC) increased likelihood of palliative principle introduction 3.4 times ($p < 0.003$) [16].

That said, when providing interdisciplinary PPC services for children, it can be expected that most children do not have a malignancy [17] and about half of the patients would be infants. Despite the great need in neonatology, more than 45% of institution in Canada and the United States not have neonatal comfort care guidelines, and of those reporting institutional neonatal comfort care guidelines, 19.1% do not address pain symptom management [18]. More than 90% of respondents in the same study felt that their institution would benefit from further education and training in neonatal EOL care. Carter elaborates on PPC for babies in his article [19] in this special edition.

3.2. Myth 2: PPC Begins when Curative Treatments Stop

Sometimes clinicians, patients and families incorrectly assume that PPC is only appropriate when all curative treatments are exhausted and discontinued and/or when a child is close to dying. In fact, PPC is recommended to commence at diagnosis of a life-threatening disease, to continue through the trajectory of the illness, and does not equal end-of-life care (but certainly includes it). PPC services extend beyond the child's death to the family during bereavement [20]. Earlier recognition by both physicians and parents that the child had no realistic chance of cure led to a stronger emphasis on treatment to lessen suffering and integrate PPC in pediatric cancer patients [21].

The overall improvement in the prognosis of serious illnesses, and the emotional involvement in trying to save the life of a child may prevent both physicians and parents from discontinuing therapies. The pursuit of such therapy modalities may overshadow attention to advanced prevention and control of distressing symptoms and to quality of life and, which unfortunately may result in increased suffering during child's end-of-life period. However, it is sometimes not possible for parents and/or the child to forgo further disease-directed treatment, and this should not be required in order to achieve optimal palliative care. The need to ensure that everything possible has been done may be the only way that some parents can live and cope with their child's death [22].

The 2010 "Concurrent Care for Children" requirement of the United States Affordable Care Act has this at heart: The 2016 briefing of the Mary J. Labyak Institute for Innovation at the National Center for Care at the End of Life [23] described concurrent care for children with serious illness as follows: "Until 2010, parents in all but a few states in the United States were faced with forgoing curative treatments for their children to be eligible for hospice services. Or conversely, they were not eligible for beneficial interdisciplinary hospice services while getting curative treatment. The Patient Protection and Affordable Care Act (ACA) changed that situation. It requires all state Medicaid programs to pay for both curative and hospice services for children under age 21 who qualify. On 23 March 2010, President Obama signed ACA into law enacting a new provision, Section 2302, termed the "Concurrent Care for Children" Requirement (CCCR). Section 2302 states that a child who is eligible for and receives hospice care must also have all other services provided, or have payment made for, services that are related to the treatment of the child's condition.1 This provision affects children who are eligible for Medicaid or the Children's Health Insurance Program (CHIP). In its simplest form, implementation of this provision could be accomplished by the state Medicaid agency eliminating any provider claims that deny or delay concurrent curative care and hospice claims [23]."

Pediatric oncology providers in a recent survey [24] issued a highly favorable opinion about their institution's PPC service and agreed that early consultation is ideal. However, they report formally consulting PPC is extremely difficult because of what the PPC symbolizes to families and the emotional labor that the oncology provider must manage in introducing them.

3.3. Myth 3: Pediatric Palliative Care Involvement Shortens Life

Clinicians trained in palliative care will never issue a statement such as "There is nothing else we can do". Quite the opposite, advanced PPC teams may say "there is always a lot we can do". Even when the underlying life-limiting disease cannot be cured, sophisticated medical technology will be utilized to improve the quality of life of the child and his and her family and to prevent and treat distressing symptom. As such, PPC is therefore a very active and advanced approach to symptom management and family support.

It appears, that a palliative care consult for patients with serious illness is associated with longer survival and better quality of life: In the ENABLE III study, patients who received early palliative oncology care had significantly longer 1-year survival rates than those who received delayed palliative care [25]. In another innovative randomized controlled trial adults with advanced lung cancer receiving a palliative care intervention (providing appropriate and beneficial treatments) at the point of diagnosis, in fact increased the quality of life, decreased depression, and led to a prolonged life (11.6 months vs. 8.9 months) [26]. These results underscore the need for palliative care early in a serious illness and refute the notion that palliative care means giving up. Patients received palliative care alongside their curative treatment. There is now emerging evidence that the inclusion of PPC specialists improves the outcome of children with advanced serious illnesses, and sometimes represents the means to allows for curative care through advanced symptom management provided by PPC [27]. Children who received pediatric palliative home care were more likely to have fun (70% versus 45%) and to experience events that added meaning to life (89% versus 63%) [9]. In addition, families who received PPC services report improved communication [28] and children receiving PPC experience shorter hospitalizations and fewer emergency department visits [29]. Parents of children with cancer who received PPC reported less distress from pain, dyspnea and anxiety during the end-of-life period [8]. Undertaking research in PPC is inherently difficult, and Nelson et al. in this special issue address this in their article [30].

The advanced pain and symptom management may explain the increase of survival in patients with serious illness enrolled into PPC. Brock et al. describe in this special edition describe emerging methods of symptom and health-related quality-of-life assessment through patient-reported outcomes tools [31]. Data has shown, that distressing pain is very common among inpatients referred to palliative care and three-quarters of patients with pain improve and improvement in pain is associated with other symptom improvement [32]. The involvement of PPC team with adolescent and young adult oncology patients is associated with the receipt of less intensive treatments during the last month of life, such as being on a ventilator, invasive procedures, and fewer deaths in the intensive care unit [33].

Advanced pain management for children with serious illness often requires multimodal analgesia. This describes an approach of utilizing multiple analgesic agents (such as basic analgesia, opioids, adjuvant analgesia), regional anesthesia (such as nerve blocks or neuroaxial analgesia), rehabilitation (such as physical therapy, motor graded imagery), psychological (such as cognitive behavioral therapy) and integrative (formally known as "non-pharmacological") therapies (such as massage, hypnosis) which usually act synergistically for more effective pediatric pain control with fewer side effects than a single analgesic or modality [34–37].

Harlow and Hain [38] explore the concept of total pain in the largest group of children with life-limiting diseases, pediatric patients with severe neurological impairment.

3.4. *Myth 4: PPC Can Only Be Provided Comprehensively within a Children's Hospital*

Currently most children in resource rich countries die in a hospital, most commonly in an intensive care unit. In a recent study [39] reviewing all pediatric intensive care unit (PICU) admissions over 15 months of 89,127 children in the United Kingdom, children with life-limiting conditions constituted 57.6% of all admissions. Of the 4821 children who died on the PICU during that period, 72.9% had a life-limiting condition. Since most of the sickest children with serious illness are being taken care of in a hospital, every children's hospital is now expected to offer an interdisciplinary palliative care service as the standard of care [40].

One of the early PPC pioneers, Dr. Ann Goldman from the Department of Hematology/Oncology at Great Ormond Street in London, UK implemented a "Symptom Care Team," a team of nurses, who were introduced at cancer diagnosis to the child and family. All children received home visits after their first discharge. Children with high-risk cancer or relapses then already knew the "Symptom Care Team", which provided a 24/7 service, from the time of diagnosis. Between 1978–1981, before the implementation of the "Symptom Care Team" only 19% of children with cancer died at home. Then, between 1989–1990, after implementation of the team 77% of the children dying from malignancies did so at home [41].

The death of a child with a serious illness at home may promote better family adjustment and healing [42,43]. This could be related to decrease helplessness and increased family intimacy by being at home. On the other hand, some have reported that family relationships appeared to be better when the child died in the hospital [44]. While it is often suggested that most children prefer to die at home, this has actually not been systematically evaluated.

Parents of terminally ill children often wish for home care [45,46], and there is a not surprisingly a positive correlation between availability of palliative home care and the number of children dying at home [9,47–49]. The interdisciplinary PPC Team involvement in compassionate extubation at home has been explored by Postier et al. in this special issue [50]. Most families regard caring for their dying child as a positive experience [45]. It is critically important to discuss preferences regarding the primary location of care as early as possible. A parental decision to care for their terminally ill child at home involves consideration of medical, psychological, social and cultural factors together with such practical considerations as the availability of respite care, physician access, and financial resources. Children with advanced cancer who also received PPC home care or hospice were significantly more likely to have fun (70% versus 45%), experience events that added meaning to life (89% versus 63%), and to die at home (93% versus 20%) [9]. Whatever the decision is regarding the primary location of care, families should be reassured that they can change from one option to another and that the primary team will remain closely involved [45].

There appears to be a growing consensus of most pediatric palliative care specialists, that advanced PPC for children with serious illness needs to be offered and coordinated primarily by an interdisciplinary team within tertiary pediatric hospitals, aided by an outpatient PPC clinic and must include a palliative home care service [51]. When these services are in place (but not instead), a freestanding hospice and respite house represents an excellent addition (but not substitution) of the services provided inpatient, in clinic, and at home. The World Health Organization (WHO) describes that palliative care can be provided in tertiary care facilities, in outpatient clinics, in community health and hospice centers, and in children's homes [52].

A key component of family support, in addition to addressing the needs of the sick child [53], must be geared toward the siblings [54,55] and parents/caregivers [56].

3.5. Myth 5: Patients and Their Parents Need to Make a Choice between "Fighting for a Cure" or "to Give up Hope"

Even when there might not be a realistic hope for cure, pediatric patients with a serious illness and their parents may opt for continued disease directed treatment [21]. This might be motivated by the desire to extend life, to palliate symptoms related to progressive disease, or the hope for a miracle. In discussions of treatment options with families, one might choose statements, as suggested by Wolfe, such as "The very nature of miracles is that they are rare. However, we have seen miracles, and they have occurred both on and off treatment" [57]. In other words, a child does not have to continue on disease-directed therapy in order to preserve hope, especially when the therapy significantly impacts the child's remaining quality of life. In fact, a large adult study could demonstrate that chemotherapy for end-stage cancer does not prolong life, however reduces the quality of life [58].

Caring for a child at end-of-life is emotionally very difficult. It may be particularly challenging for clinicians and parents to consider the early integration of PPC because this may be perceived as 'giving up'. As a result, the emotional cost of the recognition that a child may die could impede planning for optimal pain and symptom management and psycho-social-spiritual support. In fact, the "hope for cure" and "pediatric palliative care" include and complement each other. PPC translates into advanced management to maintain or improve quality of life and children can graduate from PPC. No matter the treatment goals, despite the prevailing myth, disease-directed care and excellent symptom relief must and can be provided simultaneously.

Date has shown that the integration of PPC explicitly does not result in giving up hope. Engaging in advanced care planning increases the patients knowledge without diminishing hope, increasing hopelessness, nor inducing anxiety in patients with advanced cancer [59]. The disclosure of a terminal prognosis does not mean loss of patient hope: Instead, hope was redefined on a goal other than cure [60]. In pediatrics, there is no evidence that prognostic disclosure makes parents less hopeful.

Instead, the disclosure of a prognosis by physician can support hope, even when prognosis is poor [61]. Parents who are upset by prognostic information are no less likely to want it. The upsetting nature of prognostic information does not diminish parents' desire for such information, its importance to decision making, or parents' sense of hope [62].

During a goals of care discussion with a family of child with a serious illness, a question such as "Considering what your child is up against, what are you hoping for?" may be posed by the clinician. Not surprisingly, the response may be "Cure from the disease" or "A miracle". The clinician may then respond "I hope this too. Just in case the disease cannot be cured—What else are you hoping for?" By exploring the extend of hope further, families may wish for very advanced treatment and prevention of pain and distressing symptoms, the possibility to go home, for grandmother to visit, to hold their child more often, or many other things. Blazin et al. in this special edition explore how to translate evidence into practice and communicate effectively [30]. Even when the underlying condition cannot be cured, PPC will never give up hope. Sometimes, it appears that the best chance for these children to truly live is for their parents and treating clinicians to accept the fact that this child might die [63]. Not surprisingly, data reveals, that religion, spirituality or life-philosophy play an important role in the life of most parents whose children receiving PPC [64].

3.6. Myth 6: Administering Morphine Causes Respiratory Depression and Hastens Death

To paraphrase Sykes [65] "Morphine kills the pain, not the patient. A physician killing a patient in name of pain or dyspnea relief is not merciful, just incompetent." An enduring misconception is the belief that in the management of pain and dyspnea, opioids will hasten death and should only be administered as a last resort. This was contradicted in the adult literature [66] and our PPC teams commonly observe that administering opioids and/or benzodiazepines, together with comfort care to relieve dyspnea and pain, not only improves the child's quality of life, but also prolongs life [67]. A retrospective cohort study (n = 223 adult oncologic patients) reviewing the mean survival in relation to opioid use found less than a two-fold increase in their initial opioid dose resulted in 9 days survival, and more than a two-fold increase in 22 days survival [68].

One of the most common sources of pain and distress in children is visceral hyperalgesia and feeding intolerance, addressed by Hauer in this Special Issue [69].

3.7. Myth 7: PPC Teams Are Too Expensive

A pediatric palliative care team is now expected standard of practice in every children's hospital. Every single one of the "U.S. News & World Report honor roll children's hospitals" have palliative care teams [70]. Overwhelming evidence now demonstrates, that children's hospitals in fact cannot afford to *not* have a PPC team anymore. PPC team basically "grease the wheels" of a clinical institution, such as reducing burnout and as a result staff turn-over among pediatric staff. For instance, in the United States more than 30% of all new nurses elect either to change positions or leaving nursing completely within the first 3 years of clinical practice [71]. Leading reasons include emotional distress related to patient care. The average cost of turnover for a bedside nurse ranges from $36,900 to $57,300, resulting in the average hospital losing $4.9 million–$7.6 million per year. Each percent reduction in nursing turnover will cost/safe the average hospital an additional $379,500 [72]. PPC services can help reducing turnover and improving overall job satisfaction and performance important in to assuring patient and family satisfaction while promoting quality care.

In addition to providing advanced clinical care, pediatric palliative care services are also cost-effective (although arguably not a single PPC team member worldwide provides clinical care "to safe money" to the institutions or health insurers, but rather, because it provides superior clinical care to children with advanced serious illnesses. PPC involvement results in better outcomes and lower costs: Palliative care program reduces stress, costs of care for children with life-threatening conditions [73–75]. A retrospective study of 425 children receiving pediatric palliative home care in the US comparing pediatric hospital resource utilization before and after PPC enrollment decreased in non-cancer patients the length-of-hospital-stay by 38 days and decreased hospital charges $ 275,000 per patient [76].

4. Conclusions

Despite significant growth and advances over the last two decades, a large number of children's hospitals currently either do not have a PPC service, or it significantly under-resourced and underfunded. When implementing a PPC service, the development often goes through four steps in their development. These should be anticipated, and an action plan might include

- **Denial**: Document unmet needs, undertake surveys among staff, patients and providers
- **Palliphobia**: Close collaboration with colleagues; disciplined planning, rapid conflict resolution
- **Pallilalia**: Documentation of PPC value to leadership; grand rounds by expert in field and external review
- **Palliactive**: "Do good & talk about it", perform QI, evaluate value of PPC in ACO/bundled payments environment; include clinical and administrative innovators in program development
- **Secure funding:** "Make sure your passion is connected with somebody's payment system"

High-quality pediatric palliative care for children with serious illnesses is now an expected standard of medicine. However, even in resource-rich settings, there remain significant barriers to achieving optimal care related to lack of formal education, reimbursement issues, the emotional impact of caring for a dying child, and most importantly the lack of interdisciplinary PPC teams with sufficient staffing. Whenever possible, treatment should focus on continued efforts to control the underlying illness. At the same time, children and their families should have access to interdisciplinary care aimed at promoting optimal physical, psychological and spiritual wellbeing. Persistent myths and misconceptions have led to inadequate symptom control in children with life-limiting diseases. Pediatric Palliative Care advocates the provision of comfort care, pain, and symptom management concurrently with disease-directed treatments. Families no longer have to opt for one. They can pursue both, and include integrative care to maximize the child's quality of life.

Conflicts of Interest: The authors declare no conflict of interest.

References

1. Connor, S.R.; Downing, J.; Marston, J. Estimating the Global Need for Palliative Care for Children: A Cross-sectional Analysis. *J. Pain Symptom Manag.* **2017**, *53*, 171–177. [CrossRef] [PubMed]
2. Downing, J.; Boucher, S.; Daniels, A.; Nkosi, B. Paediatric Palliative Care in Resource-Poor Countries. *Children (Basel)* **2018**, *5*, 27. [CrossRef] [PubMed]
3. Osterman, M.J.; Kochanek, K.D.; MacDorman, M.F.; Strobino, D.M.; Guyer, B. Annual summary of vital statistics: 2012–2013. *Pediatrics* **2015**, *135*, 1115–1125. [CrossRef] [PubMed]
4. Munoz-Blanco, S.; Raisanen, J.C.; Donohue, P.K.; Boss, R.D. Enhancing Pediatric Palliative Care for Latino Children and Their Families: A Review of the Literature and Recommendations for Research and Practice in the United States. *Children (Basel)* **2017**, *5*, 2. [CrossRef] [PubMed]
5. Wolfe, J.; Grier, H.E.; Klar, N.; Levin, S.B.; Ellenbogen, J.M.; Salem-Schatz, S.; Emanuel, E.J.; Weeks, J.C. Symptoms and suffering at the end of life in children with cancer. *N. Engl. J. Med.* **2000**, *342*, 326–333. [CrossRef] [PubMed]
6. Hechler, T.; Blankenburg, M.; Friedrichsdorf, S.J.; Garske, D.; Hubner, B.; Menke, A.; Wamsler, C.; Wolfe, J.; Zernikow, B. Parents' perspective on symptoms, quality of life, characteristics of death and end-of-life decisions for children dying from cancer. *Klin. Padiatr.* **2008**, *220*, 166–174. [CrossRef] [PubMed]
7. Wolfe, J.; Orellana, L.; Ullrich, C.; Cook, E.F.; Kang, T.I.; Rosenberg, A.; Geyer, R.; Feudtner, C.; Dussel, V. Symptoms and Distress in Children with Advanced Cancer: Prospective Patient-Reported Outcomes from the PediQUEST Study. *J. Clin. Oncol.* **2015**, *33*, 1928–1935. [CrossRef] [PubMed]
8. Wolfe, J.; Hammel, J.F.; Edwards, K.E.; Duncan, J.; Comeau, M.; Breyer, J.; Aldridge, S.A.; Grier, H.E.; Berde, C.; Dussel, V.; et al. Easing of suffering in children with cancer at the end of life: Is care changing? *J. Clin. Oncol.* **2008**, *26*, 1717–1723. [CrossRef] [PubMed]

9. Friedrichsdorf, S.J.; Postier, A.; Dreyfus, J.; Osenga, K.; Sencer, S.; Wolfe, J. Improved quality of life at end of life related to home-based palliative care in children with cancer. *J. Palliat. Med.* **2015**, *18*, 143–150. [CrossRef] [PubMed]
10. Bruera, E. The development of a palliative care culture. *J. Palliat. Care* **2004**, *20*, 316–319. [PubMed]
11. Friedrichsdorf, S.J.; Zeltzer, L. Palliative Care for Children with Advanced Cancer. In *Pediatric Psycho-Oncology: Psychosocial Aspects and Clinical Interventions*, 2nd ed.; Kreitler, S., Ben-Arush, M.W., Martin, A., Eds.; John Wiley & Sons, Ltd.: Hoboken, NJ, USA, 2012; pp. 160–174.
12. Friedrichsdorf, S.J. Contemporary Pediatric Palliative Care: Myths and Barriers to Integration into Clinical Care. *Curr. Pediatr. Rev.* **2017**, *13*, 8–12. [CrossRef] [PubMed]
13. Feudtner, C.; Womer, J.; Augustin, R.; Remke, S.; Wolfe, J.; Friebert, S.; Weissman, D. Pediatric palliative care programs in children's hospitals: A cross-sectional national survey. *Pediatrics* **2013**, *132*, 1063–1070. [CrossRef] [PubMed]
14. Feudtner, C. Deaths Attributed to Pediatric Complex Chronic Conditions: National Trends and Implications for Supportive Care Services. *Pediatrics* **2001**, *107*, e99. [CrossRef] [PubMed]
15. National Vital Statistics System NCfHS, CDC. 2015. Available online: https://www.cdc.gov/injury/wisqars/pdf/leading_causes_of_death_by_age_group_2015-a.pdf (accessed on 30 August 2018).
16. Weaver, M.S.; Rosenberg, A.R.; Tager, J.; Wichman, C.S.; Wiener, L. A Summary of Pediatric Palliative Care Team Structure and Services as Reported by Centers Caring for Children with Cancer. *J. Palliat. Med.* **2018**, *21*, 452–462. [CrossRef] [PubMed]
17. Siden, H. Pediatric Palliative Care for Children with Progressive Non-Malignant Diseases. *Children (Basel)* **2018**, *5*, 28. [CrossRef] [PubMed]
18. Haug, S.; Farooqi, S.; Wilson, C.G.; Hopper, A.; Oei, G.; Carter, B. Survey on Neonatal End-of-Life Comfort Care Guidelines Across America. *J. Pain Symptom Manag.* **2018**, *55*, 979–984. [CrossRef] [PubMed]
19. Carter, B.S. Pediatric Palliative Care in Infants and Neonates. *Children (Basel)* **2018**, *5*, 21. [CrossRef] [PubMed]
20. Jaaniste, T.; Coombs, S.; Donnelly, T.J.; Kelk, N.; Beston, D. Risk and Resilience Factors Related to Parental Bereavement Following the Death of a Child with a Life-Limiting Condition. *Children (Basel)* **2017**, *4*, 96. [CrossRef] [PubMed]
21. Wolfe, J.; Klar, N.; Grier, H.E.; Duncan, J.; Salem-Schatz, S.; Emanuel, E.J.; Weeks, J.C. Understanding of prognosis among parents of children who died of cancer: Impact on treatment goals and integration of palliative care. *JAMA* **2000**, *284*, 2469–2475. [CrossRef] [PubMed]
22. Vickers, J.L.; Carlisle, C. Choices and control: Parental experiences in pediatric terminal home care. *J. Pediatr. Oncol. Nurs.* **2000**, *17*, 12–21. [CrossRef] [PubMed]
23. Mary, J. Labyak Institute for Innovation at the National Center for Care at the End of Life. Pediatric Concurrent Care. 2016. Available online: https://www.nhpco.org/sites/default/files/public/ChiPPS/Continuum_Briefing.pdf (accessed on 30 August 2018).
24. Szymczak, J.E.; Schall, T.; Hill, D.L.; Walter, J.K.; Parikh, S.; DiDomenico, C.; Feudtner, C. Pediatric Oncology Providers' Perceptions of a Palliative Care Service: The Influence of Emotional Esteem and Emotional Labor. *J. Pain Symptom Manag.* **2018**, *55*, 1260–1268. [CrossRef] [PubMed]
25. Bakitas, M.A.; Tosteson, T.D.; Li, Z.; Lyons, K.D.; Hull, J.G.; Li, Z.; Dionne-Odom, J.N.; Frost, J.; Dragnev, K.H.; Hegel, M.T.; et al. Early Versus Delayed Initiation of Concurrent Palliative Oncology Care: Patient Outcomes in the ENABLE III Randomized Controlled Trial. *J. Clin. Oncol.* **2015**, *33*, 1438–1445. [CrossRef] [PubMed]
26. Temel, J.S.; Greer, J.A.; Muzikansky, A.; Gallagher, E.R.; Admane, S.; Jackson, V.A.; Dahlin, C.M.; Blinderman, C.D.; Jacobsen, J.; Pirl, W.F.; et al. Early palliative care for patients with metastatic non-small-cell lung cancer. *N. Engl. J. Med.* **2010**, *363*, 733–742. [CrossRef] [PubMed]
27. Film, L. *Kali's Story—Beyond the NICU*; Little Stars: Longford, TAS, Australia, 2015; Available online: http://littlestars.tv/short-films/beyond-the-nicu/ (accessed on 30 August 2018).
28. Kassam, A.; Skiadaresis, J.; Alexander, S.; Wolfe, J. Differences in end-of-life communication for children with advanced cancer who were referred to a palliative care team. *Pediatr. Blood Cancer* **2015**, *62*, 1409–1413. [CrossRef] [PubMed]
29. Ananth, P.; Melvin, P.; Feudtner, C.; Wolfe, J.; Berry, J.G. Hospital Use in the Last Year of Life for Children With Life-Threatening Complex Chronic Conditions. *Pediatrics* **2015**, *136*, 938–946. [CrossRef] [PubMed]
30. Blazin, L.J.; Cecchini, C.; Habashy, C.; Kaye, E.C.; Baker, J.N. Communicating Effectively in Pediatric Cancer Care: Translating Evidence into Practice. *Children (Basel)* **2018**, *5*, 40. [CrossRef] [PubMed]

31. Brock, K.E.; Wolfe, J.; Ullrich, C. From the Child's Word to Clinical Intervention: Novel, New, and Innovative Approaches to Symptoms in Pediatric Palliative Care. *Children (Basel)* **2018**, *5*, 45. [CrossRef] [PubMed]
32. Bischoff, K.E.; O'Riordan, D.L.; Fazzalaro, K.; Kinderman, A.; Pantilat, S.Z. Identifying Opportunities to Improve Pain Among Patients With Serious Illness. *J. Pain Symptom Manag.* **2018**, *55*, 881–889. [CrossRef] [PubMed]
33. Snaman, J.M.; Kaye, E.C.; Lu, J.J.; Sykes, A.; Baker, J.N. Palliative Care Involvement Is Associated with Less Intensive End-of-Life Care in Adolescent and Young Adult Oncology Patients. *J. Palliat. Med.* **2017**, *20*, 509–516. [CrossRef] [PubMed]
34. Friedrichsdorf, S.J. Cancer Pain Management in Children. In *Anaesthesia, Intensive Care, and Pain Management for the Cancer Patient*; Farquhar-Smith, P., Wigmore, T., Eds.; Oxford University Press: Oxford, NY, USA, 2011; pp. 215–227.
35. Friedrichsdorf, S.J. Prevention and Treatment of Pain in Hospitalized Infants, Children, and Teenagers: From Myths and Morphine to Multimodal Analgesia. In *Pain 2016: Refresher Courses 16th World Congress on Pain*; International Association for the Study of Pain, IASP Press: Washington, DC, USA, 2016; pp. 309–319.
36. Weekly, T.; Walker, N.; Beck, J.; Akers, S.; Weaver, M. A Review of Apps for Calming, Relaxation, and Mindfulness Interventions for Pediatric Palliative Care Patients. *Children (Basel)* **2018**, *5*, 16. [CrossRef] [PubMed]
37. Shafto, K.; Gouda, S.; Catrine, K.; Brown, M.L. Integrative Approaches in Pediatric Palliative Care. *Children (Basel)* **2018**, *5*, 75. [CrossRef] [PubMed]
38. Warlow, T.A.; Hain, R.D.W. 'Total Pain' in Children with Severe Neurological Impairment. *Children (Basel)* **2018**, *5*, 13. [CrossRef] [PubMed]
39. Fraser, L.K.; Parslow, R. Children with life-limiting conditions in paediatric intensive care units: A national cohort, data linkage study. *Arch. Dis. Child.* **2017**. [CrossRef]
40. Drake, R. Palliative Care for Children in Hospital: Essential Roles. *Children (Basel)* **2018**, *5*, 26. [CrossRef] [PubMed]
41. Goldman, A.; Beardsmore, S.; Hunt, J. Palliative care for children with cancer—Home, hospital, or hospice? *Arch. Dis. Child.* **1990**, *65*, 641–643. [CrossRef] [PubMed]
42. Lauer, M.E.; Mulhern, R.K.; Wallskog, J.M.; Camitta, B.M. A comparison study of parental adaptation following a child's death at home or in the hospital. *Pediatrics* **1983**, *71*, 107–112. [CrossRef]
43. Lauer, M.E.; Mulhern, R.K.; Schell, M.J.; Camitta, B.M. Long-term follow-up of parental adjustment following a child's death at home or hospital. *Cancer* **1989**, *63*, 988–994. [CrossRef]
44. Birenbaum, L.K.; Robinson, M.A. Family relationships in two types of terminal care. *Soc. Sci. Med.* **1991**, *32*, 95–102. [CrossRef]
45. Collins, J.J.; Stevens, M.M.; Cousens, P. Home care for the dying child. A parent's perception. *Aust. Fam. Physician* **1998**, *27*, 610–614. [PubMed]
46. Chambers, E.J.; Oakhill, A. Models of care for children dying of malignant disease. *Palliat. Med.* **1995**, *9*, 181–185. [CrossRef] [PubMed]
47. Sirkia, K.; Saarinen, U.M.; Ahlgren, B.; Hovi, L. Terminal care of the child with cancer at home. *Acta Paediatr.* **1997**, *86*, 1125–1130. [CrossRef] [PubMed]
48. Goldman, A. Home care of the dying child. *J. Palliat. Care* **1996**, *12*, 16–19. [PubMed]
49. Friedrichsdorf, B.S.; Menke, A.; Wamsler, C.; Zernikow, B. Pediatric Palliative Care Provided by Nurse-led Home Care Services in Germany. *Eur. J. Palliat. Care* **2005**, *12*, 79–83.
50. Postier, A.; Catrine, K.; Remke, S. Interdisciplinary Pediatric Palliative Care Team Involvement in Compassionate Extubation at Home: From Shared Decision-Making to Bereavement. *Children* **2018**, *5*, 37. [CrossRef] [PubMed]
51. Mherekumombe, M.F. From Inpatient to Clinic to Home to Hospice and Back: Using the "Pop Up" Pediatric Palliative Model of Care. *Children (Basel)* **2018**, *5*, 55. [CrossRef] [PubMed]
52. WHO Definition of Palliative Care. Available online: http://www.who.int/cancer/palliative/definition/en/ (accessed on 30 August 2018).
53. Sourkes, B.M. Children's Experience of Symptoms: Narratives through Words and Images. *Children (Basel)* **2018**, *5*, 53. [CrossRef] [PubMed]
54. Lovgren, M.; Jalmsell, L.; Eilegard Wallin, A.; Steineck, G.; Kreicbergs, U. Siblings' experiences of their brother's or sister's cancer death: A nationwide follow-up 2–9 years later. *Psychooncology* **2016**, *25*, 435–440. [CrossRef] [PubMed]
55. Lovgren, M.; Sveen, J.; Nyberg, T.; Eilegard Wallin, A.; Prigerson, H.G.; Steineck, G.; Steineck, G.; Kreicbergs, U. Care at End of Life Influences Grief: A Nationwide Long-Term Follow-Up among Young

Adults Who Lost a Brother or Sister to Childhood Cancer. *J. Palliat. Med.* **2018**, *21*, 156–162. [CrossRef] [PubMed]
56. Koch, K.D.; Jones, B.L. Supporting Parent Caregivers of Children with Life-Limiting Illness. *Children (Basel)* **2018**, *5*, 85. [CrossRef] [PubMed]
57. Pizzo, P.A.; Poplack, D.G. *Principles and Practice of Pediatric Oncology*, 4th ed.; Pizzo, P.A., Poplack, D.G., Eds.; Lippincott Williams & Wilkins: Philadelphia, PA, USA, 2002.
58. Prigerson, H.G.; Bao, Y.; Shah, M.A.; Paulk, M.E.; LeBlanc, T.W.; Schneider, B.J.; Garrido, M.M.; Reid, M.C.; Berlin, D.A.; Adelson, K.B.; et al. Chemotherapy Use, Performance Status, and Quality of Life at the End of Life. *JAMA Oncol.* **2015**, *1*, 778–784. [CrossRef] [PubMed]
59. Green, M.J.; Schubart, J.R.; Whitehead, M.M.; Farace, E.; Lehman, E.; Levi, B.H. Advance Care Planning Does Not Adversely Affect Hope or Anxiety Among Patients With Advanced Cancer. *J. Pain Symptom Manag.* **2015**, *49*, 1088–1096. [CrossRef] [PubMed]
60. Coulourides Kogan, A.; Penido, M.; Enguidanos, S. Does Disclosure of Terminal Prognosis Mean Losing Hope? Insights from Exploring Patient Perspectives on Their Experience of Palliative Care Consultations. *J. Palliat. Med.* **2015**, *18*, 1019–1025. [CrossRef] [PubMed]
61. Mack, J.W.; Wolfe, J.; Cook, E.F.; Grier, H.E.; Cleary, P.D.; Weeks, J.C. Hope and prognostic disclosure. *J. Clin. Oncol.* **2007**, *25*, 5636–5642. [CrossRef] [PubMed]
62. Mack, J.W.; Wolfe, J.; Grier, H.E.; Cleary, P.D.; Weeks, J.C. Communication about prognosis between parents and physicians of children with cancer: Parent preferences and the impact of prognostic information. *J. Clin. Oncol.* **2006**, *24*, 5265–5270. [CrossRef] [PubMed]
63. Friedrichsdorf, S. The End: When a Baby Dies. *The New York Times*. 16 December 2015. Available online: http://opinionator.blogs.nytimes.com/2015/12/16/when-a-baby-dies/?_r=1 (accessed on 30 August 2018).
64. Hexem, K.R.; Mollen, C.J.; Carroll, K.; Lanctot, D.A.; Feudtner, C. How parents of children receiving pediatric palliative care use religion, spirituality, or life philosophy in tough times. *J. Palliat. Med.* **2011**, *14*, 39–44. [CrossRef] [PubMed]
65. Sykes, N.P. Morphine kills the pain, not the patient. *Lancet* **2007**, *369*, 1325–1326. [CrossRef]
66. Thorns, A.; Sykes, N. Opioid use in last week of life and implications for end-of-life decision-making. *Lancet* **2000**, *356*, 398–399. [CrossRef]
67. Friedrichsdorf, S.J. Pain management in children with advanced cancer and during end-of-life care. *Pediatr. Hematol. Oncol.* **2010**, *27*, 257–261. [CrossRef] [PubMed]
68. Bengoechea, I.; Gutierrez, S.G.; Vrotsou, K.; Onaindia, M.J.; Lopez, J.M. Opioid use at the end of life and survival in a Hospital at Home unit. *J. Palliat. Med.* **2010**, *13*, 1079–1083. [CrossRef] [PubMed]
69. Hauer, J. Feeding Intolerance in Children with Severe Impairment of the Central Nervous System: Strategies for Treatment and Prevention. *Children (Basel)* **2017**, *5*, 1. [CrossRef] [PubMed]
70. Yealy, D.M. Change is hard-physician behavior and documentation guidelines. *Acad. Emerg. Med.* **2001**, *8*, 907–908. [CrossRef] [PubMed]
71. MacKusick, C.I.; Minick, P. Why are nurses leaving? Findings from an initial qualitative study on nursing attrition. *Medsurg. Nurs.* **2010**, *19*, 335–340. [PubMed]
72. NSI Nursing Solutions, Inc. 2015 National Healthcare Retention & RN Staffing Report 2015. Available online: https://docplayer.net/6163965-2015-national-healthcare-retention-rn-staffing-report.html (accessed on 30 August 2018).
73. Gans, D.; Kominski, G.F.; Roby, D.H.; Diamant, A.L.; Chen, X.; Lin, W.; Hohe, N. Better outcomes, lower costs: Palliative care program reduces stress, costs of care for children with life-threatening conditions. *Policy Brief* **2012**, *PB2012-3*, 1–8.
74. Knapp, C.; Woodworth, L.; Wright, M.; Downing, J.; Drake, R.; Fowler-Kerry, S.; Hain, R.; Marston, J. Pediatric palliative care provision around the world: A systematic review. *Pediatr. Blood Cancer* **2011**, *57*, 361–368. [CrossRef] [PubMed]

75. Pascuet, E.; Cowin, L.; Vaillancourt, R.; Splinter, W.; Vadeboncoeur, C.; Dumond, L.G.; Ni, A.; Rattray, M. A comparative cost-minimization analysis of providing paediatric palliative respite care before and after the opening of services at a paediatric hospice. In *Healthcare Management Forum/Canadian College of Health Service Executives = Forum Gestion des Soins de Sante/College Canadien des Directeurs de Services de Sante*; SAGE Publications: Los Angeles, CA, USA, 2010; Volume 23, pp. 63–66.
76. Postier, A.; Chrastek, J.; Nugent, S.; Osenga, K.; Friedrichsdorf, S.J. Exposure to home-based pediatric palliative and hospice care and its impact on hospital and emergency care charges at a single institution. *J. Palliat. Med.* **2014**, *17*, 183–188. [CrossRef] [PubMed]

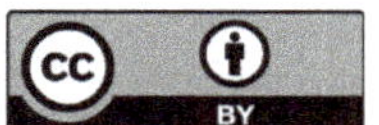

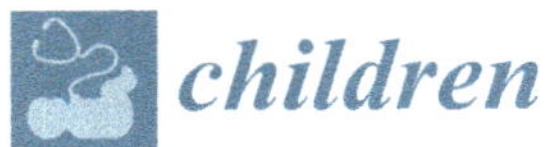

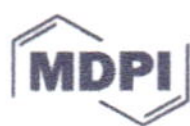

Review

Pediatric Palliative Care in Infants and Neonates

Brian S. Carter [1,2,3]

1 University of Missouri-Kansas City School of Medicine, 2411 Holmes Street, Kansas City, MO 64108, USA; bscarter@cmh.edu; Tel.: +1-816-701-5268; Fax: +1-816-302-9965
2 Children's Mercy Hospital, Kansas City, MO 64108, USA
3 Division of Neonatology and Bioethics Center, 2401 Gillham Road, Kansas City, MO 64108, USA

Received: 7 December 2017; Accepted: 1 February 2018; Published: 7 February 2018

Abstract: The application of palliative and hospice care to newborns in the neonatal intensive care unit (NICU) has been evident for over 30 years. This article addresses the history, current considerations, and anticipated future needs for palliative and hospice care in the NICU, and is based on recent literature review. Neonatologists have long managed the entirety of many newborns' short lives, given the relatively high mortality rates associated with prematurity and birth defects, but their ability or willingness to comprehensively address of the continuum of interdisciplinary palliative, end of life, and bereavement care has varied widely. While neonatology service capacity has grown worldwide during this time, so has attention to pediatric palliative care generally, and neonatal-perinatal palliative care specifically. Improvements have occurred in family-centered care, communication, pain assessment and management, and bereavement. There remains a need to integrate palliative care with intensive care rather than await its application solely at the terminal phase of a young infant's life—when s/he is imminently dying. Future considerations for applying neonatal palliative care include its integration into fetal diagnostic management, the developing era of genomic medicine, and expanding research into palliative care models and practices in the NICU.

Keywords: neonatal; palliative care; comfort care; pain

1. Introduction

The provision of palliative or hospice care for newborn infants was first introduced in the 1980s. At the time, hospice principles were being disseminated in the US and their applicability to certain newborns and young infants was noted by Whitfield et al. [1] and by Silverman [2]. Since 1982, there has been increased growth in the field of palliative care in general, and in both pediatric and neonatal palliative care specifically. Indeed, the specialty of palliative and hospice medicine has gained recognition in North America and internationally with the attendant growth of training programs in both the clinical and academic arenas.

2. Materials and Methods

A brief, but pertinent, review of the past 10 years' clinical literature was conducted to examine the breadth of neonatal palliative care as it is currently practiced. Throughout this process, additional clinical needs, potential research ideas, and future considerations were determined and are herein addressed.

3. Results

As the specialty of neonatology has grown around the world in the last three decades, the role for palliative care (PC) has likewise been recognized in the neonatal intensive care unit (NICU) and pediatric intensive care unit (ICU)—both common locales for neonatal and infant mortality [3–5]. Over the past 15 years, marked improvements have occurred around the circumstances in which newborn and young infants die in North American hospitals. There has been attention drawn to patient needs such as pain and symptom management [6,7], spiritual support [8], honoring cultural practices [5], understanding grief [9], and employing a breadth of bereavement activities and services [10,11].

Some particular features of providing PC for newborns and young infants include how pregnancy is unique among human experiences and the veritable uniqueness of each pregnancy—and child—from all others. Mothers and fathers generally enter into pregnancy with anticipation and hopefulness, having a future-oriented idea of their yet to be born infant. That a newborn may be critically ill, extremely premature, or born with significant birth anomalies that threaten his/her life and wellbeing is never truly anticipated. When discovered—at birth or even beforehand with fetal diagnostics—the pregnancy generally takes a dramatic turn as hopeful anticipation is replaced by fear, joy may be eclipsed by guilt, and the experience of pregnancy and childbirth becomes medicalized—often with obsessive thoughts surrounding each clinic visit, imaging study, or test. In addition to cure-oriented and life-extending neonatal intensive care, the provision of concurrent PC may provide supportive care for the patient and family, and may help in decision-making [12,13].

As is true in other areas of pediatric PC, neonatal PC has had a somewhat divided history. In the NICU, there have long been a number of patients who have been treated for weeks to months only to reach a plateau or stagnation in their progress toward growth and healing. They remain ventilated, perhaps dependent upon intravenous nutrition, have endured infections and maybe bowel problems, their livers are impacted by cholestasis, and they may even have parenteral nutrition-associated liver disease. Some have endured brain injury. Each day their care is challenging, and on any given day they might have an acute decompensation for which escalating support is required—often accompanied by analgesia and/or sedation to minimize cardiopulmonary instability or neurologic agitation. These infants may further decompensate or develop secondary pulmonary arterial hypertension along with their bronchopulmonary dysplasia (BPD). Any given infection may take their life. For these infants—some of whom may linger, and others may in fact be dying—neonatal PC may be an adjunctive care paradigm that is added to their continued intensive care. For some, the cure-oriented care may yield to a palliative paradigm after intensive counseling of parents, exploration of options with the interdisciplinary neonatal team, and thoughtful reflection. Psychosocial support for the family is essential and may attend to anticipatory grief; spiritual support may increase, and a decision to limit ongoing life-support may result in a mutually agreed upon redirection of care towards comfort with a reduction in vital-sign and invasive monitoring, phlebotomies, and imaging tests. In time, a compassionate withdrawal of life-supportive technology is performed, and caregivers work with families to orchestrate a meaningful time with extended family, rituals, and allow for the infant's passing. In such cases, a period of focused palliation culminates in veritable hospice care in the NICU, typically associated with the withdrawal of life-sustaining medical treatments.

As neonatal palliative care has developed, and an expanding literature is at the disposal of clinicians (Figure 1), there has been greater consideration for PC in the NICU. In recent years, especially as prenatal diagnostics have improved and life-limiting conditions are diagnosed prenatally, some newborn infants will receive concurrent palliative care (even beginning with conversations before birth) while being cared for in the NICU [14–16]. The care may be oriented toward confirming a prenatal diagnosis and exploring care options, or be directed at the baby's comfort while not taking on intensive or invasive technological care. In the latter situation, time with parents, human contact, warmth, and symptom relief may be the predominant mode of support [17]. For others, such as a newborn with hypoplastic left heart syndrome, there may be intensive care provided while the neonatal, cardiology, and cardiovascular surgical specialists confer about palliative surgical options or perhaps limits or confounders (such as prematurity, additional birth defects, or the severity of anatomical size constraints that make surgery more difficult) [18]. When concurrent palliative care is made available, the added value of an interdisciplinary team, psycho-social-spiritual support, and expert pain and symptom management are acknowledged as enhancing the baby's and family's quality of life even while cure-oriented or disease-modifying treatments are offered. The focus is on the quality of life and relationships while living with a life-limiting condition [19,20].

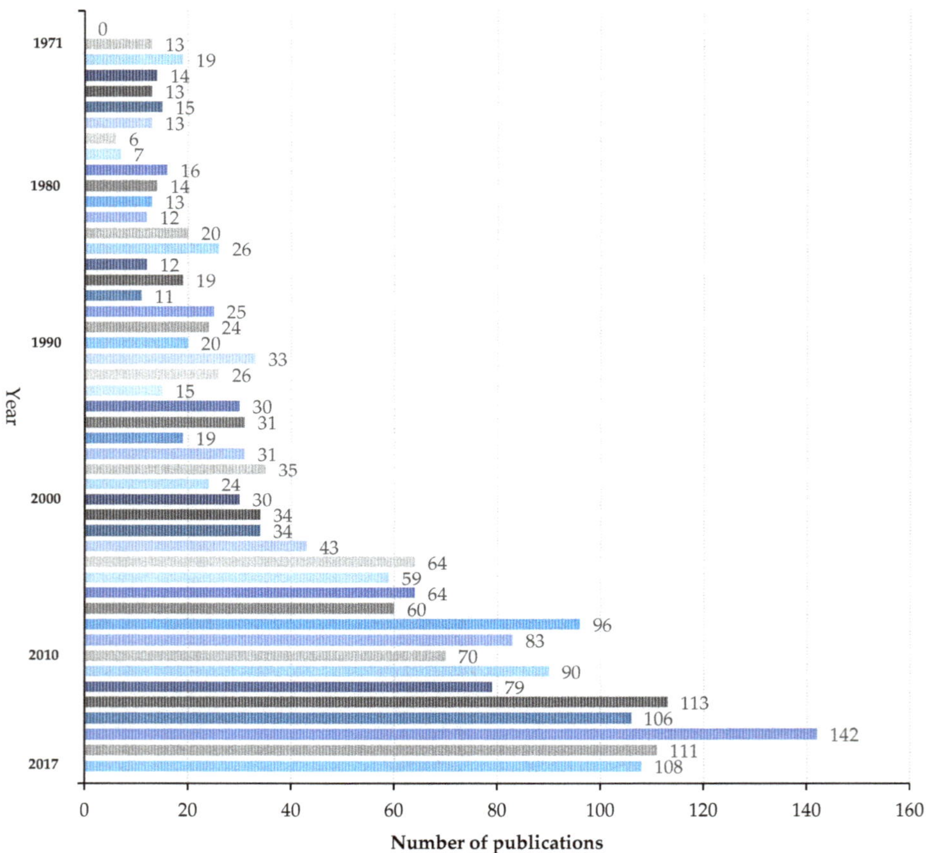

Figure 1. Increasing publications addressing neonatal palliative care.

A working definition for neonatal palliative care can be found from the organization *Together for Short Lives*, a children's palliative care group in the UK:

> "Palliative care for a fetus, neonate, or infant with a life-limiting condition is an active and total approach to care, from the point of diagnosis or recognition, throughout the child's life, at the time of death and beyond. It embraces physical, emotional, social, and spiritual elements and focuses on the enhancement of quality of life for the neonatal infant and support for the family. It includes the management of distressing symptoms, the provision of short breaks, and care through death and bereavement" [21].

Note here that this involves far more than care of the imminently dying newborn. Indeed, the many domains of PC outlined by Ferrell in 2005 [22] are present and require consideration and action in the neonatal and young infant population as much as they do in adults or older children [21]. In recent years, referrals for PC from the perinatal and newborn period have often been the starting point for long-term follow-up of children with complex chronic conditions and special health care needs by PC clinicians long after the infant has left the NICU.

The types of patients for whom PC may be anticipated and offered in the newborn period are generally in one of three categories: those born at the threshold of viability or who are similarly vulnerable by virtue of prematurity, those with birth anomalies that may threaten vital functions, and those for whom intensive care has been appropriately applied but are now burdened with interventions that no longer are deemed beneficial, but come to be seen as burdensome, inappropriate, and only prolonging the infant's dying. There are guidelines published from the National Institute of Nursing Research (NINR), National Association of Nurse Practitioners, the National Perinatal Association (NPA), the National Association of Neonatal Nurses (NANN), the National Hospice and Palliative Care Organization (NHPCO), and the Center to Advance Palliative Care (www.capc.org) that speak to these categories and potential triggers for neonatal PC [23–27]. For some of the commonly included conditions (below) a diagnosis may arise in the neonatal period and PC care may be initiated, whereas others may lead to a more long-term follow-up with PC as an adjunct to other ICU follow-up services:

- Genetic/chromosomal: Chromosomal aneuploidies with complex and life-limiting prognoses; severe metabolic, storage, or mitochondrial disorders; severe forms of skeletal dysplasia.
- Organ-system problems: Severe central nervous system (CNS) malformations (neural tube defects, migrational disorders); hypoxic-ischemic encephalopathy; spinal muscular atrophy type-1 and myotonic dystrophies; epidermolysis bullosa; Potter's syndrome, fetal oligohydramnios sequence, fetal-neonatal chronic renal failure; short-gut syndrome with parenteral nutrition dependence; multi-visceral organ transplant under consideration (e.g., liver, bowel, pancreas); biliary atresia; total aganglionosis of the bowel; severe feeding impairment with feeding tube dependence that may be permanent; complex congenital heart disease, especially if functionally univentricular; extracorporeal membrane oxygenation (ECMO) patients; severe pulmonary arterial hypertension; consideration for heart transplant; congenital diaphragmatic hernia; severe pulmonary hypoplasia; congenital central hypoventilation syndrome; asphyxiating thoracic dystrophies; multi-organ system failure.
- Infection and immune disorders: Perinatal human immunodeficiency virus infection and acquired immune deficiency syndrome (HIV/AIDS); severe combined immune deficiency (SCID); severe perinatal herpes simplex virus (HSV), cytomegalovirus (CMV), toxoplasmosis or Zika virus with meningoencephalitis or severe encephalopathy.
- Complications of prematurity: Periviable gestation; severe intraventricular hemorrhage (IVH, grade IV) or periventricular leukomalacia (PVL); refractory respiratory failure; ventilator-dependent BPD; severe necrotizing enterocolitis (NEC) with resultant short gut; liver failure.

4. Discussion

Today, newborns and young infants may receive PC that is initiated prenatally, introduced at delivery, or acquired in a consultative manner in the NICU. The acceptance of this paradigm of care, and the capacity for it to be rendered as needed, however, varies across units of care and internationally. A number of investigators have spoken to barriers to neonatal-perinatal PC such as suboptimal interdisciplinary collaboration in hospitals, unacceptance of PC broadly in society and specifically as it applies to children, poor clinician communication skills, and prognostic uncertainties among others [28–31]. Clinicians today must strive to advance PC education, employ successful models of neonatal-perinatal PC, and incorporate PC competencies into those considered fundamental in neonatal-perinatal professional education [15,32–36].

Looking ahead, I will outline what I see as three major considerations for the field of PC as it pertains to pregnancy, fetal, and neonatal patients in the next decade. First, given the improved diagnostic capabilities present with maternal-fetal imaging, and the expansion of fetal diagnostic and intervention centers, the integration of PC with prenatal counseling will likely increase. For the pediatric PC specialist familiar with neonatal-perinatal care, this will not necessarily pose concerns. However, for those unfamiliar with neonatal-perinatal care (e.g., a pediatric oncologist who has been trained in PC, or a family physician now boarded in Hospice and Palliative Medicine) there may be a learning curve to ramp up capabilities to address the often unique aspects of pregnancy and childbirth complicated by life-limiting conditions [37–39].

In such instances where a palliative medicine consultant has little experience with newborns, it will be beneficial for neonatologists, pediatricians, and hospitalist pediatricians to be identified as local "champions" for neonatal PC within a given NICU, academic faculty, or practice group. The NICU champion will likely work with unit-specific interdisciplinary staff and the local PC-trained physician or nurse practitioner to effect well-coordinated and effective PC in the NICU. The coordination of transitional care from the NICU to home-based hospice care, an inpatient hospice-house or facility, or even outpatient management anticipated to be beneficial for months to years that is shared with a primary care pediatrician, specialty clinics, and interim contact with the PC team first met in the NICU, is of added value to both NICU staff and patient families.

Related to this first consideration is the expansion of fetal and neonatal diagnostic evaluations with genomic medicine to better understand or explain multiple anomalies, metabolic disorders, or complex central nervous system dysfunction [40–43]. I foresee that pediatric (and neonatal) clinicians in general, and perhaps PC clinicians specifically, will need to develop a facility with both new diagnostic genetic tests and the cautious compilation of new diagnostic groups with yet to be determined prognoses. While some such cases may be treatable with present regimens, others may require yet to be developed, personalized pharmacogenomics-derived treatments. In the prenatal setting, genetic/genomic diagnoses that can be made from chorionic villous sampling, amniocentesis, fetal blood sampling, or even non-invasive maternal (blood) testing will likely accompany phenotypic diagnoses seen on imaging. These developments will impose the need for expanded perinatal counseling and open doors for PC clinicians to join neonatologists, geneticists, and maternal-fetal medicine specialists in contributing to perinatal and neonatal decision-making. Already, we see the possibility of expanded genome-wide newborn screening being proposed in the care of all newborns, and even if this is constrained to symptom-driven circumstances, the need to address prognostic uncertainty will call upon the superlative communication skills of trained and informed neonatologists and PC clinicians [37–39,44].

As a second consideration, PC material is increasingly being incorporated into the training and education of neonatologists. This will likely result in an enhanced momentum for PC services to be better integrated into the newborn's care concurrently with cure-oriented or life-prolonging critical care. Progress has been made in the establishment of PC teams in children's hospitals in North America. However, due to their variable staffing, composition, resource priority, and the limited number of fellowship-trained PC specialists, the ability for these teams to concurrently provide PC throughout a large children's hospital and in the NICU may be limited. This too provides an opportunity for neonatologists to become local champions for PC in their NICU—and in so doing building the capacity for PC as they partner with PC team members—until capacity is increased with more fellowship-trained pediatric or neonatal PC specialists. Given the longstanding interdisciplinary nature of the care team in the NICU, unit-specific neonatal nurse practitioners who may be PC champions, respiratory therapists, perinatal social workers, nurses, and others can work with chaplains, psychologists, and child-life specialists to create NICU-PC teams that address unit needs with input and assistance from pediatric PC specialists elsewhere in the hospital. Together these complimentary and concurrent teams can see to patients, family, and staff needs [19,37–39,44,45].

A third consideration that I would highlight in the next 10 years of PC provided for newborns is the need to conduct research, qualitative and empirical, that can advance the derivation of best practice models for neonatal PC [15,32–36]. Such research will advance the evidence base for the field, and likely result in increasing acceptance and utilization of PC in the neonatal-perinatal world. Investigations might address symptom assessment and management skills; studying commonly used, but poorly evaluated medications; looking further into the barriers and facilitators of PC in the NICU across staff/disciplines [28–31,39,44,45]; and evaluating effective communication strategies and decision-support for families and staff [46,47]. The utilization of large neonatal population databases to make inquiries and construct studies to answer common problems would seem to hold great potential [48]. What are the best ways to manage common symptoms? How should ventilator withdrawal be accomplished [49]? What do parents think about the limitation or withdrawal of medically assisted nutrition and hydration [50]? How can neonatologists, maternal-fetal medicine physicians, geneticists, and others best inform a pregnant couple of unexpected findings on fetal imaging or address prognosis in the NICU [51]? Would a complimentary presence of an ethics consultant add value anywhere along the path from diagnosis to treatment decisions or life-sustaining medical treatment withdrawal [52,53]?

5. Conclusions

The history of neonatology includes periods in which clinicians did not believe infants felt pain—now, pain assessment and management are part of standard care. Likewise, the provision of assisted ventilation, surgical interventions, and other technology at the neonatologist's disposal have all increased neonatal survival, and improved patients' quality of life through the NICU's practicing developmentally supportive care. However, when technology becomes more burdensome than beneficial, when a newborn's relational potential seems lost due to severe neurologic injury, or when being too premature and too small—or fraught with too many anomalies—confronts families and clinicians with the limits of medicine, PC should be at the ready (or already have been incorporated into a concurrent care model) to assist all stakeholders. I believe that the foundation for the integration of PC into the NICU is set, the need is present, and the progress made over the past 15 years speaks to a bright future in the practice of humane, ethical, and family-centered care for our world's tiniest and most vulnerable patients. We can meet the challenges outlined here and others with continued efforts, well-trained young leaders, forthcoming research, appropriate advocacy, and local hospital and university support.

Conflicts of Interest: The author declares no conflict of interest.

References

1. Whitfield, J.M.; Siegel, R.E.; Glicken, A.D.; Harmon, R.J.; Powers, L.K.; Goldson, E.J. The application of hospice concepts to neonatal care. *Am. J. Dis. Child.* **1982**, *136*, 421–424. [CrossRef] [PubMed]
2. Silverman, W.A. A hospice setting for humane neonatal death. *Pediatrics* **1982**, *69*, 239. [PubMed]
3. Carter, B.; Howenstein, M.; Gilmer, M.J.; Throop, P.; France, D.; Whitlock, J.A. Circumstances surrounding the deaths of hospitalized children: Opportunities for pediatric palliative care. *Pediatrics* **2004**, *114*, e361–e366. [CrossRef] [PubMed]
4. Singh, J.; Lantos, J.; Meadow, W. End-of-life after birth: Death and dying in a neonatal intensive care unit. *Pediatrics* **2004**, *114*, 1620–1626. [CrossRef] [PubMed]
5. Penn, A.A.; Paris, J.J.; Moore, M.P., Jr. Decision making for seriously compromised newborns: The importance of exploring cultural differences and unintended consequences. *J. Perinatol.* **2013**, *33*, 505–508. [CrossRef] [PubMed]
6. Carter, B.S.; Jones, P.J. Evidence-based comfort care for neonates toward the end of life. *Semin. Fetal Neonatal Med.* **2013**, *18*, 88–92. [CrossRef] [PubMed]
7. Carter, B.S.; Brunkhorst, J. Neonatal pain management. *Semin. Perinatol.* **2017**, *41*, 111–116. [CrossRef] [PubMed]

8. Meyer, E.C.; Ritholz, M.D.; Burns, J.P.; Truog, R.D. Improving the quality of end-of-life care in the pediatric intensive care unit: Parents' priorities and recommendations. *Pediatrics* **2006**, *115*, 649–657. [CrossRef] [PubMed]
9. Romesberg, T.L. Understanding grief: A component of neonatal palliative care. *J. Hosp. Palliat. Nurs.* **2004**, *6*, 161–170. [CrossRef]
10. Meert, K.L.; Donaldson, A.E.; Newth, C.J.L.; Harrison, R.; Berger, J.; Zimmerman, J.; Anand, K.J.; Carcillo, J.; Dean, J.M.; Willson, D.F.; et al. Eunice Kennedy Shriver National Institute of Child Health and Human Development Collaborative Pediatric Critical Care Research Network. Complicated grief and associated risk factors among parents following a child's death in the pediatric intensive care unit. *Arch. Pediatr. Adolesc. Med.* **2010**, *164*, 1045–1051. [PubMed]
11. McHaffie, H.E.; Laing, I.A.; Lloyd, D.J. Follow-up care of bereaved parents after treatment withdrawal from newborns. *Arch. Dis. Child. Fetal Neonatal Ed.* **2001**, *84*, F125–F128. [CrossRef] [PubMed]
12. Wool, C. State of the science on perinatal palliative care. *J. Obstet. Gynecol. Neonatal Nurs.* **2013**, *42*, 372–382. [CrossRef] [PubMed]
13. Cote-Arsenault, D.; Denney-Koelsch, E. "Have no regrets": Parents' experiences and developmental tasks in pregnancy with a lethal fetal diagnosis. *Soc. Sci. Med.* **2016**, *154*, 100–109. [CrossRef] [PubMed]
14. Rocha Catania, T.; Stein Bernardes, L.; Guerra Benute, G.R.; Bento Cicaroni Gibeli, M.A.; Bertolassi do Nascimento, N.; Aparecida Barbosa, T.V.; Jornada Krebs, V.L.; Francisco, R.P.V. When one knows a fetus is expected to die: Palliative care in the context of prenatal diagnosis of fetal malformations. *J. Palliat. Med.* **2017**, *20*, 1020–1031. [CrossRef] [PubMed]
15. Cole, J.C.M.; Moldenhauer, J.S.; Jones, T.R.; Shaughnessy, E.A.; Zarrin, H.E.; Coursey, A.L.; Munson, D.A. A proposed model for perinatal palliative care. *J. Obstet. Gynecol. Neonatal Nurs.* **2017**, *46*, 904–911. [CrossRef] [PubMed]
16. Tosello, B.; Haddad, G.; Gire, C.; Einaudi, M.A. Lethal fetal abnormalities: How to approach perinatal palliative care? *J. Matern. Fetal Neonatal Med.* **2017**, *30*, 755–758. [CrossRef] [PubMed]
17. Noseda, C.; Mialet-Marty, T.; Basquin, A.; Letourneur, I.; Bertorello, I.; Charlot, F.; Le Bouar, G.; Bétrémieux, P.; Collaborateurs. Severe hypoplastic left heart syndrome: Palliative care after prenatal diagnosis. *Arch. Pédiatr.* **2012**, *19*, 374–380. [CrossRef] [PubMed]
18. Tibballs, J.; Cantwell-Bartl, A.M. Place, age, and mode of death of infants and children with hypoplastic left heart syndrome: Implications for medical counselling, psychological counselling, and palliative care. *J. Palliat. Care* **2008**, *24*, 76–84.
19. Lemmon, M.E.; Bidegain, M.; Boss, R.D. Palliative care in neonatal neurology: Robust support for infants, families and clinicians. *J. Perinatol.* **2013**, *36*, 331–337. [CrossRef] [PubMed]
20. Parravicini, E. Neonatal palliative care. *Curr. Opin. Pediatr.* **2017**, *29*, 135–140. [CrossRef] [PubMed]
21. Together for Short Lives (2009). The Neonatal Care Pathway. Available online: http://tinyurl.com/pncuwfj (accessed on 29 November 2017).
22. Ferrell, B.R. Overview of the domains of variables relevant to end-of-life care. *J. Palliat. Med.* **2005**, *8* (Suppl. 1), S22–S29. [CrossRef] [PubMed]
23. Youngblut, J.M.; Brooten, D. Perinatal and pediatric issues in palliative and end-of-life care from the 2011 Summit on the Science of Compassion. *Nurs. Outlook* **2012**, *60*, 343–350. [CrossRef] [PubMed]
24. National Association of Neonatal Nurse Practitioners. Palliative care of newborns and infants. Position Statement #3051. *Adv. Neonatal Care* **2010**, *10*, 287–293.
25. National Perinatal Association. Position Paper on Palliative Care. 2009. Available online: www.nationalperinatal.org/Resources/PalliativeCare2012-12-13.pdf (accessed on 1 December 2017).
26. Friebert, S.; Huff, S. *Standards of Practice for Pediatric Palliative Care/Hospice*; National Hospice and Palliative Care Organization: Alexandria, VA, USA, 2009.
27. National Association of Neonatal Nurses (NANN). *Palliative and End-of-Life Care for Newborns and Infants: Position Statement #3063*; NANN: Chicago, IL, USA, 2015; Available online: http://nann.org/uploads/About/PositionPDFS/1.4.5_Palliative%20and%20End%20of%20Life%20Care%20for%20Newborns%20and%20Infants.pdf (accessed on 29 November 2017).
28. Davies, B.; Sehring, S.A.; Partridge, J.C.; Cooper, B.A.; Hughes, A.; Philp, J.C.; Amidi-Nouri, A.; Kramer, R.F. Barriers to palliative care for children: Perceptions of pediatric health care providers. *Pediatrics* **2008**, *121*, 282–288. [CrossRef] [PubMed]

29. Kain, V.; Gardner, G.; Yates, P. Neonatal palliative care attitude scale: Development of an instrument to measure the barriers to and facilitators of palliative care in neonatal nursing. *Pediatrics* **2009**, *123*, e207–e213. [CrossRef] [PubMed]
30. Kain, V.J. Palliative care delivery in the NICU: What barriers do neonatal nurses face? *Neonatal Netw.* **2006**, *25*, 387–392. [CrossRef] [PubMed]
31. Wool, C. Clinician perspectives of barriers in perinatal palliative care. *MCN Am. J. Matern. Child Nurs.* **2015**, *40*, 44–50. [CrossRef] [PubMed]
32. Marc-Aurele, K.L.; English, N.K. Primary palliative care in neonatal intensive care. *Semin. Perinatol.* **2017**, *41*, 133–139. [CrossRef] [PubMed]
33. Twamley, K.; Kelly, P.; Moss, R.; Mancini, A.; Craig, F.; Koh, M.; Polonsky, R.; Bluebond-Langner, M. Palliative care education in neonatal units: Impact on knowledge and attitudes. *BMJ Support Palliat. Care* **2013**, *3*, 213–220. [CrossRef] [PubMed]
34. Wool, C. Clinician confidence and comfort in providing perinatal palliative care. *J. Obstet. Gynecol. Neonatal Nurs.* **2013**, *42*, 48–58. [CrossRef] [PubMed]
35. Kobler, K.; Limbo, R. Making a case: Creating a perinatal palliative care service using a perinatal bereavement program model. *J. Perinat. Neonatal Nurs.* **2011**, *25*, 32–41. [CrossRef] [PubMed]
36. Balaguer, A.; Martin-Ancel, A.; Ortigoza-Escobar, D.; Escribano, J.; Argemi, J. The model of palliative care in the perinatal setting: A review of the literature. *BMC Pediatr.* **2012**, *25*. [CrossRef] [PubMed]
37. Harris, L.; Placencia, F.; Arnold, J.; Minard, C.; Harris, T.; Haidet, P. A structured end-of-life curriculum for neonatal-perinatal postdoctoral fellows. *Am. J. Hosp. Palliat. Med.* **2015**, *32*, 253–261. [CrossRef] [PubMed]
38. El Sayed, M.F.; Chan, M.; McAllister, M.; Hellmann, J. End-of-life care in Toronto neonatal intensive care units: Challenges for physician trainees. *Arch. Dis. Child. Fetal Neonatal Ed.* **2013**, *98*, F528–F533. [CrossRef] [PubMed]
39. Mancini, A.; Kelly, P.; Bluebond-Langner, M. Training neonatal staff for the future in neonatal palliative care. *Semin. Fetal Neonatal Med.* **2013**, *18*, 111–115. [CrossRef] [PubMed]
40. Petrikin, J.E.; Willig, L.K.; Smith, L.D.; Kingsmore, S.F. Rapid whole genome sequencing and precision neonatology. *Semin. Perinatol.* **2015**, *39*, 623–631. [CrossRef] [PubMed]
41. Vanderver, A.; Simons, C.; Helman, G. Whole exome sequencing in patients with white matter abnormalities. *Ann. Neurol.* **2016**, *79*, 1031–1037. [CrossRef] [PubMed]
42. Bruun, T.U.J.; DesRoches, C.L.; Wilson, D.; Chau, V.; Nakagawa, T.; Yamasaki, M.; Hasegawa, S.; Fukao, T.; Marshall, C.; Mercimek-Andrews, S. Prospective cohort study for identification of underlying genetic causes in neonatal encephalopathy using whole-exome sequencing. *Genet. Med.* **2017**. [CrossRef] [PubMed]
43. Miller, R.; Khromykh, A.; Babcock, H.; Jenevein, C.; Solomon, B.D. Putting the pieces together: Clinically relevant genetic and genomic resources for hospitalists and neonatologists. *Hosp. Pediatr.* **2017**, *7*, 108–114. [CrossRef] [PubMed]
44. Mancini, A.; Uthaya, S.; Beardsley, C.; Wood, D.; Modi, N. *Practical Guidance for the Management of Palliative Care on Neonatal Units*; Royal College of Paediatrics and Child Health, Chelsea and Westminster Hospital, NHS Foundation Trust (UK): London, UK, 2014.
45. Dean, B.; McDonald, K. Nursing Perspectives: Building an interprofessional perinatal palliative care team. *NeoReviews* **2014**, *15*, e422–e425. [CrossRef]
46. Cortezzo, D.E.; Sanders, M.R.; Brownell, E.A.; Moss, K. End-of-life care in the neonatal intensive care unit: Experiences of staff and parents. *Am. J. Perinatol.* **2015**, *32*, 713–724. [PubMed]
47. Boss, R.D.; Urban, A.; Barnett, M.D.; Arnold, R.M. Neonatal Critical Care Communication (NC3): Training NICU physicians and nurse practitioners. *J. Perinatol.* **2013**, *33*, 642–646. [CrossRef] [PubMed]
48. James, J.; Munson, D.; DeMauro, S.B.; Langer, J.C.; Dworetz, A.R.; Natarajan, G.; Bidegain, M.; Fortney, C.A.; Seabrook, R.; Vohr, B.R.; et al. Outcomes of Preterm Infants following discussions about withdrawal or withholding of life support. *J. Pediatr.* **2017**, *190*, 118–123. [CrossRef] [PubMed]
49. Abe, N.; Catlin, A.; Mihara, D. End of life in the NICU: A study of ventilator withdrawal. *MCN Am. J. Matern. Child Nurs.* **2001**, *26*, 141–146. [CrossRef] [PubMed]
50. Hellmann, J.; Williams, C.; Ives-Baine, L.; Shah, P.S. Withdrawal of artificial nutrition and hydration in the Neonatal Intensive Care Unit: Parental perspectives. *Arch. Dis. Child. Fetal Neonatal Ed.* **2013**, *98*, F21–F25. [CrossRef] [PubMed]

51. Boss, R.D.; Lemmon, M.E.; Arnold, R.M.; Donohue, P.K. Communicating prognosis with parents of critically ill infants: Direct observation of clinician behaviors. *J. Perinatol.* **2017**, *37*, 1224–1229. [CrossRef] [PubMed]
52. Rainone, F. Infants' best interests in end-of-life care for newborns. *J. Pain Sympt. Manag.* **2015**, *49*, 6505.
53. Blumenthal-Barby, J.S.; Loftis, L.; Cummings, C.L.; Meadow, W.; Lemmon, M.; Ubel, P.A.; McCullough, L.; Rao, E.; Lantos, J.D. Should neonatologists give opinions withdrawing life-sustaining treatment? *Pediatrics* **2016**, *138*, e20162585. [CrossRef] [PubMed]

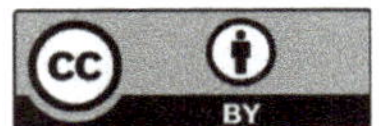

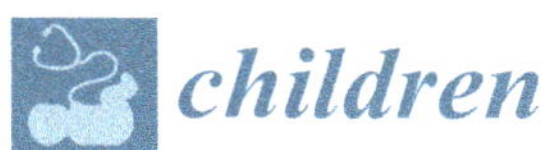

MDPI

Review

Pediatric Palliative Care for Children with Progressive Non-Malignant Diseases

Harold Siden

Canuck Place Children's Hospice, BC Children's Hospital, University of British Columbia, Vancouver, BC V6H 3N1, Canada; hsiden@cw.bc.ca; Tel.: +1-604-875-2776

Received: 22 December 2017; Accepted: 12 February 2018; Published: 20 February 2018

Abstract: A substantial number of children cared for by pediatric palliative care physicians have progressive non-malignant conditions. Some elements of their care overlap with care for children with cancer while other elements, especially prognosis and trajectory, have nuanced differences. This article reviews the population, physical-emotional and social concerns, and trajectory.

Keywords: palliative care; palliative medicine; terminal care; hospice care; metabolic diseases; inborn genetic diseases; social support; disease progression; symptom management; emotional support

1. Introduction

In industrialized countries the majority of children cared for in Pediatric Palliative Care (PPC) programs have non-malignant diseases other than cancer. This includes a very broad range of conditions affecting the brain, the muscles, the heart and lungs. Infrequently there are infectious and immunologic conditions.

In North America cancer comprises only 30–40% of the cases seen by pediatric palliative care clinical teams. This is a testimony to the overall rarity of childhood cancer and to the overarching success of current treatments. The most common of all the childhood cancers, acute lymphoblastic leukemia, also has the highest 5-year event-free survival rate, at over 90%.

Cancer is widely identified with palliative care in part for historic reasons. The first modern hospice, St. Christopher's in London, was founded by a medical oncologist, Dame Cicely Saunders. A surgical oncologist, Balfour Mount, coined the term "palliative care". It was not until some 15 years later that the first hospice for children was developed by Sister Francis Dominica with Helen House, Oxford. Helen, for whom the program is named, indeed had cancer, however it was the central nervous system sequelae of that tumor that made her a candidate for palliative care [1].

This article will describe the broad epidemiology of the non-cancer conditions seen by PPC clinicians, provide insights into aspects of care, and point out areas needing focused research.

2. Terminology and Classification

In order to understand the approach to conditions other than cancer followed by PPC teams, it helps to understand terminology and current classification schemes. All of these are continuously evolving as we come to understand the nuances of PPC.

One area of terminology that has led to some confusion is an ongoing discussion over the terms "life-limiting" and "life-threatening", as different groups use the terms differently [2]. The focus of pediatric palliative care has long been ameliorating symptoms, maintaining good quality of life, and supporting families when a child has a condition that is highly likely to end in a premature death at any time prior to adulthood. When programs, clinicians and researchers use terms such as life-threatening, life-limiting, or any other, they simply need to be explicit about the term they are using and how it is defined. This approach will be more productive than attempting to find the single unifying language, given that all of them are constructs.

The widely cited report of the U.K. charity Together for Short Lives (previously ACT) and the Royal College of Pediatrics and Child Health identified 4 groups of diseases that may receive PPC services [3]. The first of the 4 categories were those diseases where cure was generally possible but for an individual patient failed. Fortunately, the number of curable conditions is growing. The most prominent in this category is Cancer of course (congenital heart disease being a close second). This points out that the conditions seen in the other 3 categories make up the majority of diseases seen in PPC. Category 2 are conditions whereby cure is not possible, but treatments directed at the underlying disease pathophysiology greatly prolong the life-span and enable good quality of life for a long period of time. The classical example is cystic fibrosis. HIV, if full-treatment is available, is another example. In the past few years an increasing number of gene-based metabolic conditions, such as some lysosomal storage diseases, have moved into Category 2. Many of the gene-based metabolic and neurological diseases remain in Category 3. In this category, there is no cure, and no direct treatment for the disease. The focus is on treating manifestations of the disease, such as seizures, inadequate nutrition, secondary osteopenia, etc. The interventions for these conditions namely anti-convulsants, gastrostomy feeding, bisphosphonate infusion, all improve the quality of life and arguably prolong life. They do not, however, stop disease progression. Fortunately, as can now be seen with some storage diseases, and most recently with Spinal Muscular Atrophy, medical advances move diseases from Category 3 to Category 2. Lastly, Category 4 contains neurological conditions secondary to static encephalopathy. In this category we find children who have experienced hypoxic-ischemic brain injury, as well as those with congenital brain dysgenesis. Until we find ways to directly repair injured brains, the focus for care of these individuals is on symptom management and quality of life.

Another lens is to use a simple classification scheme of 7 categories of diseases seen in PPC; breaking them down into: Cancer; Primary CNS conditions; Biochemical/Metabolic diseases; Neuromuscular diseases; Cardiac and Pulmonary conditions; Infectious diseases and Immunologic diseases; Multi-Organ conditions due to chromosomal aneuploidy or gene defects. This is a simplified, practical 7 category system used for internal reporting purposes at Canuck Place Children's Hospice that has been found useful as a descriptive tool for the estimated 170 different diseases found among the children seen in the program [4]. Others include the system developed by Richard Hain and colleagues, as well as the Complex Chronic Conditions categorization developed by Chris Feudtner and colleagues [5,6]. These categorical systems enable researchers and health services planners to look for trends and evaluate different approaches to treatment.

3. Symptom Management

The principles and practice of symptom management with non-cancer conditions are similar to those for cancer, although with some nuanced differences. Attention to these differences may be important [7]. Much of what we know about symptoms in these children derives from our study of 275 children with non-curable, non-cancer conditions. In these children we tracked 7 symptoms: pain, dyspnea, nausea and vomiting, dysomnia, constipation, seizures, and changes in alertness. Strikingly on average, their parents reported 3.2 symptoms of concern for each child [8].

3.1. Pain

When discussing symptoms in PPC, attention is immediately paid to pain. Most non-cancer conditions can have pain, but generally not due to the generalized inflammation or space-occupying lesions found in cancer, nor with the marked, ongoing escalation [8,9]. Sources of pain include musculoskeletal pain secondary to weakness, bone and joint conditions, and contractures. Skin and organ pain (due to enlargement) can be found in some genetic metabolic diseases. Pain secondary to procedures and interventions is a problem. Visceral pain, especially gastro-intestinal pain arising all along the alimentary tract can be found in almost all conditions, especially if associated with non-oral feeding, reflux disease and constipation. Neuropathic pain can arise from neuropathy or in association with long-standing nociceptive, inflammatory pain. Lastly, children with central nervous system conditions can also be affected by a "central" pain or neuro-irritability that does not seem to have a nociceptive-inflammatory source [10,11]. This condition is challenging to diagnose and to manage; it is an area of active research.

Treating pain in these children, especially those who are very young or are non-verbal, requires patience, sometimes tenacity, and attention to detail [12]. One must search for readily treatable causes such as hip dysplasia, chronic constipation, or poorly adjusted seating systems [9]. When no cause is found clinicians should pursue a screening approach that takes into account silent conditions, such as renal stones, especially with a young or non-verbal patient. In this circumstance pain is relieved when the underlying cause is directly addressed. The treatment of pain (and many other symptoms described in this article) often requires the input of many disciplines. Medical and surgical interventions are only two components. The involvement of physiotherapists, occupational therapists, and speech-language pathologists is often required to address pain and/or other symptoms.

If no cause is identified, then families and clinicians are faced with "pain-like" behaviors that look like what happens with nociception or inflammation but may be induced by activation of internal central nervous circuits alone. One then undertakes empiric treatment with environmental modifications (e.g., swaddling, massage) and with medications (e.g., gabapentin trial) [13]. A step-wise, trial and error approach using validated assessment tools is needed, along with close communication between clinicians and patients/family members. The nature of this central pain—irritability and approaches to its treatment are areas of active research.

3.2. Dysomnia

The second most common symptom in our study was dysomnia. Disturbances of sleep in children can be multi-dimensional and include problems with delayed onset, frequent awakening with fragmented sleep, inadequate sleep duration, and daytime sleepiness (so called "day-night reversal"). For some children many of these features are mixed together. Singly or combined they can pose a major challenge to the child's health and to the family's overall wellbeing. They are very common in children with neurological conditions, comprising a large number of the children followed in PPC [14,15]. There are many potential causes that need to be considered in the evaluation including physical health conditions such as upper airway obstruction; poorly-treated pain leading to poor sleep, and environmental factors. Some conditions, such as Rett Syndrome and Mucopolysaccharidosis Type III are well known to have sleep disturbances, probably on a primary neurological basis [16–18].

Treatment is highly empirical, and evidence is mostly based on either surveys of current practices (by both clinicians and parents), or on case reports. There is a widespread agreement that environmental and behavioral interventions are worth under-taking. Examples include structured bedtime routines, dark and quiet rooms, avoiding pre-bedtime stimulation with videos. The drawback is that such interventions need to be individualized for each patient's particular circumstance and therefore it can be time-consuming to find the interventions that work best. Similarly, there needs to be consistency in implementing them. There is evidence, albeit not very strong, for the use of melatonin [14]. Melatonin appears to assist with sleep onset but may lead to a shortened total duration of sleep; using a combination of immediate-acting and long-acting melatonin may avoid this problem. The environmental interventions and melatonin are considered to be safe. Other medications used are a wide variety of drugs with sedation effects—these include anti-histamines, chloral hydrate and benzodiazepines. Chloral hydrate's only indication is sedation but there are concerns about its long-term use and side effects, especially the effect on the liver. The other medications, as well as a variety of anti-depressants and anti-psychotics, are all sedating but sedation/hypnosis is not their main indication. Specialists however find them useful, and the non-expert prescriber should become familiar with their use and side effects and not hesitate to ask for expert input. Almost every review of dysomnia in children with severe diseases emphasizes the need for family support, especially practical support such as having a night-time nurse or sitter.

3.3. Feeding Difficulties and Constipation

In children with non-cancer, life-threatening conditions the 3rd and 4th most common troubling symptoms were feeding difficulties and constipation [8]. The evaluation and treatment of feeding difficulties in children who receive artificial enteral nutrition has been well described. Similarly, there are a number of approaches to treating constipation that can be considered. There are two points worth noting: one is that treating feeding intolerance requires a step-wise, patient approach. Similarly, treating constipation involves more than simply prescribing a stool softener and assuming the problem is resolved. It requires ongoing assessment of the situation. The second is that in some circumstances feeding intolerance, especially intolerance of elemental formulas and electrolyte solutions in the absence of signs of malabsorption, may be a harbinger of terminal decline. This has been reported but not widely studied [19].

Due to the preponderance of neurological disorders found in children with non-cancer diagnoses, artificial enteral nutrition is a common feeding approach. Not only can these children have difficulties secondary to reflux, delayed gastric emptying and constipation, but their parents also report a higher prevalence of pain and respiratory problems. Pain may be a component of the gastrointestinal symptoms, or another manifestation of the overall disease condition. Respiratory difficulties again may be due to reflux, perhaps exacerbated by the addition of a feeding tube, or it may be se secondary to inadequate airway protection and ongoing aspiration of saliva and bronchial secretions. In some centers this may be an indication for tracheostomy, but it has not been the practice at our institution.

3.4. Dyspnea

Dyspnea, the sensation of breathlessness, was also found in our longitudinal study. Dyspnea is a symptom best studied in the context of adult cancers, especially those involving the lungs, the airway, or the muscle system. While the sensation is well described, there are few commonly used tools to assess it, and a minimal literature on treatment—the literature emphasizes the use of airflow across the face, and opioids to alter the CO_2 ventilation threshold so that there is reduced stimulus towards compensatory hyperventilation.

Dyspnea is primarily understood in the context of adult cancer and cardio-respiratory medicine. Scales have been developed in children, such as the Dalhousie Dyspnea Scales [20]. These scales were developed with verbal, cooperative children over 8 years of age, in situations such as severe asthma and cystic fibrosis. There has not been a similar scale developed for non-verbal, non-cooperating children. Overall there is a paucity of research [21]. Clinically there is a challenge in determining whether a child with severe neurological impairment, from whatever cause, is experiencing dyspnea. Clinicians may assume that the child with tachypnea, use of accessory respiratory muscles, decreased oxygen saturation and other sings of respiratory distress are experiencing dyspnea. They may empirically utilize dyspnea plans with interventions such as airflow, opioids and benzodiazepines with the expectation of benefit.

3.5. Neurological Symptoms

There are other symptoms of concern that must be addressed in children with non-cancer, life-threatening illnesses, especially neurological symptoms [22]. First among these are seizures. Closely working with the child's neurologist will be the best step towards determining an optimal plan for seizure control. In some cases, full control cannot be achieved. Developing both an optimal target and a rescue plan for prolonged or frequent seizures is critical.

Along these lines dystonia is a challenging symptom to contend with [23]. The first step in treating dystonia is to recognize that it is distinct from seizures, although to the uninformed observer, and especially with a non-verbal patient, the uncoordinated movements may suggest a convulsion.

Children may also have co-existing dystonia and seizure disorder, further complicating the picture. Diagnostic evaluation needs to include an EEG to evaluate and delineate seizure-related movements and to treat those. While treatment of dystonia may involve muscle relaxants such as baclofen, parasympathetic inhibitors (trihexyphenidyl), benzodiazepines and dopamine agonists are often tried; these all depend on knowing the etiology of the condition.

Two other symptoms warrant consideration as parents may raise them, although very little is actually known about them. One is lack of arousal or easy fatigability, while the other is temperature dysregulation (cold or hot extremities). These two symptoms have appeared in reports by parents as troubling to them [24]. The lack of arousal is suggested when a parent notes that the child "is no longer him/herself" at times, or less interactive than usual. While the children are in many cases very impaired in language, parents and other caregivers who know the child well learn the individual signals that indicate preferences and emotions. When these are absent, it is clear to the family and close caregivers that something is different. There may be many causes to be investigated, including the introduction of new medications, neurological changes—for example more seizures, or fatigue due to lack of good sleep. More ominously, it may indicate progression of an underlying disease, especially for metabolic conditions related to energy or storage diseases. Some clinicians have speculated that a change in arousal might be related to a psychiatric depression; our current state of understanding the emotional life of a child with neurological impairment is very limited, so we must consider these speculations with reservation.

Temperature dysregulation is also reported by parents, especially in reference to cold and hot extremities. This is also an area that has not received much attention in the literature. One reason that hands and feet may be cold is that the child may lack large muscle mass due to inactivity, resulting in decreased thermal production. When the extremities alternate between being hot and cold, then centrally based autonomic dysfunction may be the etiology. We are learning more about the role that the autonomic nervous system plays in children and this may lead to useful interventions [25]. In the short term, simple environmental measures are useful paying attention to cold and hot hands and feet and changing clothing accordingly.

4. Emotional Support

It is fundamental that emotional support for the affected child is a responsibility of pediatric palliative care. In this regard there is no difference between children experiencing cancer and those with non-cancer diagnoses. In both situations the range of services must be broad and robust. There needs to be capacity to provide many different modalities adjusted to age, developmental capacity, and child/youth preferences. Modalities employed include play-based therapy, art therapy, music therapy, and standard talk-based approaches such as cognitive-behavior therapy.

Just because a child is very young or non-verbal it is wrong to assume that they are not experiencing feelings that need to be addressed. Many parents of non-verbal children provide consistent descriptions of their child's understanding that usually exceeds what a brief observation in a clinic will demonstrate to a clinician. Prolonged interaction and observation of a child by nurses, physical and occupational therapists, and others generally confirms the parents' assessment. Therefore, taking the lead from parents and developing a strategy to address a child's depression, anxiety, and fears, regardless of perceived developmental stage is important.

5. Social Issues

It is here that we consider the family beyond the affected child; parents and siblings, and in many cases, grandparents, aunts and uncles and other extended members. Foremost is addressing their questions that may focus on prognosis; this will be covered further on under the Trajectory section. Social support for family includes both care for their emotional needs—anxiety, depression, guilt—but also the practical issues of daily life that are complicated by having a child with a life-threatening condition.

Some observations about how non-cancer conditions can be different are warranted here. One is that while "cancer" is not a single diagnosis, the care of children with cancer is often provided by a unified team at a single center. Parents then benefit from services available at a single site under the banner of cancer care; this may include mental health services for themselves and for siblings, family support through activities such as camps, and a communal experience with other families encountered in the clinic and hospital. Simply having a recognizable condition such as cancer, as difficult as that is, may create a framework for social understanding.

Non-cancer diagnoses number in the hundreds and cover a wide variety of organ systems [26]. There is no single team or clinic that may follow these children. There is often not a support system for parents or siblings provided in an ongoing, organized fashion, and families may feel highly isolated. As most of these conditions are very rare, families may struggle to explain to others what exactly is going on in their lives.

A particular challenge for families are one of a kind diagnoses where there are no other children with a similar condition, and similarly where a child lacks a diagnosis. In both cases families are left without information, increasing the uncertainty. New techniques in genome analysis, such as Whole Exome Sequencing and Whole Genome Sequencing are now available at both the clinical and research level. However, not all gene-based conditions can be identified as due to a single gene mutation. In some cases, there are multiple gene interactions that lead to a phenotype. Understanding how the protein product of a gene creates the condition is a necessary piece of information. Recent studies suggest that families' value a "diagnosis" even when it does not lead to any treatment [27].

Regardless of having the gene explanation, families with children whose condition is either very rare or non-diagnosed can feel isolated. This can occur both in their family and community as well as with interactions in the health system. It is not unusual for families to report confusion by health care providers and sometimes reluctance to provide care. It is important for clinicians to understand that in the absence of a life-prolonging or curative treatment, the focus on symptom management will rely on basic principles that are similar across conditions, until we learn otherwise.

Because of their expertise in symptom management, familiarity with rare and undiagnosed conditions, and family-centered approach, pediatric palliative care teams can be important to families, sometimes akin to a "medical home" for families if they are resourced accordingly. If not that well resourced, they can still be valuable as consultants to primary teams caring for these children.

6. Trajectory

In the model we teach to trainees and use day-to-day in practice, following the sequence outlined as Physical, Emotional (child), Social (family), Spiritual (religion and meaning), and Trajectory, the last item keying into advance care planning. Trajectory is a topic that uncovers child and family goals, hopes and concerns. Based on these elements we then develop alternative pathways using a "what if" approach. This is an iterative process.

As described in the previous sections, non-malignant conditions are often hard to characterize as they are rare, not well studied, and with a resulting low level of evidence. As many of these conditions have a genetic basis, the nature of the gene defect, balancing and unbalancing genetic factors, and interaction with the environment all play a role in phenotype and therefore clinical course. These factors all combine to make disease course and prognostication very difficult. A high degree of clinical expertise, experience, careful communication, and a healthy dose of skepticism are all needed.

Figure 1 gives insight into an interesting finding; the majority of children followed at any given time on the Canuck Place program have non-cancer diseases, whereas mortality rates show a high incidence of cancer deaths.

This pattern suggests that there are differences in the way that, and the timing of, engagement of children and their families with PPC services at least in one well-established program. Similar data is found when examining timing of death in relationship to referral, broken down by disease category as shown in Figure 2. Children with cancer may die sooner after referral as curative attempts continue well into the disease course. For many patients with non-cancer, non-curable conditions, clinicians and families are seeking hospice, medical respite, and palliative care support earlier in the disease, and therefore constitute a larger proportion of patients on program at any given time. This is one hypothesis to explain the differences. In addition, the services accessed for patients and families with cancer as compared to a non-cancer diagnosis may differ. Care intensity may be high in children and families living with cancer, although for a shorter period of time. In contrast, children with non-cancer diagnoses, especially those with static encephalopathy (Together for Short Lives Category 4), received care intermittently but over longer-time periods [28].

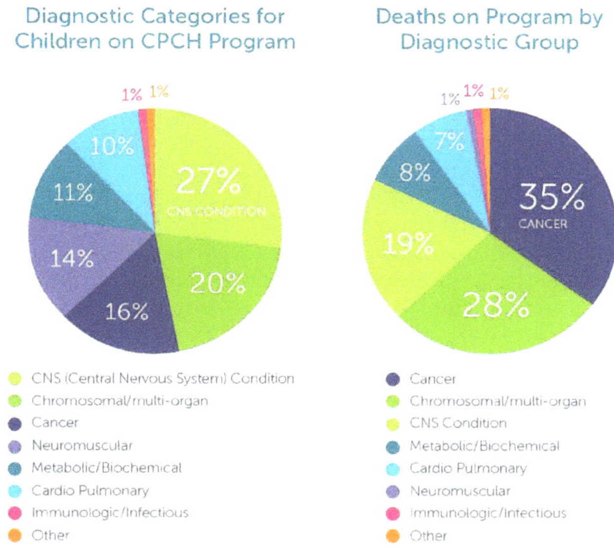

Figure 1. Children on Program and Deaths on Program Canuck Place Children's Hospice.

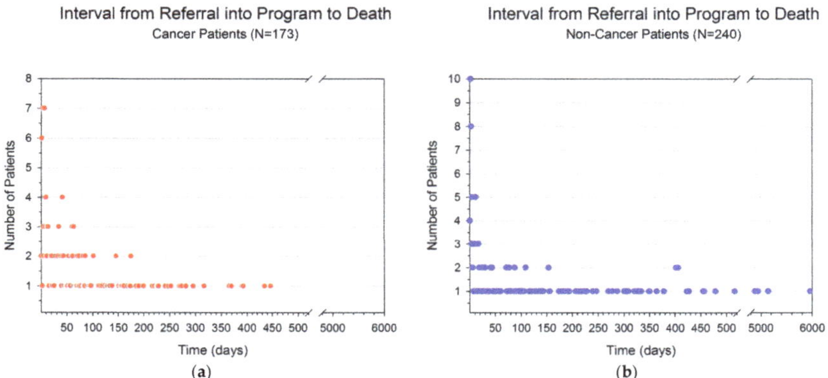

Figure 2. (**a**) Intervals from referral to palliative care until death for cancer patients; (**b**) Intervals from referral to palliative care until death for patients with non-cancer conditions.

As was shown in Figure 2 the unpredictable pattern of time from referral to death, observed in several studies, confirms that the best approach is to prepare families, and oneself, both for sudden terminal events and simultaneously for a protracted course. Preparing families involves both education and careful planning. One mother aptly describes this as "only a (parent in a pediatric palliative care program) meets their kindergarten principal and funeral director in the same week".

In addition to discussing advance care planning and advance directives with families as ongoing discussion, it is also advisable to explore scenarios. Completing paperwork, for example a letter to be used in the Emergency Room, is also advisable so that one is prepared for the unexpected.

The pediatric palliative care program at Canuck Place does not require an advance directive document or Do Not Attempt Resuscitation order. It is practice however to have advance care planning discussions with families on an annual basis, at minimum. In these discussions it may be sufficient to simply review the relevant concepts and terminology that families may encounter (e.g., what is a "Code Blue"), without requiring any specific decision-making. As we found in a retrospective review, this kind of conversation supports family decision-making, and one result is that even among the families who self-described as choosing all resuscitation measures, at the time of their child's death almost none asked for intervention.

7. Future Directions

As the field of pediatric palliative care matures more attention is being paid to the non-malignant conditions in research and knowledge translation. An understanding that cross-communication among several fields and subspecialties in medicine and other disciplines needs to occur in order to develop a more comprehensive (holistic) understanding of how these conditions are experienced by affected children and their families, and in turn to design interventions that support quality of life.

Immediate targets include epidemiological and health services research studies to better delineate the population of interest and their service use; clinical intervention studies of physical symptoms, children's emotional wellbeing, and family psycho-social health; and basic physiology and pharmacology studies to enhance our understanding of symptoms and symptom treatment.

Children and their families with non-malignant conditions are a substantial proportion of the work of pediatric palliative care and will potentially increase in number in the future with advances in life-prolonging treatments. This is an area that deserves our attention especially for on-going research.

Conflicts of Interest: The author declares no conflict of interest.

References

1. Worswick, J. *A House Called Helen: The Development of Hospice Care for Children*, 2nd ed.; Oxford University Press: Oxford, UK, 2000; ISBN 978-0-19-263235-7.
2. Spicer, S.; Macdonald, M.; Davies, D.; Vadeboncoeur, C.; Siden, H. Introducing a Lexicon of Terms for Pediatric Palliative Care. *Paediatr. Child Health* **2015**, *20*, 155–156. [CrossRef] [PubMed]
3. ACT (The Association for Children's Palliative Care). *RCPCH A Guide to the Development of Children's Palliative Care Services: Report of the Joint Working Party of the Association for Children with Life-Threatening or Terminal Conditions and Their Families (ACT) and the Royal College of Paediatrics and Child Health (RCPCH)*; ACT: Bristol, UK, 1997.
4. Chavoshi, N.; Miller, T.; Siden, H. Resource utilization among individuals dying of pediatric life-threatening diseases. *J. Palliat. Med.* **2013**, *16*, 1210–1214. [CrossRef] [PubMed]
5. Bergstraesser, E.; Hain, R.D.; Pereira, J.L. The development of an instrument that can identify children with palliative care needs: The Paediatric Palliative Screening Scale (PaPaS Scale): A qualitative study approach. *BMC Palliat. Care* **2013**, *12*, 20. [CrossRef] [PubMed]
6. Feudtner, C.; Christakis, D.A.; Connell, F.A. Pediatric Deaths Attributable to Complex Chronic Conditions: A Population-Based Study of Washington State, 1980–1997. *Pediatrics* **2000**, *106*, 205–209. [PubMed]
7. Malcolm, C.; Hain, R.; Gibson, F.; Adams, S.; Anderson, G.; Forbat, L. Challenging symptoms in children with rare life-limiting conditions: Findings from a prospective diary and interview study with families. *Acta Paediatr.* **2012**, *101*, 985–992. [CrossRef] [PubMed]
8. Steele, R.; Siden, H.; Cadell, S.; Davies, B.; Andrews, G.; Feichtinger, L.; Singh, M. Charting the territory: Symptoms and functional assessment in children with progressive, non-curable conditions. *Arch. Dis. Child.* **2014**, *99*, 754–762. [CrossRef] [PubMed]

9. Siden, H.; Oberlander, T. Pain management for children with a developmental disability in a primary care setting. In *Pain in Children: A Practical Guide for Primary Care*; Humana Press: New York, NY, USA, 2008.
10. Oberlander, T.F.; O'Donnell, M.E. Beliefs about pain among professionals working with children with significant neurologic impairment. *Dev. Med. Child Neurol.* **2001**, *43*, 138–140. [CrossRef] [PubMed]
11. Oberlander, T.F.; Symons, F.; Van Dongen, K.; Abu-Saad, H.H. Pain in Individuals with Developmental Disabilities: Challenges for the Future. *Prog. Pain Res. Manag.* **2003**, *24*, 705–724.
12. Siden, H.B.; Carleton, B.C.; Oberlander, T.F. Physician variability in treating pain and irritability of unknown origin in children with severe neurological impairment. *Pain Res. Manag. J. Can. Pain Soc. J. Soc. Can. Pour Trait. Douleur* **2013**, *18*, 243–248. [CrossRef] [PubMed]
13. Hauer, J.M.; Wical, B.S.; Charnas, L. Gabapentin Successfully Manages Chronic Unexplained Irritability in Children with Severe Neurologic Impairment. *Pediatrics* **2007**, *119*, e519–e522. [CrossRef] [PubMed]
14. Braam, W.; Didden, R.; Smits, M.; Curfs, L. Melatonin treatment in individuals with intellectual disability and chronic insomnia: A randomized placebo-controlled study. *J. Intellect. Disabil. Res.* **2008**, *52*, 256–264. [CrossRef] [PubMed]
15. Jan, J.E.; Freeman, R.D. Melatonin therapy for circadian rhythm sleep disorders in children with multiple disabilities: What have we learned in the last decade? *Dev. Med. Child Neurol.* **2004**, *46*, 776–782. [CrossRef] [PubMed]
16. Piazza, C.C.; Fisher, W.; Kiesewetter, K.; Bowman, L.; Moser, H. Aberrant sleep patterns in children with the Rett syndrome. *Brain Dev.* **1990**, *12*, 488–493. [CrossRef]
17. Mariotti, P.; Della Marca, G.; Iuvone, L.; Vernacotola, S.; Ricci, R.; Mennuni, G.F.; Mazza, S. Sleep disorders in Sanfilippo syndrome: A polygraphic study. *Clin. EEG Electroencephalogr.* **2003**, *34*, 18–22. [CrossRef]
18. Zucconi, M.; Bruni, O. Sleep disorders in children with neurologic diseases. *Semin. Pediatr. Neurol.* **2001**, *8*, 258–275. [CrossRef] [PubMed]
19. Siden, H.; Tucker, T.; Derman, S.; Cox, K.; Soon, G.S.; Hartnett, C.; Straatman, L. Pediatric enteral feeding intolerance: A new prognosticator for children with life-limiting illness? *J. Palliat. Care* **2009**, *25*, 213–217. [PubMed]
20. Pianosi, P.; Smith, C.P.; Almudevar, A.; McGrath, P.J. Dalhousie dyspnea scales: Pictorial scales to measure dyspnea during induced bronchoconstriction. *Pediatr. Pulmonol.* **2006**, *41*, 1182–1187. [CrossRef] [PubMed]
21. Craig, F.; Henderson, E.M.; Bluebond-Langner, M. Management of respiratory symptoms in paediatric palliative care. *Curr. Opin. Support. Palliat. Care* **2015**, *9*, 217–226. [CrossRef] [PubMed]
22. Rasmussen, L.A.; Gregoire, M.-C. Challenging neurological symptoms in paediatric palliative care: An approach to symptom evaluation and management in children with neurological impairment. *Paediatr. Child Health* **2015**, *20*, 159–165. [CrossRef] [PubMed]
23. Allen, N.M.; Lin, J.-P.; Lynch, T.; King, M.D. Status dystonicus: A practice guide. *Dev. Med. Child Neurol.* **2014**, *56*, 105–112. [CrossRef] [PubMed]
24. Hunt, A.M. A Survey of Signs, Symptoms and Symptom Control in 30 Terminally Ill Children. *Dev. Med. Child Neurol.* **1990**, *32*, 341–346. [CrossRef] [PubMed]
25. Rees, C.A. Lost among the trees? The autonomic nervous system and paediatrics. *Arch. Dis. Child.* **2014**, *99*, 552–562. [CrossRef] [PubMed]
26. Hain, R.; Devins, M.; Hastings, R.; Noyes, J. Paediatric palliative care: Development and pilot study of a "Directory" of life-limiting conditions. *BMC Palliat. Care* **2013**, *12*, 43. [CrossRef] [PubMed]
27. Makela, N.L.; Birch, P.H.; Friedman, J.M.; Marra, C.A. Parental perceived value of a diagnosis for intellectual disability (ID): A qualitative comparison of families with and without a diagnosis for their child's ID. *Am. J. Med. Genet. A* **2009**, *149A*, 2393–2402. [CrossRef] [PubMed]
28. Bender, H.U.; Riester, M.B.; Borasio, G.D.; Führer, M. "Let's Bring Her Home First." Patient Characteristics and Place of Death in Specialized Pediatric Palliative Home Care. *J. Pain Symptom Manag.* **2017**, *54*, 159–166. [CrossRef] [PubMed]

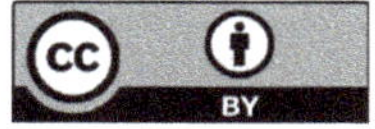

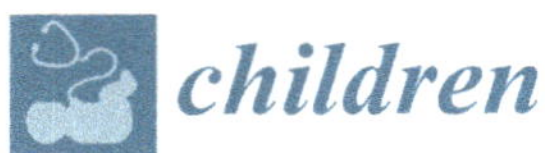

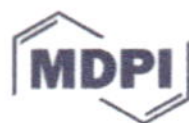

Review

Feeding Intolerance in Children with Severe Impairment of the Central Nervous System: Strategies for Treatment and Prevention

Julie Hauer [1,2]

[1] Boston Children's Hospital, Division of General Pediatrics, Harvard School of Medicine, 300 Longwood Ave, Boston, MA 02115, USA; julie.hauer@childrens.harvard.edu; Tel.: +1-978-448-3388

[2] Seven Hills Pediatric Center, 22 Hillside, Groton, MA 01450, USA

Received: 1 December 2017; Accepted: 21 December 2017; Published: 22 December 2017

Abstract: Children with severe impairment of the central nervous system (CNS) experience gastrointestinal (GI) symptoms at a high rate and severity, including retching, vomiting, GI tract pain, and feeding intolerance. Commonly recognized sources of symptoms include constipation and gastroesophageal reflux disease. There is growing awareness of sources due to the impaired nervous system, including visceral hyperalgesia due to sensitization of sensory neurons in the enteric nervous system and central neuropathic pain due to alterations in the thalamus. Challenging the management of these symptoms is the lack of tests to confirm alterations in the nervous system as a cause of symptom generation, requiring empirical trials directed at such sources. It is also common to have multiple reasons for the observed symptoms, further challenging management. Recurrent emesis and GI tract pain can often be improved, though in some not completely eliminated. In some, this can progress to intractable feeding intolerance. This comprehensive review provides an evidence-based approach to care, a framework for recurrent symptoms, and language strategies when symptoms remain intractable to available interventions. This summary is intended to balance optimal management with a sensitive palliative care approach to persistent GI symptoms in children with severe impairment of the CNS.

Keywords: pediatric; neurological impairment; feeding intolerance; retching; visceral hyperalgesia; central neuropathic pain; autonomic dysfunction; disability; pediatric palliative care; symptom management

1. Introduction

Retching, vomiting, and gastrointestinal (GI) pain are frequent and significant problems experienced by children with severe impairment of the central nervous system (CNS), often referred to as children with severe neurological impairment (SNI) [1–9]. The GI tract is one of the most frequent sources of pain in children with SNI despite treatment of common sources such as gastroesophageal reflux disease (GERD) and constipation [2–6,10]. Pain attributed to the GI tract is noted to have a high pain intensity of 7.5 (from a 0–10 scale), second only to pain of unknown cause, with significantly higher rates of pain in children already receiving treatment for GERD or impaired GI tract motility [2,5,10]. Many continue to have recurrent symptoms despite evaluation and treatment directed at such problems, and such children may experience repeated testing in search of a cause.

These problems can result in feeding intolerance that for some can become a recurrent and persistent problem despite management of commonly recognized sources. This was identified as one of the most common problems in children with progressive genetic, metabolic, or neurologic conditions with no cure, with pain, sleep, and feeding difficulties identified by parents as the three most common problems, with symptoms often not well controlled [11].

This article will focus on GI symptoms that are recurrent and persistent in children with SNI. The goal of this article is to provide evidence-based suggestions to guide empirical treatment trials. This includes a review of how the altered CNS can contribute to such symptoms and interventions to modify how these symptoms are generated.

2. A Framework

Children with SNI and recurrent retching, emesis, and feeding intolerance often have multiple sources that contribute to these symptoms. As a starting framework, some are common management issues such as constipation and minimizing excessive calories, some are due to the altered CNS, and some are acute problems that can worsen the chronic symptoms. Further considerations include:

- Problems with tests that are "fixable": urinary tract infection (UTI), acute pancreatitis, cholecystitis, nephrolithiasis, volvulus, helicobacter pylori.
- Problems with tests that can be modified and empirically managed: GERD, dysmotility.
- Problems without tests due to the altered nervous system that can be modified, require empirical trials, and can remain intractable: autonomic dysfunction, altered enteric nervous system, visceral hyperalgesia, central neuropathic pain, altered vomiting center in the medulla.
- Problems due to a wide range of needs in the same group of children: calorie and fluid estimates.

3. Testable Causes

Causes of acute emesis and abdominal pain typically have a diagnostic test to then guide treatment. Causes to consider include acute gastroenteritis, urinary tract infection, acute pancreatitis, nephrolithiasis, cholecystitis, volvulus, superior mesenteric artery syndrome, or adhesions. When symptoms persist, causes due to the altered nervous system (Table 1) are important to consider in a child with negative tests and insufficient benefit from treatment for such problems as GERD.

4. Causes Due to the Altered Nervous System

4.1. Visceral Hyperalgesia and Central Neuropathic Pain

Visceral hyperalgesia is an altered threshold to pain generation in response to a stimulus in the GI tract [12]. As a result, a normal stimulus, such as distention and pressure within the GI tract, can result in pain. Alternatively, tissue inflammation or injury, such as from GERD or surgery to the GI tract, may result in sensitization of visceral afferent pathways, with resulting visceral hyperalgesia.

Central neuropathic pain can develop when injury or disease of the CNS involves the thalamus or spinothalamic tract [13–15]. Symptoms due to this cause of pain include visceral pain associated with distention of the GI tract and bladder, described by one adult as feeling "like my bowels will explode" [16].

Both are reviewed together given the inability to know when GI tract pain is due to sensitization of sensory neurons in the enteric nervous system or a result of altered descending inhibitory control. Both can be suggested by (1) pain, retching and vomiting associated with gastrostomy tube (G-tube) feedings as a result of decreased gastric volume threshold to symptom generation; (2) pain associated with intestinal gas and jejunostomy tube (J-tube) feedings, suggesting pain with intestinal distention; (3) pain associated with flatus and bowel movements suggesting pain associated with colonic distention; and (4) persistent symptoms despite treatment of an identified problem such as GERD. The inability to tolerate a reasonable feeding rate may indirectly indicate a decreased threshold to symptom generation from GI tract distention.

Table 1. Chronic sources of retching, emesis, and visceral pain.

Cause	Management Options	Comments
Constipation	Polyethylene glycol Lactulose Milk of Magnesia Senna	Colonic distention from constipation can trigger pain symptoms due to visceral hyperalgesia and central neuropathic pain
GERD, motility disorders	H-2 blockers and PPIs Protective barrier: sucralfate Promotility drugs: erythromycin, metoclopramide Jejunostomy feeding tube	Motility disorders can be a result of impaired input from the CNS to the enteric nervous system Suggested by bloating, distension, retching, vomiting, discomfort Other problems can contribute, including constipation and pain
Vomiting reflex	Medications that block the 5HT-2, 5HT-3, H-1, Ach, and D-2 receptors Cyproheptadine (5HT-2, H-1, Ach) Ondansetron (5HT-3)	Suggested by retching, forceful vomiting, and associated symptoms of sweating, pale skin, and appearing distressed
Visceral hyperalgesia, central neuropathic pain	Gabapentin Pregabalin Tricyclic antidepressants	Suggested by pain, retching, and emesis associated with feedings, intestinal gas, flatus, and bowel movements
Autonomic dysfunction	Gabapentin Pregabalin Clonidine	Suggested by pain and emesis associated with tachycardia, hyperthermia, diaphoresis, and skin flushing
Pseudo-obstruction	Conservative management Erythromycin Neostigmine or pyridostigmine	Suggested by recurrent episodes of abdominal distension, pain, emesis, and severe constipation, in the absence of mechanical obstruction

Ach: acetylcholine; CNS: central nervous system; D: dopamine; H: histamine; 5HT: serotonin; GERD: gastroesophageal reflux disease; PPI: proton pump inhibitor.

Two considerations to management are: interventions that lessen GI tract distention and medications that lessen symptom generation. The former includes alterations in feeding volume rate, a review of calorie estimates, and G-tube venting, as examples. The later can include medication trials directed at visceral hyperalgesia and central neuropathic pain (Table 1).

Medication options for both include gabapentin and tricyclic antidepressants (TCAs) [13–19]. In addition, use of gabapentin for persistent pain in children with SNI resulted in a significant reduction of associated GI symptoms, including decreased emesis and retching, improved feeding tolerance, weight gain, and change from J-tube to G-tube feedings [17,20,21]. Clonidine also has suggested benefit in reducing pain perception during gastric and colonic distension [22].

4.2. Autonomic Dysfunction

Autonomic dysfunction, also called dysautonomia, paroxysmal sympathetic hyperactivity, autonomic storming, or sympathetic storming, can be due to alterations in the hypothalamus in children with SNI. Symptoms include tachycardia, hyperthermia, flushing of skin, abdominal pain, vomiting, bowel dysmotility, constipation, urinary retention, excessive sweating, increased salivation, posturing, and agitation [23–25].

Literature is limited to case reports, predominantly in patients with hypoxic and traumatic brain injury, with mixed results for interventions reported including benzodiazepines, bromocriptine, clonidine, oral and intrathecal baclofen (ITB), beta antagonists, and morphine sulfate [26–29]. More recently reported interventions include gabapentin and pregabalin [25,30]. In addition to scheduled gabapentinoid or clonidine, children with intermittent "autonomic storms" may benefit from as needed clonidine, benzodiazepine, or morphine sulfate during these episodes.

4.3. Emetic Reflex and Vomiting Center

The emetic reflex is the mechanism by which the CNS protects the body from potentially toxic substances. This complex reflex involves input to the vomiting center (VC), the final pathway. Receptors in the VC include histamine (H-1), acetylcholine (Ach), and serotonin (5HT-2) [31]. Alterations in the GI tract can stimulate the VC, predominantly mediated through the vagus and sympathetic nerves. The receptors involved include various serotonin (5HT) receptors in the GI tract including 5HT-4 prokinetic receptors and dopamine (D-2) receptors in the gastric wall. Substance P has also been identified in the GI tract, a neurotransmitter that induces vomiting through stimulation of the neurokinin (NK-1) receptors located in the chemoreceptor trigger zone.

Stimulation of these receptors can involve either distention or inflammation in the GI tract. Distention is detected by mechanoreceptors and inflammation by chemoreceptors. The goal is to treat sources when possible and block triggered receptors when the source cannot be fully eliminated. As an example, altered motility can result in recurrent distention of the intestines and colon. Treatment to modify motility is intended to minimize development of symptoms, with medications that target involved receptors then lessening symptom generation.

Medications that block these receptors include cyproheptadine and ondansetron (Table 2). Some medications, such as cyproheptadine, block more than one receptor involved with triggering the emetic reflex. Cyproheptadine has been identified to improve feeding tolerance, decrease emesis, and decrease retching including after fundoplication [32,33].

Table 2. Interventions for chronic retching, vomiting, and visceral pain.

Intervention	Comments
Treat constipation	Minimizes colonic distension and further slowing of motility
Assess for over-feeding	Children at highest risk: intermittent hypothermia, minimal movement of extremities, decreased movement following symptom reduction, gradual health decline Initiate 30% reduction and monitor for 2–4 weeks
Review bolus volume and feed rate	Suggested guidelines: bolus < 15 mL/kg per bolus, continuous rate < 8 mL/kg/h [34]
Review osmolarity of feeds	Minimize use of elemental formulas or dilute, use additives to add calories without adding osmotic load (microlipid)
Gastric acid reduction and protective barrier: H-2 blockers, PPIs, sucralfate, antacids	Consider 8–12 weeks treatment course: chronic use of PPIs associated with *Clostridium difficile*, small bowel bacterial overgrowth, pneumonia, bone fracture, and hypomagnesemia Anticipate gastric acid rebound when a PPI is stopped; consider managing with short-term use of antacids or H-2 blocker
Gabapentin, pregabalin	Treatment of visceral hyperalgesia and dysautonomia
Tricyclic antidepressant	Treatment of visceral hyperalgesia and central neuropathic pain
Clonidine	Treatment of symptoms due to dysautonomia
Cyproheptadine	Blocks receptors that trigger the VC (5HT-2, H-1, and Ach)
Ondansetron	Blocks receptors that trigger the emetic reflex (5HT-3)
Erythromycin Metoclopramide	May improve gastric emptying and intestinal motility No clear benefit of one over the other Limit use of metoclopramide due to risk of dystonic reaction and lower seizure threshold
G-tube venting and equipment that allows venting during feedings	Minimizes gastric distension and associated discomfort
Gastrojejunal tube (GJ-tube)	Lessens gastric distension G-tube venting possible while feeding through the J-tube GI pain may not improve with J-tube feedings
Soy, partially hydrolyzed, or elemental formula	Management of protein hypersensitivity Higher omolarity with elemental formula
Select antibiotics	For *Helicobacter pylori* identified by stool antigen or endoscopy, or empirical trial for small bowel bacterial overgrowth
Anti-reflux surgery (fundoplication)	Consider empirical medication trials for problems outlined above before elective surgery Some children will develop retching, bloating, and pain following fundoplication

G-tube: gastrostomy tube; GJ-tube: gastrojejunal tube; TCA: tricyclic antidepressant; VC: vomiting center.

5. Over-Feeding

Over-feeding was identified as the third most common contributor to feeding intolerance, behind formula osmolarity and feeding rate [34]. Children with SNI have significantly lower energy expenditure as assessed by indirect calorimetry [35,36]. Calorie estimates using guidelines for children with cerebral palsy (CP) can over-estimate energy requirements in children with SNI by 30–40% [36–39]. Factors that contribute to this over-estimation include that children with SNI often have decreased muscle mass, which can account for 20–30% of resting energy expenditure [35]. Other factors that also decrease energy expenditure by approximately 25% include limited movement of extremities and hypothermia [36,40].

Guidelines for energy requirements have been established for children with CP. Using length, energy requirements are typically 12–15 kcal/cm for those who are ambulatory and 10–11 kcal/cm for those who are non-ambulatory, with some needing only 6–9 kcal/cm or less as a result of those factors that further lower energy expenditure [38,39]. Energy expenditure can also be determined by estimating the physical activity coefficient factor to use with the resting energy expenditure (REE, in kcal/day). Many children with SNI require a factor of 0.8 (kcal/day = REE × 0.8), with some as low as 0.5–0.6 [38]. This is in contrast to a factor of 1.5 to 1.6 for a typically developing, healthy child and a factor of 1.1 for a child who is non-ambulatory due to CP.

The goal in children with feeding tubes who remain life-long dependent on others to estimate calorie intake is to avoid excessive weight gain and to minimize associated symptoms of over-feeding, including retching, emesis, and GI tract pain. Children at highest risk for over-estimating intake include children with:

- Limited movement of extremities at baseline.
- A decrease in movement following improvement in symptoms (increase in baseline tone and movement are common features associated with pain) [20].
- Hypothermia due to impaired central regulation of body temperature.
- Gradual decline in activity when there is a decline in function and health over months to years.

Fluid needs can also be overestimated in children with a low metabolic rate, given that energy expenditure accounts for a portion of fluid needs. Of note, fluid requirement calculations based on weight were developed in ambulatory individuals with higher metabolic rates. This recognition allows a feed reduction trial without a need to maintain the same total fluid volume, when the goal of the trial is to determine if this will reduce emesis and GI tract pain.

A discussion regarding a reduction in calories is best approached gently, given the symbolic nature of feeding and nutrition. Language that may benefit families is an acknowledgment that it can seem counter intuitive to suggest a reduction in feeds as potentially beneficial for a child. Taking time to reflect on information can lessen associated fear and allow concerns to be adequately explored.

Some children will benefit from a feeding reduction trial when emesis, retching, or pain localized to the GI tract persists, following a comprehensive assessment for testable/treatable sources and management of common problems such as GERD and constipation. A 30% reduction of feeds is suggested to ensure an adequate trial while monitoring for benefit. A dietician can determine the need for micronutrient and protein supplementation when feeds are decreased. Along with monitoring weight, parents can monitor for changes in how clothing is fitting. This author has observed children with minimal to no change in weight when symptoms are improved following a reduction in feeds. This may reflect improved retention of intake due to decreased emesis and decreased metabolic expenditure due to a decrease in tone and movement when pain is reduced [20,38].

6. Empirical Trials

Many of the interventions listed in Table 2 require an empirical trial, including medications directed at causes due to the altered nervous system given the lack of diagnostic tests. Information regarding empirical trials directed at these problems, including dosing guidelines, is reviewed in detail in this clinical report from the American Academy of Pediatrics [16].

6.1. Medication Trials

Recurrent emesis and GI tract pain can often be improved, though in some not completely eliminated. The optimal plan can involve significant time and effort in those with recurrent symptoms and is best guided by broader considerations [16]. Information to consider when starting an empirical medication trial includes (1) response to previous medications; (2) interaction with other drugs; (3) initial dose; (4) the need for titration to minimize adverse effects; (5) the minimal initial dose; and (6) adverse effects [16]. Monitoring will determine whether there is adequate benefit and, if not, if a second medication will be added while continuing the first medication. As an example, the use of two or more medications with different mechanisms of action may reduce symptoms generated by neuropathic pain and reduce adverse effects if synergistic benefit allows for dose reduction [16].

6.2. Home Care Plans

Medications can modify symptoms generated by the altered nervous system, though breakthrough symptoms can occur due to the inability to eliminate the cause. Parents can be empowered with care plans to utilize for breakthrough symptoms. Interventions can be tried and then the care plan modified as information is gained. As an example, some children will benefit from use of an as needed suppository when retching or GI tract pain recurs, with such a trial determining if this is helpful for a specific child. Such an intervention can lessen colonic distention if the intervention results in a bowel movement, given the inability to know if there was incomplete evacuation with the last bowel movement.

Information to consider and document in a care plan includes:

- Presenting symptoms (vomiting, retching, pain).
- Initial routine interventions (vent G-tube).
- Interventions for triggers due to GI tract distention (use as-needed suppository, use enema if no results within 1-h of suppository, hold feeds for 2 h, hold feeds and give electrolyte replacement overnight, reduce total feeds/fluids).
- Use of as-needed medications (options include as needed antacid, ondansetron, clonidine, or benzodiazepine).
- When to call (call the clinic during the day or the on-call clinician after hours if symptoms persist despite use of the interventions outlined).

As an example, this was a beneficial strategy for an 18-year-old with SNI, thought to be due to birth anoxia, with recurrent episodes of abdominal distention and pain. Through trial and error, the following care plan was developed. This allowed care during events to remain at home and lessened repeat testing.

Initiate care plan for the following symptoms: persistent abdominal distention with discomfort or vomiting.

- Vent G-tube, hold use × 2 h.
- If no stool that day, give fleet enema.
- Give pedialyte at 40 mL/h × 4 h, then 70 mL/h × 24–36 h.
- Give acetaminophen every 4–6 h × 3–4 doses.
- Use morphine as needed, as often as every 4 h.
- Update team.

7. Acute on Chronic Symptom Events

If the frequency or severity of events increases, there is a balance between two considerations: assessment for a new acute source while considering a modification to a medication dose or an additional empirical medication trial directed at the sources due to the altered nervous system. Past experience, along with parental preference, will guide this balance. In a child with repeated negative tests, there may be a shared decision to focus on modifying the chronic care plan, given the decreased likelihood of the same tests identifying a new problem. A supportive and flexible approach can guide decisions in the child with recurrent symptoms. Language at such times might include the following:

- "Most recent tests have been negative, and I have the option of increasing the dose of his gabapentin or clonidine (I have the option to add a medication that targets the same symptoms in a different way). It might make sense to adjust medications while considering tests. You know your son best and I want you to feel comfortable with the plan. What makes best sense to you at this time?"
- "I imagine this is hard as I talk about sources that can be improved but not fixed".

- "It must be hard as I talk about his nervous system being a reason for these symptoms when I don't have a test to tell you with certainty. What are your thoughts as we discuss this information?"

8. Intractable Feeding Intolerance and Features at End of Life

Persistent feeding intolerance following various interventions is an intensely stressful experience for families of children with SNI. The assessment and management often reflect months of repeated studies and various interventions. Though intractable feeding intolerance is not common, the inherent challenges deserve consideration.

It can be beneficial, as further interventions outlined in Table 2 are considered, to simultaneously be mindful that this may be part of an irreversible decline. Language at such times can include, "I hope for as much benefit from this next trial, although I also want you to be prepared that we might not have the hoped-for benefit. What is important to you as we consider these possibilities?" [41].

This can be challenging, as children with SNI often experience decline over a long period, increasing the likelihood of testing and intervention trials of an irreversible problem. Alterations in GI tract function that is under the control of the CNS [42,43] may be a result of ongoing neuronal apoptosis. Changes in the CNS may account for why some children with SNI develop feeding intolerance that is not amenable to medical interventions [44]. Other features that can suggest changes in CNS function include altered alertness (pathways involved with arousal), altered regulation of body temperature and heart rate (autonomic function), frequency of seizures, level of comfort (thalamus), and altered vasomotor tone resulting in peripheral edema (hypothalamus and medulla), along with the regulation of GI tract function (hypothalamus and medulla). The development of persistent peripheral edema is the most likely to indicate irreversible changes, reported as a feature in the last weeks to months of life in children with SNI, and as a terminal feature in adults with multiple sclerosis and CNS tumors [45,46].

These considerations are important for parents to minimize over-testing at a time of diminishing benefit. Palliative care teams can provide support and guidance throughout this process. Suggested language includes: "These features can be due to changes in the brain. This means that the problems we are seeing might not improve with available treatment. As we try the next intervention we discussed, what is most important to you at this time?", "I know that comfort is an important goal. I worry that it has been difficult to meet this goal or that it will only be possible with increased sedation or a decrease in total feeds. What are your thoughts?" [41]. Discussions may result in a shared decision to redirect goals and change care plans, such as reconsidering the role of further testing, resuscitation, and hospitalization.

The use of medical fluids and nutrition can be reviewed when there is persistent symptom burden due to tube feedings that is not alleviated with available interventions. At such times the use of a feeding tube can be viewed as a life-sustaining technology that may be prolonging suffering. This allows one to consider the amount of benefit and harm when technology is becoming more burdensome, even when that technology is "routine" to use. This is also a time to celebrate the years of benefit that were provided by the feeding tube as development of harm from this intervention is considered.

The process of considering peripheral nutrition as an alternative means of providing medical nutrition and hydration in children with SNI can be considered in the context of how a child is doing overall. Peripheral nutrition has greater likelihood of harm in the child with a variety of features that might be due to alterations in the CNS. A family may view such technology as burdensome and as prolonging suffering, when a child has experienced a decline in other areas of health and function. It is also helpful to consider what goal is intended by the intervention. Examples of goals are to improve comfort, to restore health, or to maintain life.

Discontinuing medical nutrition and hydration remains challenging and controversial, because of the symbolic significance of nutrition, the myths about dehydration and "starvation," and the under-recognition of symptoms that can be due to medical nutrition and hydration. It is ethically permissible to discontinue medical nutrition and hydration that is contributing to suffering and prolonging the dying process [47]. Parents interviewed about their decision to forgo artificial nutrition and hydration (FANH) did not regret their decision [48]. This represented the paradoxical experience of not wanting their child to die yet concluding that FANH was the best of all options available, even viewed "as the only thing that made any sense". The decision to FANH included that all children were viewed to have a significant alteration in quality of life due to pain and suffering and a decline in health that was not viewed as likely to improve. Family members also wrote about their experience regarding the harm they perceived when medical nutrition and hydration was used for their child with a neurodegenerative condition [49]. At such times, an approach of feeding to an amount that allows comfort can be beneficial and allow time to reflect on information while ensuring the child's comfort. This topic is reviewed in greater detail elsewhere [47,48,50].

9. Conclusions

Vomiting, GI tract pain, and feeding intolerance are common problems in children with SNI. Awareness of sources with tests, sources due to the altered nervous system and risk for over-estimating calorie needs can then guide management strategies and lessen symptom burden in many. Some will progress to intractable feeding intolerance, likely due to further alterations in the CNS. Using the information in this review can improve comfort throughout life and lessen suffering at the end of life for children with SNI.

Conflicts of Interest: The author declares no conflict of interest.

References

1. Stallard, P.; Williams, L.; Velleman, R.; Lenton, S.; McGrath, P.J. Brief report: Behaviors identified by caregivers to detect pain in noncommunicating children. *J. Pediatr. Psychol.* **2002**, *27*, 209–214. [CrossRef] [PubMed]
2. Breau, L.M.; Camfield, C.S.; McGrath, P.J.; Finley, A. The incidence of pain in children with severe cognitive impairments. *Arch. Pediatr. Adolesc. Med.* **2003**, *157*, 1219–1226. [CrossRef] [PubMed]
3. Carter, B.; McArthur, E.; Cunliffe, M. Dealing with uncertainty: Parental assessment of pain in their children with profound special needs. *J. Adv. Nurs.* **2002**, *38*, 449–457. [CrossRef] [PubMed]
4. Hunt, A.; Mastroyannopoulou, K.; Goldman, A.; Seers, K. Not knowing—The problem of pain in children with severe neurological impairment. *Int. J. Nurs. Stud.* **2003**, *40*, 171–183. [CrossRef]
5. Houlihan, C.M.; O'Donnell, M.; Conaway, M.; Stevenson, R.D. Bodily pain and health-related quality of life in children with cerebral palsy. *Dev. Med. Child Neurol.* **2004**, *46*, 305–310. [CrossRef] [PubMed]
6. Hunt, A.; Goldman, A.; Seers, K.; Crichton, N.; Mastroyannopoulou, K.; Moffat, V.; Oulton, K.; Brady, M. Clinical validation of the paediatric pain profile. *Dev. Med. Child Neurol.* **2004**, *46*, 9–18. [CrossRef] [PubMed]
7. Sullivan, P.B. Gastrointestinal disorders in children with neurodevelopmental disabilities. *Dev. Disabil. Res. Rev.* **2008**, *14*, 128–136. [CrossRef] [PubMed]
8. Stallard, P.; Williams, L.; Lenton, S.; Velleman, R. Pain in cognitively impaired, non-communicating children. *Arch. Dis. Child.* **2001**, *85*, 460–462. [CrossRef] [PubMed]
9. Del Giudice, E.; Staiano, A.; Capano, G.; Romano, A.; Florimonte, L.; Miele, E.; Ciarla, C.; Campanozzi, A.; Crisanti, A.F. Gastrointestinal manifestations in children with cerebral palsy. *Brain Dev.* **1999**, *21*, 307–311. [CrossRef]
10. Breau, L.M.; Camfield, C.S.; McGrath, P.J.; Finley, G.A. Risk factors for pain in children with severe cognitive impairments. *Dev. Med. Child Neurol.* **2004**, *46*, 364–371. [CrossRef] [PubMed]
11. Steele, R.; Siden, H.; Cadell, S.; Davies, B.; Andrews, G.; Feichtinger, L.; Singh, M. Charting the territory: Symptoms and functional assessment in children with progressive, non-curable conditions. *Arch. Dis. Child.* **2014**, *99*, 754–762. [CrossRef] [PubMed]
12. Delgado-Aros, S.; Camilleri, M. Visceral hypersensitivity. *J. Clin. Gastroenterol.* **2005**, *39*, S194–S203. [CrossRef] [PubMed]

13. Nicholson, B.D. Evaluation and treatment of central pain syndromes. *Neurology* **2004**, *62*, S30–S36. [CrossRef] [PubMed]
14. Frese, A.; Husstedt, I.W.; Ringelstein, E.B.; Evers, S. Pharmacologic treatment of central post-stroke pain. *Clin. J. Pain* **2006**, *22*, 252–260. [CrossRef] [PubMed]
15. Klit, H.; Finnerup, N.B.; Jensen, T.S. Central post-stroke pain: Clinical characteristics, pathophysiology, and management. *Lancet Neurol.* **2009**, *8*, 857–868. [CrossRef]
16. Hauer, J.; Houtrow, A.J.; Section on Hospice and Palliative Medicine, Council on Children with Disabilities. Pain Assessment and Treatment in Children with Significant Impairment of the Central Nervous System. *Pediatrics* **2017**, *139*, E20171002. [CrossRef] [PubMed]
17. Zangen, T.; Ciarla, C.; Zangen, S.; Di Lorenzo, C.; Flores, A.F.; Cocjin, J.; Reddy, S.N.; Rowhani, A.; Schwankovsky, L.; Hyman, P.E. Gastrointestinal motility and sensory abnormalities may contribute to food refusal in medically fragile toddlers. *J. Pediatr. Gastroenterol. Nutr.* **2003**, *37*, 287–293. [CrossRef] [PubMed]
18. Hasler, M.L. Pharmacotherapy for intestinal motor and sensory disorders. *Gastroenterol. Clin. N. Am.* **2003**, *32*, 707–732. [CrossRef]
19. Lee, K.J.; Kim, J.H.; Cho, S.W. Gabapentin reduces rectal mechanosensitivity and increases rectal compliance in patients with diarrhoea-predominant irritable bowel syndrome. *Aliment. Pharmacol. Ther.* **2005**, *22*, 981–988. [CrossRef] [PubMed]
20. Hauer, J.; Solodiuk, J. Gabapentin for Management of Recurrent Pain in 22 Nonverbal Children with Severe Neurological Impairment: A Retrospective Analysis. *J. Palliat. Med.* **2015**, *18*, 453–456. [CrossRef] [PubMed]
21. Hauer, J.; Wical, B.; Charnas, L. Gabapentin successfully manages chronic unexplained irritability in children with severe neurologic impairment. *Pediatrics* **2007**, *119*, e519–e522. [CrossRef] [PubMed]
22. Kuiken, S.D.; Tytgat, G.N.; Boeckxstaens, G.E. Review article: Drugs interfering with visceral sensitivity for the treatment of functional gastrointestinal disorders—The clinical evidence. *Aliment. Pharmacol. Ther.* **2005**, *21*, 633–651. [CrossRef] [PubMed]
23. Chelimsky, G.; Chelimsky, T. Familial association of autonomic and gastrointestinal symptoms. *Clin. Auton. Res.* **2001**, *11*, 383–386. [CrossRef] [PubMed]
24. Chelimsky, G.; Hupertz, V.F.; Chelimsky, T.C. Abdominal Pain as the Presenting Symptom of Autonomic Dysfunction in a Child. *Clin. Pediatr. (Phila)* **1999**, *38*, 725–729. [CrossRef] [PubMed]
25. Axelrod, F.B.; Berlin, D. Pregabalin: A New Approach to Treatment of the Dysautonomic Crisis. *Pediatrics* **2009**, *124*, 743–746. [CrossRef] [PubMed]
26. Baguley, I.J.; Cameron, I.D.; Green, A.M.; Slewa-Younan, S.; Marosszeky, J.E.; Gurka, J.A. Pharmacological management of Dysautonomia following traumatic brain injury. *Brain Inj.* **2004**, *18*, 409–417. [CrossRef] [PubMed]
27. Diesing, T.S.; Wijdicks, E.F. Arc de cercle and dysautonomia from anoxic injury. *Mov. Disord.* **2006**, *21*, 868–869. [CrossRef] [PubMed]
28. Baguley, I.J. Autonomic complications following central nervous system injury. *Semin. Neurol.* **2008**, *28*, 716–725. [CrossRef] [PubMed]
29. Mehta, N.M.; Bechard, L.J.; Leavitt, K.; Duggan, C. Severe weight loss and hypermetabolic paroxysmal dysautonomia following hypoxic ischemic brain injury: The role of indirect calorimetry in the intensive care unit. *J. Parenter. Enter. Nutr.* **2008**, *32*, 281–284. [CrossRef] [PubMed]
30. Baguley, I.J.; Heriseanu, R.E.; Gurka, J.A.; Nordenbo, A.; Cameron, I.D. Gabapentin in the management of dysautonomia following severe traumatic brain injury: A case series. *Neurol. Neurosurg. Psychiatry* **2007**, *78*, 539–541. [CrossRef] [PubMed]
31. Antonarakis, E.S.; Hain, R.D. Nausea and vomiting associated with cancer chemotherapy: Drug management in theory and in practice. *Arch. Dis. Child.* **2004**, *89*, 877–880. [CrossRef] [PubMed]
32. Rodriguez, L.; Diaz, J.; Nurko, S. Safety and efficacy of cyproheptadine for treating dyspeptic symptoms in children. *J. Pediatr.* **2013**, *163*, 261–267. [CrossRef] [PubMed]
33. Merhar, S.L.; Pentiuk, S.P.; Mukkada, V.A.; Meinzen-Derr, J.; Kaul, A.; Butler, D.R. A retrospective review of cyproheptadine for feeding intolerance in children less than three years of age: Effects and side effects. *Acta Paediatr.* **2016**, *105*, 967–970. [CrossRef] [PubMed]
34. Cook, R.C.; Blinman, T.A. Alleviation of retching and feeding intolerance after fundoplication. *Nutr. Clin. Pract.* **2014**, *29*, 386–396. [CrossRef] [PubMed]

35. Gale, R.; Namestnic, J.; Singer, P.; Kagan, I. Caloric Requirements of Patients With Brain Impairment and Cerebral Palsy Who Are Dependent on Chronic Ventilation. *J. Parenter. Enter. Nutr.* **2017**, *41*, 1366–1370. [CrossRef] [PubMed]
36. Dickerson, R.N.; Brown, R.O.; Hanna, D.L.; Williams, J.E. Energy requirements of non-ambulatory, tube-fed adult patients with cerebral palsy and chronic hypothermia. *Nutrition* **2003**, *19*, 741–746. [CrossRef]
37. Vernon-Roberts, A.; Wells, J.; Grant, H.; Alder, N.; Vadamalayan, B.; Eltumi, M.; Sullivan, P.B. Gastrostomy feeding in cerebral palsy: Enough and no more. *Dev. Med. Child Neurol.* **2010**, *52*, 1099–1105. [CrossRef] [PubMed]
38. Hauer, J.; Yip, D.O. Feeding Intolerance and Edema in Children and Adults with Severe Neurological Impairment: Features in the Last Year of Life (TH306). *J. Pain Symptom Manag.* **2016**, *51*, 318. [CrossRef]
39. Pohl, J.F.; Cantrell, A. Gastrointestinal and nutritional issues in cerebral palsy. *Pract. Gastroenterol.* **2006**, *29*, 14–22.
40. Dickerson, R.N.; Brown, R.O.; Hanna, D.L.; Williams, J.E. Effect of upper extremity posturing on measured resting energy expenditure of nonambulatory tube-fed adult patients with severe neurodevelopmental disabilities. *J. Parenter. Enter. Nutr.* **2002**, *26*, 278–284. [CrossRef] [PubMed]
41. Hauer, J.; Wolfe, J. Supportive and Palliative Care of Children with Metabolic and Neurological Diseases. *Curr. Opin. Support. Palliat. Care* **2014**, *8*, 296–302. [CrossRef] [PubMed]
42. Altaf, M.A.; Sood, M.R. The nervous system and gastrointestinal function. *Dev. Disabil. Res. Rev.* **2008**, *14*, 87–95. [CrossRef] [PubMed]
43. Browning, K.N.; Travagli, R.A. Central nervous system control of gastrointestinal motility and secretion and modulation of gastrointestinal functions. *Compr. Physiol.* **2014**, *4*, 1339–1368. [CrossRef] [PubMed]
44. Siden, H.; Tucker, T.; Derman, S.; Cox, K.; Soon, G.S.; Hartnett, C.; Straatman, L. Pediatric enteral feeding intolerance: A new prognosticator for children with life-limiting illness? *J. Palliat. Care* **2009**, *25*, 213–217. [PubMed]
45. Bramow, S.; Faber-Rod, J.C.; Jacobsen, C.; Kutzelnigg, A.; Patrikios, P.; Sorensen, P.S.; Lassmann, H.; Laursen, H. Fatal neurogenic pulmonary edema in a patient with progressive multiple sclerosis. *Mult. Scler.* **2008**, *14*, 711–715. [CrossRef] [PubMed]
46. Macleod, A.D. Neurogenic pulmonary edema in palliative care. *J. Pain Symptom Manag.* **2002**, *23*, 154–156. [CrossRef]
47. Diekema, D.S.; Botkin, J.R.; Committee on Bioethics. Clinical report: Forgoing medically provided nutrition and hydration in children. *Pediatrics* **2009**, *124*, 813–822. [CrossRef] [PubMed]
48. Rapoport, A.; Shaheed, J.; Newman, C.; Rugg, M.; Steele, R. Parental perceptions of forgoing artificial nutrition and hydration during end-of-life care. *Pediatrics* **2013**, *131*, 861–869. [CrossRef] [PubMed]
49. Marcovitch, H. Artificial feeding for a child with a degenerative disorder: A family's view. The mother and grandmother of Frances. *Arch. Dis. Child.* **2005**, *90*, 979.
50. Hauer, J. Care at the End of Life. In *Caring for Children Who Have Severe Neurological Impairment: A Life with Grace;* Johns Hopkins University Press: Baltimore, MD, USA, 2013; pp. 413–429, ISBN 1421409372.

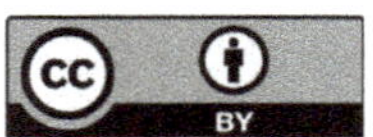

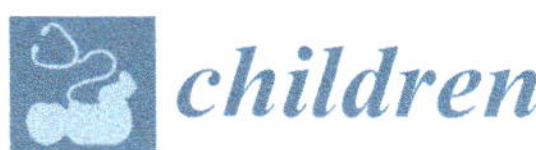

MDPI

Review

'Total Pain' in Children with Severe Neurological Impairment

Timothy A. Warlow * and Richard D.W. Hain

All Wales Paediatric Palliative Care Managed Clinical Network, University Hospital of Wales, Heath Park, Cardiff CF14 4XW, UK; richard.hain@wales.nhs.uk

* Correspondence: twarlow@doctors.org.uk; Tel.: +44-773-739-4757

Received: 28 November 2017; Accepted: 12 January 2018; Published: 18 January 2018

Abstract: Many children with palliative care needs experience difficulty in managing pain. Perhaps none more so than those with severe neurological impairment. For many years; behaviours in these children were misunderstood. As a result; pain was poorly recognised and inadequately managed. Significant advances have been made in the assessment and management of pain in this challenging group of patients. We summarise these advances; drawing on our own experience working with infants; children and young adults with palliative care needs within a UK tertiary paediatric palliative care service. We expand on the recent understanding of 'Total Pain'; applying a holistic approach to pain assessment and management in children with severe neurological impairment.

Keywords: 'Total Pain'; paediatric palliative care; chronic pain; persistent pain; cerebral palsy; cognitive impairment; neurological impairment

---

1. What Is 'Total Pain'?

The internationally accepted definition of pain is:

> An unpleasant sensory and emotional experience associated with actual or potential tissue damage, or described in terms of such damage (International Association of the Study of Pain (IASP) 1973). [1]

This definition makes two specific points. Firstly, the pain experience is an inherently subjective one. It can only be described accurately by the person experiencing it, and sometimes not even by them. Secondly, pain is not just a physical experience. The relationship between physical tissue damage and patient experience of pain is highly complex. Long gone are the days when pain was described as in a purely linear relationship with nociceptive input. With our understanding of the complex integration of these inputs with cortical networks, and supraspinal modulation of pain through descending pathways, even suggestions of pain as either mental or physical are a thing of the past [2]. Cicely Saunders in the 1960s saw a broader view than the IASP definition, acknowledging the impact of spiritual and psychosocial aspects on the pain experience, coining the term 'Total Pain' [3]. Pain is experienced as an overall feeling state with multiple layers of meaning. This is particularly true for children with palliative care needs, for whom the onset of pain may represent the relentless progression of a life limiting or life-threatening disease. Table 1 lists some of the key factors identified as impacting the experience of pain in children.

Table 1. Factors contributing to experience of pain in children.

Cognitive Appraisal of Pain [2,3]
Context of disease trajectory [3]
Beliefs about pain [2]
Existential meanings attached to pain [4]
Social abandonment [3]
Anxiety [2]
Depression [2]
Fear of implications of pain on disease [2]
Memories of prior pain [1]
Distress of prior pain [1]
Mental isolation [3]
Boredom [3]
Fatigue [3]
Grieving [3]
Pain tolerance [3]
Coping ability/strategies [3]
Cultural implications of pain and associated functional limitations [2]
Degree of tissue damage
Central excitation and inhibition of afferent signals [1]

2. Total Pain in Children with SNI

For children with severe neurological impairment (SNI), our definition of pain becomes fraught with difficulty. How can we assess and manage the individual pain of children who cannot verbally communicate their experience? When cognitive appraisal is the most significant factor in the affective and spiritual dimension of pain, how can we understand their unique experience in order to holistically assess and manage their pain? [3].

2.1. Physical Aspects of the Pain Experience

90% of children with SNI experience recurrent pain for more than a year during childhood [5]. For 75% this is on at least a weekly basis and for 50% the pain episodes last longer than 9 h [6]. These children experience more episodes of nociceptive pain and a greater number of pain sources than those with mild to moderate impairment [6]. Table 2 highlights some of the sources of pain identified in children with SNI.

Table 2. Sources of nociceptive pain in children with severe neurological impairment (SNI).

Common	Less Common
Musculoskeletal (osteopenia, scoliosis, hip subluxation, pathological fractures)	Dental caries
Hypertonia (spasticity, dystonia)	Non-specific back pain
Muscle fatigue and immobility	Renal stones and urinary tract infections (UTI) (topiramate, ketogenic diet)
Constipation	Pancreatitis (valproate and hypothermia)
Gastro-oesophageal reflux disease (GORD)	Cholecystitis (tube feeding)
Gastrointestinal dysmotility (autonomic and post-surgical e.g., fundoplication)	Ventricular shunt blockage, infection
Iatrogenic (investigations, surgery)	Headache [5,7]
Sources common to all children (e.g., Otitis media, dysmenorrhoea, appendicitis)	

Children with SNI experience pain more intensely than children with normal neurological function. They are also vulnerable to intensely distressing episodes of pain without identifiable cause, and abdominal pain despite optimal treatment of constipation and gastro-oesophageal reflux disease (GORD). In addition to the breadth of nociceptive sources of pain, there are three physical processes contributing to this increased pain experience, all with their origins in the central nervous system (CNS).

2.1.1. Central Neuropathic Pain

Riquelme et al. studied proprioception, touch and pain pressure thresholds in 15 children with cerebral palsy and found significantly increased sensitivity to painful stimuli. Children with CNS damage display altered excitability in the somatosensory cortex [5,8]. Nociceptive processing at a molecular, cellular and circuit level are altered, leading to system wide changes in neuroexcitability that ultimately lead to an amplified pain experience [5].

2.1.2. Autonomic Dysfunction

Damage to the autonomic nervous system is common in children with SNI. It can result in abdominal pain, retching and constipation, due in part to gastrointestinal dysmotility [5]. Key features include flushing or pallor, heart rate changes, increased saliva production alongside abdominal symptoms.

2.1.3. Sensitisation to Pain

Children with SNI may have experienced many painful procedures early on in life, from blood tests on the neonatal unit, through to invasive investigations and surgery. GORD, constipation, and insertion of gastrostomy tubes also provide repeated mechanical and chemical stimulation to what is already in many children a dysmotile gastrointestinal tract. These repeated nociceptive inputs lead spinal afferent neurones to become sensitised peripherally [9,10].

Nociceptive signals from sensitised spinal afferents are repeatedly received at the dorsal horn of the spinal cord. This can lead to a progressive build-up in amplitude of action potentials and cumulative depolarisation known as the 'wind-up phenomenon' [11,12]. As nociceptive fibres continue to be activated, children experience a progressively intense sensation of pain, out of proportion with the original stimulus. In addition, low-level signals from peripheral nociceptors can lead to increased synaptic efficacy of spinal cord neurones. As a result, exaggerated nociceptive signals are produced long after the pain stimulus has gone. Non-nociceptive input from other neurones, (such as those produced by normal gut movements or light touch), become amplified, and trigger action potentials in spinal pain pathways. The resulting process of central sensitisation is one of disproportionately widespread pain which persists for longer and at greater intensity than is expected from the original stimulus [5,11,13]. Visceral hypersensitivity describes these peripheral and central sensitisation processes when the stimulus originates in from the body viscera, especially the gastrointestinal tract.

A further degree of modulation occurs at the point of cognitive and emotional processing, leading to interpretation of non-noxious sensations as noxious. This leads to hypervigilance [14]. This can amplify the pain experience further. It therefore becomes clear that even at a neuronal network level, psychosocial and spiritual factors are fundamentally entwined with physical aspects of pain.

Contribution from these neuropathic elements is suspected when children have higher baseline pain ratings and significant intensity and duration of pain attributed to experiences that are not normally painful. In children with abdominal pain, features include a history of pain with tube feeds, bowel gas and before bowel movements. Pain relieved by slowing or cessation of feeds, or substitution of feed for electrolyte solution is also suggestive [5].

In addition to the above, seizures, dystonia and contractures due to spasticity may cause pain, be triggered by pain from other sources, or become involved in the expression of pain behaviours. In reality, most children with SNI have more than one cause of pain, and a mixture of nociceptive and neuropathic pain elements [5].

2.2. Psychosocial and Spiritual Aspects of the Pain Experience

It is clear that the perception of pain is a function of a child's cognitive and emotional development [1]. While affective and spiritual dimensions of suffering must depend to a certain extent on cognitive ability, it would be wrong to assume that only patients with fully developed cognition can experience existential distress. Children with SNI are in fact more susceptible to psychosocial problems. There is an increased prevalence of emotional and behavioural difficulties that significantly impact the quality of life for them and their families. In a study by Dolapo et al. of 22 children with dystonic cerebral palsy, they were found to have more difficulty understanding their own mental states when compared to the group of 20 control subjects. In addition, they had a reduced ability to manage and monitor their emotion [15]. Patients, especially those who are very young or who have a more significant degree of cognitive impairment, may perceive pain to be a form of punishment, and find it difficult to rationalise its cause, recognise that it will come to an end or anticipate the impact of analgesia. In children with SNI, chronic or recurrent pain can lead to outburst of aggression, withdrawal from the world socially, reduced adaptive abilities in communication, and have a significant impact on function in daily life [1,6,16]. Emotionally they may have little in the way of coping strategies [1]. Fear, sadness and anger are the dominant emotions [1]. These factors all amplify the pain experience.

Spirituality for the child can be best defined as 'how they make sense of the world and their place in it' [16]. The spiritual experience of pain in children with SNI is also therefore grounded in their cognitive and emotional development. James Fowler suggests that for children of a developmental age akin to those with SNI, an appreciation of meaning is made from the bonds of attachment and mutual relationship experienced by the child [16]. The ability of the parent or carer to appraise the experience of the child and respond appropriately makes it possible for the child to trust and therefore hope, a definitively spiritual concept [4]. Children with SNI may be limited in their ability to give signals and respond reciprocally to the signals of others [2]. Atypical behaviours in response to pain may be misinterpreted or unrecognised by caregivers. This breakdown in mutual experience between the child and carer can lead to existential distress, further exacerbating the pain experience [2]. Children with SNI are completely reliant on caregivers in their immediate environment to be sensitive and to recognise their distress, the urgency of their distress signal, and to take action to decrease it. The parental response not only determines whether pain is identified and whether steps are taken to relieve it, but also shapes the child's experience and expression of pain [17]. Pain distress is either magnified or moderated by the carers response. A parent experiencing significant anxiety or existential distress associated with an infant's pain may be less emotionally available to the child during periods of distress [17]. Emotional availability encompasses sensitivity to the child's cues, and responses that are appropriately non-intrusive, non-hostile and structured to meet their need. Din et al. identified that in a group of infants undergoing vaccination, poor emotional availability is not only associated with increased pain reactivity, but increased pain expression also [18]. Osmun et al. explored this concept further with a similar cohort of infants identifying that over time, caregivers who are consistently emotionally available had infants who learned to better regulate negative emotion around future episodes of pain [19].

Maternal anxiety has independently been shown to reduce sensitivity in interactions with children and their ability to regulate the child's distress [20]. This sensitivity is vital for assessing the impact of various soothing behaviours and developing a repertoire of individualised soothing techniques for their child.

Positive caregiver behaviours shown to improve distress during pain include vocalisations, proximal soothing such as rocking, stroking, kissing, and sensitivity to the individual preferences of the child as various comforting behaviours by the caregiver are tried [17,20]. Interventions for carers encouraging these positive behaviours should include carer coping strategies such as self-talk and distraction, encouraging positive carer affect, improving carer self-efficacy, and encouraging a sense of control during pain episodes [17,20]. These may improve the emotional availability of the carer to the child with SNI in pain, ameliorating pain related distress for both.

3. The Assessment of 'Total Pain'

Assessing the experience of pain in children with SNI and distinguishing it from other causes of distress is extremely challenging. As a result, pain often goes unrecognised, with only 50% of those with persistent pain receiving analgesia [5,16].

A thorough pain assessment includes a comprehensive history to identify sites of pain, timing, onset, character, associated features, and response to previous pain relief. Table 3 outlines important and often overlooked aspects of the physical examination to identify sources of pain in these children.

Table 3. Examination for nociceptive causes of pain in children with SNI.

Eyes—corneal abrasion
Mouth, and throat—dental caries and abscess, gingivitis, tonsillitis
Central lines, implanted devices, shunt catheter sites—malfunction, infection
Gastrostomy tube—gastrostomy tube tension, site infection
Abdomen—constipation, distention
Skin—hair tourniquet or pressure ulcer
Extremities and joints—occult fracture, subluxation [5]

It is vital to explore the context, and take into account the psychosocial and spiritual factors discussed above. Impact on sleep and carer response to episodes of pain should be considered. These assessments are best completed using a multi-disciplinary approach, including professionals skilled in psychological and spiritual assessment. In our service, play specialists and hospice family support practitioners, in addition to our chaplaincy service play a vital role in building a picture of the pain experience of our children and families. A period of observation at our local hospice for prolonged assessment and comparison of symptoms outside of the patient's usual psychosocial context can be extremely helpful. Investigations should be directed by history and examination, co-ordinated by the primary medical team looking after the child. In a palliative population, the appropriateness of invasive investigations should be carefully considered in discussion with the family and all teams involved, with the aim of minimising harm and maximising quality of life for the child and family.

Difficulty encoding expressive behaviour means children with SNI display behaviours that may represent pain or primitive reflexes or abnormal movements. Some display atypical responses to pain, such as sudden stillness (freezing phenomenon), smiling, laughter or self-harming [5]. Parents may misinterpret pain behaviours as part of their usual condition. Despite this, observed pain behaviours are considered a valid approach to assessment of pain in those unable to self-report, and there is now much consensus on pain cues expressed by these patients [2,21]. A myriad of pain tools exist to assess children with SNI. A recent systematic review identified 15 tools of high reliability, validity, comprehensiveness and usability [22]. Of these, three were recommended for children with SNI (Gross Motor Function Classification System Grading IV-V). Two main rating scales were the Paediatric Pain Profile (PPP) and Non-Communicating Children's Pain Checklist-Revised Version (NCCPC-RV) [23,24]. These both assess a wide range of behaviours, including those pertaining to the psychosocial and spiritual distress associated with the pain experience [22]. A body-map tool is recommended for use alongside these to aid with intensity and location of pain [22]. Tertiary training centres in Paediatric Palliative Care in the UK uniformly use another tool, the Face Legs Activity Cry Consolability (FLACC) tool, revised for children with SNI [25]. Our experience is that using a range of tools enables a more individualised approach to pain assessment. The PPP and NCCPC-RV provide a broader and more information rich assessment of pain during periods of significant instability or diagnostic uncertainty, whereas the FLACC provides a simpler more flexible assessment for contexts and time periods when this is required. A summary of these tools with additional critique can be seen in Table 4.

Table 4. Pain assessment tools in children with severe neurological impairment (SNI).

Tool Name	Description	Process of Validation	Key Interpretation	Positive Features	Negative Features
Paediatric Pain Profile (PPP) [23]	20 Item behaviour scale.	Interviews 21 children, 26 professionals + Questionnaire 121 parents to develop scale. Children with severe cognitive impairment.	Robustly developed and validated in real world setting.	Designed specifically for non-verbal children with SNI.	Lengthy compared to FLACC scale.
	Four-point scale for each item.	Interrater reliability acceptable for combined item score.	Clear difference in pain scores between when in pain and no pain with narrow confidence interval.	Can compare scores with a baseline score. Completed in 2–3 min.	
	Assess pain at baseline, then repeatedly for regular monitoring or to monitor intervention.	Correlation between raters of 0.75.	Reliable between raters.	Descriptors of more than one pain type.	Many behaviours open to significant interpretation.
	Designed to be parent held.	Sensitivity of 1.0 and Specificity of 0.91 for moderate/severe pain at PPP score of 14.	Very sensitive and specific for detecting pain.	Takes into account psychosocial aspects.	
Face Legs Activity Cry Consolability (FLACC) [25]	Five-items behaviour scale.	Validated on children with varying degrees neurological impairment.	Small sample size of 50 patients in validation study.	Can add individual behaviours to the pain scale for each child.	Validated in a post-surgical population only.
	Three-point scale per item (0–2).				
	Option for individualised items to be included.	Validated in 52 children with 80 observations per-operatively including video assessment by experts.		Quick, un-ambiguous tool to use.	
	Mild pain = 0–3.		Correlations of scores to parental perceived pain good, but cut-offs defined for mild/moderate/severe are not validated.		Fewer behaviours assessed so data less rich to inform assessment.
	Moderate pain = 4–6.	Good inter-rater correlations of total score (0.90 (0.87–0.92)) between nurse observations.		Very high interrater correlations of total score.	
	Severe pain = 7–10.				
Non-Communicating Children's Pain Checklist—Revised [24]	30 items behaviour scale.	71 children assessed. Daily 2 h observation for 1 week. Repeated 3 monthly.	Thorough validation of pain tool.	Many behaviours assessed over long assessment period so rich data for pain assessment.	2 h observation period may be impractical for many carers.
	Four-point scale per item (0–4).	Inter-rater correlation for total score of 0.46, statistically significant but not strong correlation. Correlation between numerical pain score of parent and pain scale was 0.64 and for researcher and parent pain score 0.72.	High specificity and sensitivity at score cut-off.		
	2 h observation period required per scoring.	Score of 7 or greater had Sensitivity 84% and Specificity 68% for pain.	Weaker correlations between raters and parent rating than other scales.	Behaviours clearly described and unambiguous.	

4. An Approach to Managing 'Total Pain'

Once a thorough assessment of the causes and experience of pain are complete, a holistic, multidisciplinary plan should be put in place to manage the pain, support the family, and monitor and evaluate the impact of interventions.

Management of dystonia and spasticity should be optimised in accordance with national guidance [7,26]. This includes monitoring for hip subluxation and managing orthopaedic complications alongside appropriate specialist teams. For children with undiagnosed pain or abdominal pain, gastro-oesophageal reflux and constipation should be aggressively treated, and the impact of analgesic medications on these symptoms reviewed regularly [5,7]. Bone health and fracture prevention should be considered by maximising mobility, optimising vitamin D and calcium intake, and use of bisphosphonates as required [6]. Medication should be rationalised to limit side effects and interactions which may result in exaggerated symptom experience.

In addition to treatment directed at identified causes of pain, optimal pain management requires a comprehensive approach using opioid, adjuvant and non-pharmacological strategies [27]. Non-pharmacological strategies include swaddling, rocking, repositioning and massage [5,28]. There is limited evidence for the use of music and audiotherapy, acupuncture, aromatherapy, vibratory therapy and weighted blankets in this population [5,28]. Employing the skills of therapists including physiotherapy, occupational therapy and orthotics is vital for children with musculoskeletal pain and disorders of increased tone.

The basis for a logical approach to using opioids in palliative care has been the World Health Organization (WHO) 'pain ladder' [21]. In the past, the ladder had three steps: simple analgesia on step 1, 'weak' or 'minor' opioids on step 2 and 'strong' or 'major' opioids on step 3. There is, however, no pharmacological basis for making a distinction between 'weak' and 'strong' opioids. Furthermore, the two most common opioids prescribed on step 2 were codeine and tramadol, both of which are now felt to be potentially hazardous, especially in children [21]. This has led the WHO to describe a two-step analgesia ladder that consists of simple analgesia on the first 'rung' and opioids on the second [27]. Hain points out, however, that optimal use of opioids in severe pain is distinctly different from their use in moderate pain. Opioids for severe pain should be given regularly and should be at a higher dose than those for moderate pain. There is therefore still value in separating the use of opioids for moderate pain (Step 2) and that for severe pain (Step 3) [21]. Treatment should be tailored to the individual child, using the least invasive route possible [21]. Additional doses of short acting analgesia should be provided for episodes of predictable (incident) and unpredictable (breakthrough) pain [29].

Central neuropathic causes of pain that play a significant role in children with SNI typically do not respond completely to opioid therapy [5]. Mediations directed at these CNS sources may have a preferential role in children with SNI [5]. Recent guidance by the American Academy of Paediatrics recommends the use of empirical trials of neuropathic agents in children with SNI and persistent pain behaviours. First-line agents include gabapentinoids and tricyclic antidepressants (TCAs), with Clonidine, Methadone, Ketamine and Cannabinoids considered if initial therapy fails [5,30]. Recent Cochrane reviews of antiepileptic and antidepressant medications for non-cancer pain in children found insufficient evidence to formally recommend any of these medications for pain. However, adverse effects with gabapentin, pregabalin and TCAs were uncommon [31]. From adult experimental studies, the number needed to treat to improve pain for TCAs is slightly lower than for gabapentin. However, when quality of life is considered alongside pain severity as an outcome, gabapentin is preferred due to an improved side effect profile [32,33]. From observational paediatric data, gabapentin significantly reduced unexplained irritability related to bowel symptoms in a retrospective observational study of 9 children with SNI [34]. In a further case series, 21 out of 22 children (95%) with SNI demonstrated a significant decrease (greater than 50%) in frequency and severity of pain episodes with gabapentin, with many demonstrating improved feed tolerance [35]. Gabapentin reduces the release of neuroexcitatory neurotransmitters implicated in central neuropathic pain and visceral hyperalgesia. It also inhibits central sensitisation in animals and human studies [32]. Gabapentin is less sedating than TCAs, and may also improve dystonia which so significantly exacerbates pain in many children with SNI [36]. In a retrospective review of 69 children with dystonia, most of whom had SNI, Liow et al. identified significant improvements in sleep, mood, pain, general muscle tone, involuntary muscle contractions and seating tolerance with gabapentin [36]. In light of the above, the authors first choice for an empirical trial would be gabapentin followed by a TCA if treatment failed or was not tolerated. In our experience gabapentin is generally well tolerated, although the sedative effects can be profound in some patients. These patients may benefit from a slower titration to therapeutic doses [5]. While no official dosing guidance exists in this patient group for pain, studies typically started with doses of gabapentin between 2 and 6 mg/kg/day in three divided doses, increasing every few days by 5 mg/kg/day until a response is achieved [5,35]. Therapeutic doses were noted to be between 15–45 mg/kg/day with a maximum suggested dose of 70 mg/kg/day advised by both the American Academy of Pediatrics and National Institute of Health and Care Excellence in the UK [5,37]. Clear goals must be set with families, ensuring a clear plan for dosing, duration of the treatment trial, monitoring, and gradual withdrawal if no improvement is seen [5,30].

5. Conclusions

Our understanding of children with SNI, their expression of pain, and the processes underpinning their pain experience have improved dramatically in recent years. The assessment and management of pain in children with SNI, while challenging, is possible with the use of a holistic approach to the physical, psychosocial and spiritual aspects of the pain experience for the child and family. Only by addressing each of these areas in both the assessment and treatment stages, will care teams be able to achieve maximum relief of pain and improvement in quality of life for this patient group.

Author Contributions: T.A.W. with support from R.D.W.H. identified the topic for review. T.A.W. researched and wrote the paper. R.D.W.H. revised the initial and final draft prior to final editing by T.A.W.

Conflicts of Interest: The authors declare no conflict of interest.

References

1. Bioy, A.; Wood, C. Introduction to pain. In *Oxford Textbook of Palliative Care for Children*, 2nd ed.; Goldman, A., Hain, R., Liben, S., Eds.; Oxford University Press: Oxford, UK, 2012.
2. Hunt, A. Pain assessment. In *Oxford Textbook of Palliative Care for Children*, 2nd ed.; Goldman, A., Hain, R., Liben, S., Eds.; Oxford University Press: Oxford, UK, 2012.
3. Twycross, R. *Introducing Palliative Care*, 5th ed.; Twycross, R., Wilcock, A., Eds.; Palliativedrugs.com: Amersham, UK, 2016.
4. Macauley, R.; Hylton-Rushton, C. Spirituality and meaning for children, families and clinicians. In *Oxford Textbook of Palliative Care for Children*, 2nd ed.; Goldman, A., Hain, R., Liben, S., Eds.; Oxford University Press: Oxford, UK, 2012.
5. Hauer, J.; Houtrow, A.J. Pain assessment and treatment in children with significant impairment of the central nervous System. *Pediatrics* **2017**, *139*. [CrossRef] [PubMed]
6. Breau, L.M.; Camfield, C.S.; McGrath, P.J.; Finley, G.A. The incidence of pain in children with severe cognitive impairments. *Arch. Pediatr. Adolesc. Med.* **2003**, *157*, 1219–1226. [CrossRef] [PubMed]
7. National Institute for Health and Care Excellence. Cerebral Palsy in under 25s: Assessment and Management. 2017. Available online: https://www.nice.org.uk/guidance/ng62 (accessed on 20 October 2017).
8. Riquelme, I.; Montoya, P. Developmental changes in somatosensory processing in cerebral palsy and healthy individuals. *Clin. Neurophysiol.* **2010**, *121*, 1314–1320. [CrossRef] [PubMed]
9. Camilleri, M.; Coulie, B.; Tack, J.F. Visceral hypersensitivity: Facts, speculations, and challenges. *Gut* **2001**, *48*, 125–131. [CrossRef] [PubMed]
10. Grundy, D. Neuroanatomy of visceral nociception: Vagal and splanchnic afferent. *Gut* **2002**, *51*, i2–i5. [CrossRef] [PubMed]

11. McCulloch, R. Pharmacological approaches to pain. Adjuvants for neuropathic and bone pain. In *Oxford Textbook of Palliative Care for Children*, 2nd ed.; Goldman, A., Hain, R., Liben, S., Eds.; Oxford University Press: Oxford, UK, 2012.
12. Herrero, J. Wind-up of spinal cord neurones and pain sensation: Much ado about something? *Prog. Neurobiol.* **2000**, *61*, 169–203. [CrossRef]
13. Woolf, C.J. Central sensitization: Implications for the diagnosis and treatment of pain. *Pain* **2011**, *152*, S2–S15. [CrossRef] [PubMed]
14. Woolf, C.J. Windup and central sensitization are not equivalent. *Pain* **1996**, *66*, 105–108. [CrossRef] [PubMed]
15. Adegboye, D.; Sterr, A.; Lin, J.P.; Owen, T.J. Theory of mind, emotional and social functioning, and motor severity in children and adolescents with dystonic cerebral palsy. *Eur. J. Paediatr. Neurol.* **2017**, *21*, 549–556. [CrossRef] [PubMed]
16. Massaro, M.; Pastore, S.; Ventura, A.; Barbi, E. Pain in cognitively impaired children: A focus for general paediatricians. *Eur. J. Pediatr.* **2013**, *172*, 9–14. [CrossRef] [PubMed]
17. Riddell, R.P.; Racine, N. Assessing pain in infancy: The Caregiver Context. *Pain Res. Manag.* **2009**, *14*, 27–32. [CrossRef]
18. Din, L.; Pillai Riddell, R.; Gordner, S. Brief report: Maternal emotional availability and infant pain-related distress. *J. Pediatr. Psychol.* **2009**, *34*, 722–726. [CrossRef] [PubMed]
19. Din Osmun, L.; Pillai Riddell, R.; Flora, D.B. Infant Pain-Related Negative Affect at 12 months of Age: Early Infant and Caregiver Predictors. *J. Pediatr. Psychol.* **2013**, *39*, 23–34. [CrossRef] [PubMed]
20. Rosenberg, R.E.; Clark, R.A.; Chibbaro, P.; Hambrick, H.R.; Bruzzese, J.; Feudtner, C.; Mendelsohn, A. Factors predicting parenting anxiety around infant and toddler postoperative pain. *Hosp. Pediatr.* **2017**, *7*, 313–319. [CrossRef] [PubMed]
21. Hain, R.D.W.; Friedrichsdorf, S.J. Pharmacological approaches to pain. 'By the ladder'—The WHO approach to management of pain in palliative care. In *Oxford Textbook of Palliative Care for Children*, 2nd ed.; Goldman, A., Hain, R., Liben, S., Eds.; Oxford University Press: Oxford, UK, 2012.
22. Kingsnorth, S.; Orava, T.; Provvidenza, C.; Adler, E.; Ami, N.; Gresley-Jones, T.; Mankad, D.; Slonim, N.; Fay, L.; Joachimides, N.; et al. Chronic pain assessment tools for cerebral palsy: A systematic Review. *Pediatrics* **2016**, *136*, e947–e960. [CrossRef] [PubMed]
23. Hunt, A. Clinical validation of the Paedaitric Pain Profile. *Dev. Med. Child Neurol.* **2004**, *46*, 9–18. [CrossRef] [PubMed]
24. Malviya, S.; Voepel-Lewis, T.; Burke, C.; Merkel, S.; Tait, A.R. The revised FLACC observational pain tool: Improved reliability and validity for pain assessment in children with cognitive impairment. *Pediatr. Anaestesia* **2006**, *16*, 258–265. [CrossRef] [PubMed]
25. Breau, L.M. Psychometric properties of the non-communicating children's pain checklist-revised. *Pain* **2002**, *99*, 349–357. [CrossRef]
26. National Institute for Health and Care Excellence. Spasticity in under 19s. 2012. Available online: https://www.nice.org.uk/guidance/cg145 (accessed on 20 October 2017).
27. World Health Organization. *WHO Guidelines on the Pharmacological Treatment of Persisting Pain in Children with Medical Illness*; WHO Press: Geneva, Switzerland, 2012.
28. Novak, I.; McIntyre, S.; Morgan, C.; Campbell, L.; Dark, L.; Morton, N.; Stumbles, E.; Wilson, S.A.; Goldsmith, S. A Systematic review of interventions for children with cerebral palsy: State of the evidence. *Dev. Med. Child Neurol.* **2013**, *55*, 885–910. [CrossRef] [PubMed]
29. Hain, R.; Jassal, S.S. *Paediatric Palliative Medicine*; Oxford University Press: Oxford, UK, 2010.
30. International Association for the Study of Pain. Pharmacological management of neuropathic pain. *Pain Clin. Updates* **2010**, *9*, 1–9.
31. Cooper, T.E.; Wiffen, P.J.; Heathcote, L.C.; Clinch, J.; Howard, R.; Krane, E.; Lord, S.M.; Sethna, N.; Schechter, N.; Wood, C. Antiepileptic drugs for chronic non-cancer pain in children and adolescents (review). *Cochrane Database Syst. Rev.* **2017**, *8*, CD012536. [PubMed]
32. Finnerup, N.B.; Otto, M.; McQuay, H.J.; Jensen, T.S.; Sindrup, S.H. Algorithm for neuropathic pain treatment: An evidence based proposal. *Pain* **2005**, *118*, 289–305. [CrossRef] [PubMed]
33. Beecham, E.; Candy, B.; Howard, R.; McCulloch, R.; Laddie, J.; Rees, H.; Vickerstaff, V.; Bluebond-Langner, M.; Jones, L. Pharmacological interventions for pain in children and young people with life-limiting conditions. *Cochrane Database Syst. Rev.* **2015**, *3*, CD010750.

34. Hauer, J.M.; Wical, B.S.; Charnas, L. Gabapentin successfully manages chronic unexplained irritability in children with severe neurological impairment. *Pediatrics* **2007**, *119*, e519–e522. [CrossRef] [PubMed]
35. Hauer, J.M.; Solodiuk, J.C. Gabapentin for management of recurrent pain in 22 nonverbal children with severe neurological impairment: A retrospective analysis. *J. Palliat. Med.* **2015**, *18*, 453–456. [CrossRef] [PubMed]
36. Liow, N.Y.; Gimeno, H.; Lumsden, D.E.; Marianczak, J.; Kaminska, M.; Tomlin, S.; Lin, J.P. Gabapentin can significantly improve dystonia severity and quality of life in children. *Eur. J. Paediatr. Neurol.* **2016**, *20*, 100–107. [CrossRef] [PubMed]
37. Joint Formulary Committee. *British National Formulary*; BMJ Group and Pharmaceutical Press: London, UK, 2017.

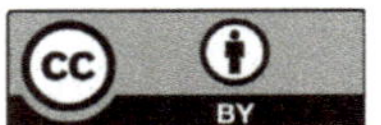

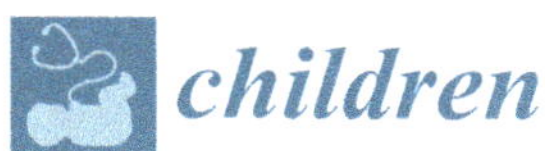

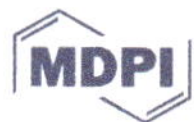

Review

Paediatric Palliative Care in Resource-Poor Countries

Julia Downing *, Sue Boucher, Alex Daniels and Busi Nkosi

International Children's Palliative Care Network, Assagay 3624, South Africa; sue.boucher@icpcn.org (S.B.); education@icpcn.org (A.D.); busi.nkosi@icpcn.org (B.N.)
* Correspondence: julia.downing@icpcn.org

Received: 30 November 2017; Accepted: 12 February 2018; Published: 19 February 2018

Abstract: There is a great need for paediatric palliative care (PPC) services globally, but access to services is lacking in many parts of the world, particularly in resource-poor settings. Globally it is estimated that 21.6 million children need access to palliative care, with 8.2 needing specialist services. PC has been identified as important within the global health agenda e.g., within universal health coverage, and a recent Lancet commission report recognised the need for PPC. However, a variety of challenges have been identified to PPC development globally such as: access to treatment, access to medications such as oral morphine, opiophobia, a lack of trained health and social care professionals, a lack of PPC policies and a lack of awareness about PPC. These challenges can be overcome utilising a variety of strategies including advocacy and public awareness, education, access to medications, implementation and research. Examples will be discussed impacting on the provision of PPC in resource-poor settings. High-quality PPC service provision can be provided with resource-poor settings, and there is an urgent need to scale up affordable, accessible, and quality PPC services globally to ensure that all children needing palliative care can access it.

Keywords: palliative care; paediatric/pediatric/children; low-resource settings; advocacy; education; access to medicines

---

1. Introduction

There is a need for paediatric palliative care (PPC) services around the world, yet access to services remains intermittent and at times non-existent, particularly in many Lower- and Middle-Income Countries (LMICs). However, there are various good quality services in LMICs that have successfully overcome some of the challenges to provision. This paper will explore the need for PPC globally, and particularly in LMICs, along with challenges to service provision and how these challenges can be overcome through advocacy and public awareness, education, access to medications, implementation and research.

2. The Need for Paediatric Palliative Care

At least 26% of the global population is under 15 years of age, rising to up to 40% in low-resourced settings such as sub-Saharan Africa [1]. Yet, the need for PPC has not been recognised in many LMICs, where development has lagged behind that of palliative care for adults. The World Health Organization (WHO) [2] states that *"palliative care for children represents a special, albeit closely related field to adult palliative care"*.

Palliative care for children is the active, total care of the child's body, mind and spirit, and also involves giving support to the family.

- It begins when illness is diagnosed and continues regardless of whether or not a child receives treatment directed at the disease.
- Health providers must evaluate and alleviate a child's physical, psychological and social distress.

- Effective palliative care requires a broad multidisciplinary approach that includes the family and makes use of available community resources; it can be successfully implemented even if resources are limited.
- It can be provided in tertiary care facilities, in community health centres and even in children's homes.

Other definitions exist, such as that from Together for Short Lives [3], which states that "palliative care for children and young people with life-limiting conditions is an active and total approach to care, from the point of diagnosis or recognition, embracing physical, emotional, social and spiritual elements through to death and beyond. It focuses on enhancement of quality of life for the child/young person and support for the family and includes the management of distressing symptoms, provision of short breaks and care through death and bereavement." Whilst the Lancet Commission on Pain and Palliative Care built on the WHO definition and adopted the term 'Serious Health Related Suffering' (SHS) [4], the WHO definition is that which is generally used within most resource-poor settings, and in many key documents, such as the 2014 World Health Assembly (WHA) Resolution on Palliative Care [5] and within the WHO definition of Universal Health Coverage (UHC) [6].

The Global Atlas of Palliative Care at the End of Life [7] estimates that globally, more than seven million children need palliative care at the end of life. Out of these seven million, nearly half of them (49%) are in Africa with 97% of all children needing palliative care at the end of life living in low-resourced settings, i.e., LMICs. Importantly, the Global Atlas notes that of the seven million needing palliative care at the end of life, 67.7% will die from perinatal conditions, 9.8% from congenital anomalies, 6.5% from Human Immunodeficiency Virus (HIV)/Acquired Immune Deficiency Syndrome (AIDS) and only 3.1% from malignant neoplasms. Thus, despite external perceptions, within PPC the majority of children needing palliative care will not have cancer, but other life-limiting and life-threatening conditions. Work has been carried out, mainly in well-resourced settings to look at the types of children requiring palliative care, with Hain et al. [8] identifying more than 376 conditions from death certificates in the UK, with 32% of deaths being from the ten most common diagnosis. In addition, Together for Short Lives [9] has developed a classification system of four categories of life-limiting and life-threatening conditions in childhood that would benefit from palliative care service provision, based largely on disease trajectories, to facilitate service provision provided around need (Table 1). Wood et al. [10] have further built on these categories by the inclusion of two further categories—that of neonates with limited life expectancy and family members who have unexpectedly lost a child. However, there is ongoing discussion as to whether extra categories are needed, for example, whilst bereavement care is important, bereavement in itself is not a life-limiting category. Whilst this debate may continue, the important thing is not the category, but whether all children who need palliative care, and their families, can access it regardless of their condition.

Table 1. Categories of life-limiting and life-threatening conditions [9].

Category 1	Those children with life-threatening conditions for which curative treatment may be feasible but can fail. e.g., cancer, irreversible organ failure
Category 2	Those children with conditions in which there may be long phases of intensive treatment aimed at prolonging life, but premature death is still possible e.g., cystic fibrosis, Duchenne muscular dystrophy
Category 3	Those children with progressive conditions without curative treatment. e.g., batten disease, mucopolysaccharidoses
Category 4	Those children with conditions with severe neurological disability, which may deteriorate unpredictably, but are not considered progressive.

More recently, a study published in 2017 [11] looked beyond the end-of-life and mortality figures and estimated the global need for PPC to be 21.6 million, with 8.2 million children needing access to specialist palliative care service provision. Need ranged between countries from 21 per 10,000 to >100 per 10,000 [11–13] with the greatest need being seen in low-resourced settings and those with high rates of HIV. The Lancet Commission report [4] addressed the issue of Serious Health-related Suffering (SHS) noting that one third of children aged 15 years or younger who died in 2015 (almost 2.5 million) experienced SHS and >98% of these lived in LMICs. However, a review of PPC services in 2011 [14] found that despite need, 65.6% of countries had no known PPC activity, with only 5.7% having provision reaching mainstream providers and these were well-resourced countries. Likewise, the APCA Atlas of Palliative Care in Africa [15], and the Atlas of Palliative Care in the Eastern Mediterranean Region [16] both demonstrated this ongoing lack of PPC service provision (Figure 1).

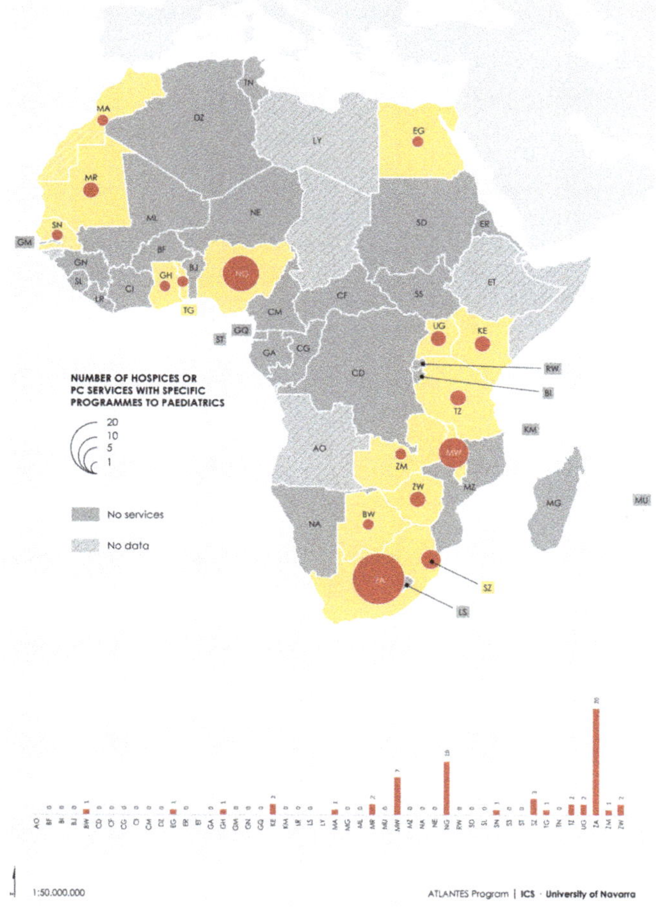

Figure 1. Number of Paediatric Palliative Care (PPC) programmes across Africa ([15] p. 37).

Studies have shown that strengthening palliative care is a key component of strengthening healthcare systems more generally, as the impact of changing attitudes, skills and knowledge extends beyond that of palliative care itself [17]. The Sustainable Development Goals (SDGs) set out 17 goals and 168 targets to end extreme poverty, fight inequalities and injustice, and protect our planet by

2030 [18]. SDG 3 is about 'Good health and well-being' with palliative care fitting well under this goal, although not specifically identified as a target. However, the recent emphasis on UHC, arguably one of the most pressing issues in healthcare today [19], has brought the spotlight on palliative care. Palliative care is being seen as a component of the essential and needed spectrum of health services as defined within UHC by the WHO [6]. UHC is about providing everyone with adequate health services, which must include palliative care services to seriously ill children, who are arguably some of the most vulnerable people within a population. This was emphasised in the Lancet Commission report 'Alleviating the access abyss in palliative care and pain relief—an imperative of UHC.' [4]. Whilst recognising that children who need palliative care face tremendous barriers to accessing it, and removing these barriers must be a priority, and providing some child related recommendations, they call on a future Lancet Commission to focus on the issue of palliative care for children, acknowledging that the area could not be fully covered within the scope of the existing commission. This would open ongoing opportunities for prioritising the global health agenda on PPC.

3. Challenges to PPC Development in LMICs

There are a variety of challenges to developing PPC services, the majority of which impact disproportionately on LMICs [4,20,21]. Whilst exact statistics may not be known due to limitations in data collection, the burden of life-limiting and life-threatening conditions in LMICs is high. For example, in 2016 in sub-Saharan Africa there were 160,000 children <15 years of age infected with HIV [22]. Likewise, the rate of non-communicable diseases, both in adults and children, is set to increase exponentially in LMICs by 2030 [23]. The incidence of childhood cancers globally is also increasing, with 215,000 cases reported in children <14 years in 2016 with many more remaining unreported due to a lack of childhood cancer registries in many countries [24]. Other conditions requiring PPC, such as Multi-drug-resistant tuberculosis (MDR-TB) [25], malaria and perinatal and congenital conditions, are also on the increase; therefore, the need for PPC in LMICs is set to increase, whilst provision remains poor. Alongside this, resources remain limited, both in terms of access to treatments, medications, finances and trained personnel, to name but a few.

Access to treatment can be a challenge. For example, in Eastern and Southern Africa only 63% of children <15 years living with HIV are accessing antiretroviral therapy [22]. Chemotherapy and other medications for the treatment and management of cancer are limited and at times not available. Across sub-Saharan Africa there are a significant number of countries with no radiotherapy machines, so children needing radiotherapy treatment have to travel outside of their country to access this treatment [26]. Access to analgesics, such as oral morphine, also remains a challenge as highlighted in the Lancet Commission report [4]. There are many children globally who are suffering needlessly due to pain and distressing symptoms because the essential medicines for palliative care are not available [27,28]. For children, it is also important that paediatric formulations are available, along with immediate-release liquid oral morphine [20]. It is important to note that despite current poor access, the cost to cover morphine-equivalent pain treatment for all children <15 years with SHS in low income countries would only be $1 million per year [4]. However, even when oral morphine is available, access can be hindered by 'opiophobia'. Opiophobia, the fear individuals (both health and non-health care professionals) have about prescribing/using opioids, exists in many parts of the world, with beliefs ranging from there being a maximum dose of morphine that can be given safely, the fear of addiction, of tolerance, of issues of respiratory depression, and of the possibility of misuse, to name but a few [29], with these fears frequently being heightened in PPC, alongside many commonly held myths about pain in children, such as babies not experiencing pain [20].

More barriers to the development of PPC include a lack of related policies and guidelines. Whilst countries will have policies for HIV and Non Communicable Diseases (NCDs), these may or may not include the provision of palliative care, and the majority of LMICs do not have a specific palliative care policy. While there has been some progress in this area, with countries such as Botswana, South Africa, Rwanda, Malawi, Uganda and Kenya leading the way, without specific policies, palliative care for a population, including children, may not appear in a government's work plan or budget. It is therefore essential that PPC is integrated into a broad range of national policies as well as in specific national palliative care policies. Clinical guidelines also need to be available for use in LMICs, utilising appropriate and available medications, without compromising the quality of the care provided.

The lack of trained health and social care workers in PPC is another issue that needs to be addressed. Whilst the WHA resolution [5], along with the European Association of Palliative Care (EAPC) core competencies for PPC [30,31], recognise the need for education in PPC at three levels, such training is not available in the majority of LMICs, with the lack of education and trained professionals being a major barrier to care provision [32,33]. Alongside this, there is a general lack of awareness of what palliative care entails, the impact it can have, and insufficient acknowledgement of the need for PPC, both at the community and the policy levels. Finally, lack of financial resources, in terms of education, research and clinical care, remains a significant barrier to the growth of PPC provision [20]. Funding for PPC in LMICs is limited and donors willing to fund this type of service have reduced over the past few years, making the situation even more critical [4].

4. Overcoming Barriers and Challenges to PPC Provision

4.1. Advocacy and Public Awareness

Advocacy is a key component of any development work for PPC. Advocacy is needed at all levels of the health system: from within local communities, at hospitals and health centres, at governmental level, within law enforcement agencies, with policy makers, and internationally in order to ensure that there is an urgent and universal agenda promoting the ongoing development of PPC service provision.

Examples of such advocacy work for PPC is seen throughout LMICs where PPC is developing. Advocacy at the community level allows the community, including patients and families, to become aware of what palliative care is and how it can support and help them when it is needed and also gives guidance on how they can become involved. This is an essential element of advocacy work which will assist in overcoming challenges such as a lack of community ownership for PPC programmes, challenging the myths about opioid use and enabling home care support. Community ownership is key and was recognised as one of the core components of a successful model of PPC in sub-Saharan Africa [34].

At the national level, work is ongoing with governments, law enforcement agencies and multi-lateral and national organisations. Recognition of PPC at the national level is essential if there is to be ongoing planning and support (both in terms of resources, personnel and finances) for PPC service provision. Likewise, holding governments to account for some of the international resolutions and treaties they have signed, such as the WHA Resolution on PC [5] and Cancer Care [35], is important and can be a way to hold governments to account while offering to support them to fulfil their obligations and having something to report back on at the next WHA.

Regional and international palliative care organisations are committed to advocating for the development of PC and PPC services. Leading the advocacy activities within the regions are the APCA, the EAPC, the Asia Pacific Hospice and Palliative Care Network (APHN) and the Latin American Association for Palliative Care (ALCP), all of which have key roles in bringing together the thoughts of the region, and bringing their concerns and interests to the international level. They are an important forum in supporting national palliative care associations to advocate with governments and encouraging them to support different motions and resolutions at key meetings. The International Children's Palliative Care Network (ICPCN), the Worldwide Hospice Palliative Care Alliance (WHPCA) and the International Association of Hospice and Palliative Care (IAHPC) collaborate at the international level to bring the global voice of palliative care to the table, with the ICPCN advocating for the voice of the child and PPC. Bringing together the collaborative voice has been successful in supporting side-events at the WHA, the WHA resolution on Palliative care [5] and the WHA resolution on cancer care [35], to name but a few.

Working with multi-lateral organisations such as the WHO and the United Nations Children's Fund (UNICEF) is also important, ensuring that the palliative care voice is heard within issues such as UHC [6], the SDGs [18] and efforts to improve access to medications [4]. Work has been undertaken with human rights organisations such as Human Rights Watch [36] to ensure that access to medications is on the global agenda, with access to pain control and palliative care being seen as an essential human right [37,38]. Thus, the development of palliative care should be seen as a public health and human rights priority. Other important documents and advocacy activities include World Hospice and Palliative Care Day, celebrated on the second Saturday in October each year, with emphasis being placed on key global issues such as the lack of access to UHC [19]. Work has also been undertaken on developing a PC essential medicines list [27,28], essential practices for primary palliative care [39] and the recent Lancet Commission report on an essential package of health care interventions [4].

4.2. Education

Education at all levels of health and social care professional training is essential for the ongoing development of PPC. In line with recent recommendations, such as those within the WHA resolution [5] and the Lancet Commission report [4], education on PPC should be provided across three levels of training: (a) the Palliative Care Approach; (b) General PPC; and (c) Specialist PPC [30,31]. The EAPC developed core competencies for PPC training which were aimed at these three levels and are useful across a range of different settings and countries [30,31].

The first level of training is that of the palliative care approach, which is aimed at educating undergraduate/pre-registration students as well as qualified professionals so that they can integrate PPC in non-specialist settings [30,31]. A variety of competency documents e.g., the EAPC Guide for the Development of Palliative Nurse Education [40], the APCA Core competencies document [41], have been developed to support this level of education. Examples of integrating PC generally, and PPC as appropriate, can be seen from a variety of different LMICs such as in Uganda [42] and Serbia [43]. If PPC can be integrated at this level, then all future health and social care professionals will qualify with an element of PPC knowledge.

General PPC training is for those who are more frequently involved in PPC but do not provide it as the main part of their work [30,31]. A wide variety of curricula and programmes have been developed for this level of training, which is essential to overcome some of the myths and barriers to PPC provision. Examples of such training include the ICPCN elearning programmes [44], the Education in Palliative and End-of-Life Care (EPEC) Paediatric curriculum [45], the PC toolkit training materials [46], the ecancer elearning programmes focused on sub-Saharan Africa and India [47], along with a wide range of locally developed courses. Ensuring that individuals are provided with this level of training will help in providing the continuum of care for individuals, and will support those providing specialist PPC services. For example, the link nurse programme developed at Mulago Hospital in Uganda, and now expanded to other hospitals, ensures that nurses on the wards throughout the hospital can provide a generalist level of PC provision, including PPC, and thus support the specialist team, with 80% of patients being seen by the link nurses and 20% by the specialist team [48].

Specialist palliative care education is aimed at those for whom the provision of PPC is their core activity. Programmes at this level may be focused specifically on different cadres e.g., doctors or nurses, or they may be multi-professional. There are limited numbers of specialist training programmes available in LMICs for PPC, although examples include paediatric PC training for doctors in Argentina, the Masters/Postgraduate Diploma in PC (Paediatric) provided through the University of Cape Town and the Diploma in PPC from Mildmay Uganda [42]. There is a great need to increase specialist level training—ensuring that it is both accessible and affordable, as well as culturally appropriate, thus increasing the number of PPC specialists in LMICs. An essential ingredient of any training, regardless of at which level, is that of clinical modelling so that professionals can see PPC in practice. However, there remain limited environments where this is possible.

Much of the provision of PPC in LMICs is done in the community, so it is also important to train community health workers on PPC. An example of such training has been in South Africa where training for community health workers on PPC has enabled the expansion of PPC provision. Likewise, parents and family members need training in order to support them to look after their child.

4.3. Access to Medications

Access to essential palliative care medicines, such as oral morphine, is limited in many countries and indeed the recent Lancet Commission report focused on this and the disparities seen throughout the world in terms of both availability and price variations [4]. Both the WHO [28] and the IAHPC [27] have accepted essential medicines lists of palliative care, and the Lancet report also recommends an essential package that includes medications; however, this remains an issue in many places. In addition, some countries may have secured access to medications for adults but paediatric formulations are not yet available. There is ongoing work at the international, regional and national levels to address the issue of access to medications, ensuring that they will be both available, but also accessible to all children who need them, regardless of where they live. The ICPCN, IAHPC and WHPCA continue to try and address this issue, working closely with some of the key stakeholders, including the International Narcotics Control Board, the United Nations (UN) Councils, the WHO, etc. This situation has been impacted by the current situation in the United States of America (USA) regarding the misuse of medications, which was highlighted in the Lancet Commission report. There are examples in a wide range of LMICs of how access to essential medicines for PPC has been improved e.g., in Kenya, in South Africa and in Zambia.

4.4. Implementation of PPC

A variety of models of PPC delivery exist within LMICs, covering the continuum of care. Home-based care is important, enabling families to care for their children at home, in their own environment, with the support of community health workers and volunteers. Rachael House in Indonesia is a good example of how a team can work within the existing health care structure to support children with palliative care needs, and their families, at home [20]. However, home-based care is just one model of providing PPC and it is important that care is provided across different settings, in accordance to need, and the WHO definition of PPC. Other models include hospital PPC teams, outpatient care, day care and inpatient care [49,50]. Examples of each of these exist with the LMIC setting, for example Mildmay Uganda have an inpatient as well as day care and outpatient services [51], Umodzi, at Queen Elizabeth Hospital in Blantrye, in Malawi is an example of a specialist PPC hospital team [20,52].

Significant challenges exist to the provision of PPC in remote rural areas, and work has been done looking at the provision of such services in different settings in order to draw on the lessons learnt [53]. Centres of Excellence or Beacon Centres are being developed in different settings in order to not only provide PPC services, but also to provide an environment for clinical placements and learning [54]. Some work was undertaken across sub-Saharan Africa to identify the key areas for an effective PPC programme (Figure 2) and to try and understand the challenges faced by different PPC service providers. Challenges to service provision included a lack of financial resources; the high disease burden; lack of collaboration, PPC not being a priority; poor integration into the formal health services; and staffing issues. It was found that whilst sharing common core elements, each service had unique aspects that were important and ensured they were appropriate and embedded into their local community and context. Successful PPC services could also be integrated into or run parallel with existing structures, depending on the system in which they are operating [34].

- Clear and strong leadership
- Focused on the vision
- Linked to what makes the programme unique
- Different components of care
- Holistic approach to care
- Clear strategy
- In touch with changes in the environment
- Adaptable (but not losing focus)
- Consistency in approach
- Acceptance by the community and collaboration
- Access to a variety of education programmes

Figure 2. Key elements of an effective PPC programme [34].

4.5. Research

Whilst originally not seen as a priority, the importance of research has been recognised in developing the evidence base, and seen as a key pillar in palliative care development [55] alongside policy, drug availability, education and implementation [56]. Whilst resources for service delivery may be limited in many LMICs, it is essential that we undertake research to ensure that we are using those resources wisely, and adapting them as required. However, there has been a lack of research in palliative care generally [57], and more specifically in PPC. In 2010, just five peer-reviewed papers were found on PPC in sub-Saharan Africa, and a report on the status of PPC across the region highlighted that the evidence base for PPC had not progressed, there were no measurement tools, few models were discussed and that there was an urgent need for research within the field [58].

This lack of research has been identified on many occasions over the years [4,58–62]. The WHO guidelines on the pharmacological management of persisting pain in children with medical illnesses [63] highlight how this lack of evidence has impacted on the development of evidence-based guidelines, and therefore the management of pain within PPC, and proceed to make a call for the expansion of the evidence base within the field [62]. Global priorities for research on PPC have been identified which encompass holistic care, education, interventions and models, legislation and ethics and policies and procedures (Figure 3). Thus, the generation of evidence needs to be recognised as an integral part of PPC service provision to ensure that we can deliver evidence-based, cost-effective and equitable PPC, not just in LMICs, but globally [61].

- Children's understanding of death and dying
- Managing pain in children where there is no morphine
- Funding for and the cost of PPC
- Training needs for PPC
- Assessment of the 2-step analgesic ladder
- Pain management for children with diseases other than cancer
- Interventions and models of care
- Outcomes of care
- Integration of PPC into core curriculum
- Use of opioids in children
- The global need for PPC
- Ethical issues in PPC

Figure 3. Global Priorities for PPC Research [61].

5. Conclusions

Many examples of high-quality PPC service provision within LMICs exist; however, these remain few and far between, with an urgent need to scale up affordable, accessible and quality PC services for children globally. Whilst challenges exist inhibiting the ongoing development of PPC, these have been identified, and work is ongoing in different contexts and at different levels, to try and overcome these barriers. Strategies should be put in place to continue to scale up PPC service provision in LMICs, so that access is assured for all children who need palliative care, and their families, regardless of where they live.

Acknowledgments: Figure 1 is reprinted with permission from the International Association for Hospice and Palliative Care.

Author Contributions: J.D. drafted the paper with input from S.B., A.D. and B.N. All authors commented on the draft and inputted into the final version of the paper.

Conflicts of Interest: The authors declare no conflict of interest.

References

1. Population Reference Bureau. 2017. Available online: http://www.prb.org/pdf17/2017_World_Population.pdf (accessed on 30 November 2017).
2. WHO Definition of Palliative Care for Children. Available online: www.who.int/cancer/palliative/definition/en/ (accessed on 25 November 2017).
3. Together for Short Lives. Children's Palliative Care Definitions. Available online: http://www.togetherforshortlives.org.uk/professionals/childrens_palliative_care_essentials/definitions (accessed on 25 November 2017).
4. Knaul, F.M.; Farmer, P.E.; Krakauer, E.L.; De Lima, L.; Bhadelia, A.; Kwete, X.J.; Arreola-Ornelas, H.; Gómez-Dantés, O.; Rodriguez, N.M.; Alleyne, G.A.O.; et al. Alleviating the access abyss in palliative care and pain relief—An imperative of universal health coverage: The Lancet Commission report. *Lancet* **2017**. published online October 12. [CrossRef]
5. World Health Assembly. *Strengthening of Palliative Care as a Component of Integrated Treatment within the Continuum of Care. 134th Session*; EB134.R7; World Health Organization: Geneva, Switzerland, 2014.
6. World Health Organization. Health Financing for Universal Health Coverage. Available online: http://www.who.int/health_financing/universal_coverage_definition/en/ (accessed on 25 November 2017).
7. Connor, S.R.; Sepulveda Bermedo, M.C. *Global Atlas of Palliative Care at the End of Life*; Worldwide Palliative Care Alliance: London, UK, 2014.

8. Hain, R.; Devins, M.; Hastings, R.; Noyes, J. Paediatric palliative care: Development and pilot study of a 'Directory' of life-limiting conditions. *BMC Palliat. Care* **2013**, *12*, 43. [CrossRef] [PubMed]
9. Together for Short Lives. Key Information. Available online: http://www.togetherforshortlives.org.uk/professionals/childrens_palliative_care_essentials/approach (accessed on 25 November 2017).
10. Wood, F.; Simpson, S.; Barnes, E.; Hain, R. Disease trajectories and ACT/ RCPCH categories in paediatric palliative care. *Palliat. Med.* **2010**, *24*, 796–806. [CrossRef] [PubMed]
11. Connor, S.R.; Downing, J.; Marston, J. Estimating the global need for palliative care for children: A cross-sectional analysis. *J. Pain Symptom Manag.* **2017**, *53*, 171–177. [CrossRef] [PubMed]
12. Connor, S.R.; Sisimayi, C.; Downing, J.; King, E.; Lim Ah Ken, P.; Yates, R.; Ikin, B.; Marston, J. Assessment of the need for palliative care for children in South Africa. *Int. J. Palliat. Nurs.* **2014**, *20*, 130–134. [CrossRef] [PubMed]
13. Connor, S.R.; Sisimayi, C. *Assessment of the Need for Palliative Care for Children: Three Country Report: South Africa, Kenya and Zimbabwe*; UNICEF; ICPCN: London, UK, 2013.
14. Knapp, C.; Woodworth, L.; Wright, M.; Downing, J.; Drake, R.; Fowler-Kerry, S.; Hain, R.; Marston, J. Paediatric palliative care provision around the world: A systematic review. *Pediatr. Blood Cancer* **2011**, *57*, 361–368. [CrossRef] [PubMed]
15. Rhee, J.Y.; Luyirika, E.; Namisango, E.; Powell, R.A.; Garralda, E.; Pons, J.J.; De Lima, L.; Centeno, C. *APCA Atlas of Palliative Care in Africa*; IAHPC Press: Houston, TX, USA, 2017.
16. Osman, H.; Rihan, A.; Garralda, E.; Rhee, J.Y.; Pons, J.J.; De Lima, L.; Tfayli, A.; Centeno, C. *Atlas of Palliative Care in the Eastern Mediterranean Region*; IAHPC Press: Houston, TX, USA, 2017.
17. Grant, L.; Downing, J.; Luyirika, E.; Murphy, M.; Namukwaya, L.; Kiyange, F.; Atieno, M.; Kemigish-Ssali, E.; Hunt, J.; Snell, K.; et al. Integrating palliative care into national health systems in Africa: A multi-country intervention study. *J. Glob. Health* **2017**, *7*, 010419. [CrossRef] [PubMed]
18. The United Nations Development Programme (UNDP). *Sustainable Development Goals*; UNDP: Geneva, Switzerland, 2000.
19. Jackson, K.; Morris, C.; Thomas, S. *Universal Health Coverage and Palliative Care—Don't Leave Those Suffering Behind*; World Hospice and Palliative Care Day Toolkit 2017; WHPCA: London, UK, 2017.
20. Downing, J.; Powell, R.A.; Marston, J.; Huwa, C.; Chandra, L.; Garchakova, A.; Harding, R. Children's palliative care in low and middle-income countries. *Arch. Dis. Child.* **2015**, *101*, 85–90. [CrossRef] [PubMed]
21. Downing, J.; Birtar, D.; Chambers, L.; Drake, R.; Gelb, B.; Kiman, R. Children's palliative care: A global concern. *Int. J. Palliat. Nurs.* **2012**, *18*, 109–114. [CrossRef] [PubMed]
22. UNAIDS Fact Sheet—World AIDS Day. 2017. Available online: http://www.unaids.org/sites/default/files/media_asset/UNAIDS_FactSheet_en.pdf (accessed on 25 November 2017).
23. World Health Organization. Chapter 1—Burden: Mortality, morbidity and risk factors. In *Global Status Report on Noncommunicable Diseases 2010*; World Health Organization: Rome, Italy, 2011; pp. 9–31.
24. Childhood Cancer International. International Childhood Cancer Day. 2017. Available online: http://www.internationalchildhoodcancerday.org (accessed on 30 November 2017).
25. Mariandyshew, A.; Eliseev, P. Drug-resistant tuberculosis threatens WHO's End-TB strategy. *Lancet Infect. Dis.* **2017**, *17*, 674–675. [CrossRef]
26. Zubizarreta, E.H.; Fidarova, E.; Healy, B.; Rosenblatt, E. Need for radiotherapy in low and middle income countries—The silence crisis continues. *Clin. Oncol.* **2015**, *27*, 107–114. [CrossRef] [PubMed]
27. De Lima, L.; Krakauer, E.L.; Lorenz, K.; Praill, D.; Macdonald, N.; Doyle, D. Ensuring palliative medicine availability: The development of the IAHPC list of essential medicines for palliative care. *J. Pain Symptom. Manag.* **2007**, *33*, 521–526. [CrossRef] [PubMed]
28. World Health Organization. *WHO Essential Medicines in Palliative Care*; IAHPC Press: Houston, TX, USA, 2013.
29. Bennett, D.S.; Carr, D.B. Opiophobia as a barrier to the treatment of pain. *J. Pain Palliat. Care Pharmacother.* **2002**, *16*, 105–109. [CrossRef] [PubMed]
30. Downing, J.; Ling, J.; Benini, F.; Payne, S.; Papadatou, D. A summary of the EAPC White Paper on core competencies for education in paediatric palliative care. *Eur. J. Palliat. Care* **2014**, *21*, 245–249.
31. Downing, J.; Ling, J.; Benini, F.; Payne, S.; Papadatou, D. *EAPC Core Competencies for Education in Paediatric Palliative Care*; Report of the EAPC children's palliative care education task force; European Association for Palliative Care: Milano, Italy, 2013.

32. Downing, J.; Ling, J. Education in children's palliative care across Europe and internationally. *Int. J. Palliat. Nurs.* **2012**, *18*, 115–120. [CrossRef] [PubMed]
33. Mwangi-Powell, F.N.; Downing, J.; Powell, R.A.; Kiyange, F.; Ddungu, H. Chapter 76: Palliative care in Africa. In *Oxford Textbook of Palliative Nursing*, 4th ed.; Ferrell, B.R., Coyle, N., Paice, J.A., Eds.; Oxford University Press: Oxford, UK, 2015.
34. Downing, J.; Kieffer, S.; Marston, J.; Taglieri, J.; Sullivan, G. An evaluation of models of children's palliative care in sub Saharan Africa. Abstract Book. Differentiated care for diverse communities. In Proceedings of the 5th International African Palliative Care Conference, Kampala, Uganda, 16–19 August 2016.
35. World Health Assembly. Cancer prevention and control. In Proceedings of the 58th World Health Assembly, Geneva, Switzerland, 16–25 May 2005.
36. Human Rights Watch. *Global State of Pain Treatment: Access to Medicines and Palliative Care*; Human Rights Watch: New York, NY, USA, 2011.
37. Brennan, F.; Carr, D.; Cousins, M. Access to Pain Management—Still Very Much a Human Right. *Pain Med.* **2016**, *17*, 1785–1789. [CrossRef] [PubMed]
38. Gwyther, L.; Brennan, F.; Harding, R. Advancing palliative care as a human right. *J. Pain Symptom Manag.* **2009**, *38*, 767–774. [CrossRef] [PubMed]
39. De Lima, L.; Bennett, M.I.; Murray, S.A.; Hudson, P.; Doyle, D.; Bruera, E.; Grande-Cameron, C.; Strasser, F.; Downing, J.; Wenk, R. International Association for Hospice and Palliative Care (IAHPC) List of Essential Practices in Palliative Care. *J. Pain Palliat. Care Pharmacother.* **2012**, *26*, 118–122. [CrossRef] [PubMed]
40. De Vlieger, M.; Gorchs, N.; Larkin, P.J.; Porchet, F. *A Guide for the Development of Palliative Nurse Education in Europe*; Palliative Nurse Education: Report of the EAPC Task Force; EAPC: Milano, Italy, 2004.
41. APCA. *African Palliative Care Association Core Competencies: A Framework of Core Competencies for Palliative Care Providers in Africa*; APCA: Kampala, Uganda, 2012.
42. Rawlinson, F.; Gwyther, L.; Kiyange, F.; Luyirika, E.; Meiring, M.; Downing, J. The current situation in education and training of health-care professionals across Africa to optimise the delivery of palliative care for cancer patients. *Ecancermedicalscience* **2014**, *8*, 492. [CrossRef] [PubMed]
43. Milicevic, N.; Haraldsdottir, E.; Lukic, N.; Baskott, J.; Rayment, C.; Downing, J. Palliative care development in Serbia. *Eur. J. Palliat. Care* **2015**, *22*, 30–33.
44. Downing, J.; Boucher, S.; Nkosi, B.; Steel, B.; Marston, J. Transforming children's palliative care through the International Children's Palliative Care Network. *Int. J. Palliat. Nurs.* **2014**, *20*, 109–114. [CrossRef] [PubMed]
45. Northwestern Medicine (2017) Pediatrics. Available online: http://bioethics.northwestern.edu/programs/epec/curricula/pediatrics.html (accessed on 25 November 2017).
46. Lavy, V. *Palliative Care Toolkit Trainers Manual*; WHPCA: London, UK, 2009.
47. Ecancer Palliative Care e-learning Course for Healthcare Professionals in Africa. Available online: http://ecancer.org/education/course/1-palliative-care-e-learning-course-for-healthcare-professionals-in-africa.php (accessed on 25 November 2017).
48. Downing, J.; Batuli, M.; Kivumbi, G.; Kabahweza, J.; Grant, L.; Murray, S.A.; Namukwaya, E.; Leng, M. Evaluation of a palliative care link nurse programme in Mulago hospital, Uganda: An evaluation using mixed methods. *BMC Palliat. Care* **2016**, *15*, 40. [CrossRef] [PubMed]
49. Downing, J.; Powell, R.A.; Mwangi-Powell, F. Home-based palliative care in sub-Saharan Africa. *Home Healthc. Nurse* **2010**, *28*, 298–307. [CrossRef] [PubMed]
50. Mwangi-Powell, F.N.; Powell, R.A.; Harding, R. Models of delivering palliative and end-of-life care in sub-Saharan Africa: A narrative review of the evidence. *Curr. Opin. Support Palliat. Care* **2013**, *7*, 223–228. [CrossRef] [PubMed]
51. Downing, J.; Nakawesi, J.; Kiwanuka, R. Chapter 4. Paediatric Palliative Care in Uganda. In *Pediatric Palliative Care: Global Perspectives*; Knapp, C., Madden, V., Fowler-Kerry, S., Eds.; Springer: New York, NY, USA, 2012; pp. 41–64.
52. Chiputula, F.; Palmer, Z. Chapter 2—Pediatric Palliative Care in Malawi. In *Pediatric Palliative Care: Global Perspectives*; Knapp, C., Madden, V., Fowler-Kerry, S., Eds.; Springer: New York, NY, USA, 2012; pp. 17–26.
53. Downing, J.; Jack, B.A. End-of-life care in rural areas: What is different? *Curr. Opin. Support Palliat. Care* **2012**, *6*, 391–397. [CrossRef] [PubMed]
54. Downing, J.D.; Marston, J.; Selwyn, C.; Ross-Gakava, L. Developing children's palliative care in Africa through beacon centres: lessons learnt. *BMC Palliat. Care* **2013**, *12*. [CrossRef] [PubMed]

55. Harding, R.; Selman, L.; Powell, R.A.; Namisango, E.; Downing, J.; Merriman, A.; Ali, Z.; Gikaara, N.; Gwyther, L.; Higginson, I. Cancer Control in Africa 6. Research into palliative care in sub-Saharan Africa. *Lancet Oncol.* **2013**, *14*, e183–e188. [CrossRef]
56. Stjernsward, J.; Foley, K.M.; Ferris, F.D. The public health strategy for palliative care. *J Pain Symptom Manag.* **2007**, *33*, 486–493. [CrossRef] [PubMed]
57. Grant, L.; Downing, J.; Namukwaya, E.; Leng, M.; Murray, S.A. Palliative care in Africa since 2005: Good progress, but much further to go. *BMJ Support Palliat. Care* **2011**, *1*, 118–122. [CrossRef] [PubMed]
58. Harding, R.; Albertyn, R.; Sherr, L.; Gwyther, L. Pediatric palliative care in Sub-Saharan Africa: A systematic review of the evidence for care models, interventions and outcomes. *J. Pain Symptom Manag.* **2014**, *47*, 642–651. [CrossRef] [PubMed]
59. Downing, J. Editorial: To research or not to research—An important question in paediatric palliative care. *Palliat. Med.* **2016**, *30*, 902–903. [CrossRef] [PubMed]
60. Beecham, E.; Hudson, B.F.; Oostendorp, L.; Candy, B.; Jones, L.; Vickerstaff, V.; Lakhanpaul, M.; Stone, P.; Chambers, L.; Hall, D.; et al. A call for increased paediatric palliative care research: Identifying barriers. *Palliat. Med.* **2016**, *30*, 979–980. [CrossRef] [PubMed]
61. Downing, J.; Knapp, C.; Mukaden, M.A.; Fowler-Kerry, S.; Marston, J. ICPCN Scientific Committee. Priorities for global research into children's palliative care: Results of an International Delphi Study. *BMC Palliat. Care* **2015**, *14*, 36. [CrossRef] [PubMed]
62. Milani, B.; Magnini, N.; Gray, A.; Wiffen, P.; Scholten, W. WHO Calls for Targeted research on the Pharmacological Treatment of Persisting Pain in Children with Medical Illnesses. *Evid. Based Child Health* **2011**, *6*, 1017–1020. [CrossRef]
63. World Health Organization. *WHO Guidelines on the Pharmacological Treatment of Persisting Pain in Children with Medical Illnesses*; WHO: Geneva, Switzerland, 2012.

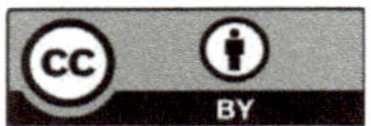

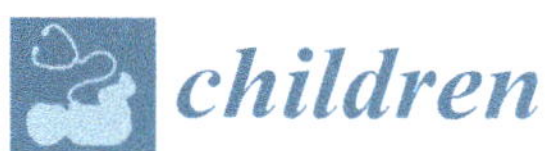
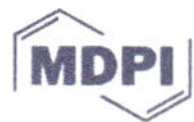

Review

Palliative Care for Children in Hospital: Essential Roles

Ross Drake

Starship Children's Health, Park Road, Grafton, Auckland 1023, New Zealand; rossd@adhb.govt.nz

Received: 30 November 2017; Accepted: 12 February 2018; Published: 19 February 2018

Abstract: Palliative care for children in pediatric hospitals is a vital part of the network of services supporting children with severe illness. This has been recognized, with a trend over the past decade for an increased number of pediatric palliative care (PPC) services established in pediatric hospitals. The inpatient team is in the unique position of influencing the early identification of children and their families, across the age and diagnostic spectrum, which could benefit from palliative care. These services have an opportunity to influence the integration of the palliative approach throughout the hospital, and in so doing, have the capacity to improve many aspects of care, including altering an increasingly futile and burdensome treatment trajectory, and ensuring improved symptom (physical and psychological) management.

Keywords: pediatrics; infant; children; adolescent; hospitals; inpatient; hospital-specific palliative care issues; pediatric palliative care; end-of-life care; life-limiting conditions; chronic disease

1. Introduction

Pediatric palliative care (PPC) services have been in development since England led the way with the founding of the first children's hospice, Helen House, in 1982 and the pioneering hospital-based palliative care team in 1986 at Great Ormond Street Hospital. Internationally, the establishment of PPC services has been variable and largely restricted to countries with a very high human development index. However, the location of these services—whether in the hospital versus the community—has often been imbalanced, with capacity gradually built in the contrasting area over time. For example, the United Kingdom (UK) has had a focus on residential hospice teams, while the United States (USA) has concentrated on hospital-based teams.

The hospital-based PPC service is an important part of the network of care for children with serious illness. The experience of the USA has been detailed in a 2012 survey [1], which indicated a creditable 72% of respondents had a PPC program, with the majority having been launched since 2005. The most common service offered was consultation (88%), with the majority providing this throughout the hospital (87%) and across the age range (>90%). In terms of community capacity, all of the programs reported having developed a relationship with a hospice program, with 80% working with one or more independent hospice organization, and close to 20% working in a hospital that operated its own hospice program.

Regardless of location of care, the philosophy of palliative care remains the same. However, there are some requirements of a hospital-based team over and above that of a community-based service. They hospital service plays an essential role in identifying children and families in need, which includes integrating the palliative approach within the hospital, liaising effectively with community-based services, and providing impeccable assessment and treatment of pain and other problems to the betterment of the mind, body, and spirit of children and their families.

2. Identification

Being situated in a children's hospital, particularly a tertiary facility, means that PPC clinicians are more likely to be exposed to children with rare disorders [2], many of whom have an uncertain or guarded prognosis [3]. This provides an opportunity for the hospital-based service to identify children who could benefit from a palliative approach or palliative care, and relay this to the primary pediatric service engaged in the child's care. This charges the PPC service to be effective communicators and educators, both formally and informally, to all of the pediatric services, not just the "big three" of oncology, neurology, and cardiology.

The neonatal unit is likely to see the largest number of deaths in a children's hospital, while the pediatric intensive care unit (PICU) is likely to admit children with a serious illness at their most vulnerable. In a national cohort study [4] of children admitted to a PICU in England over an 11-year period, 57.6% (n = 89,127) of admissions and 72.9% (n = 4,821) of deaths were of an individual with a potentially life-shortening medical condition. The mortality rate in the PICU for these children was double compared with those who did not have such a diagnosis (5.4% versus 2.7%), and a child with a life-limiting condition was 75% more likely to die in the PICU once all of the factors had been taken into account (OR 1.75; 95% CI 1.64 to 1.87).

Case 1. "A" was born by emergency cesarean section at term after placental abruption. She required extensive resuscitation at birth and mechanical ventilation for six days. Magnetic resonance imaging showed severe cerebral edema consistent with severe hypoxic ischemic encephalopathy. She developed seizures, and her electroencephalogram was profoundly abnormal. In discussion with her parents, mechanical ventilation was withdrawn, with the expectation that she would not survive. Surprisingly, she established spontaneous respirations after extubation, and a referral was made to the hospital PPC team. She was seen by the PPC service, and a discussion was held with the family around their goals and expectations of care, and an advance care plan was completed. In line with their wishes, "A" was discharged home once community pediatric support had been arranged. At home, she began feeding orally; she thrived, and medical care was increasingly provided by the developmental pediatric service.

In-depth information on the demographic profile and clinical characteristics of children requiring palliative care has been a relatively recent event. In 2011, a prospective cohort study [5] of 515 children cared for by six hospital-based PPC teams in the United States and Canada was published. The study reported an age range of less than one year (17.3%) to 19 years or older (15.5%), with non-cancer conditions dominating. The single largest group was children with a genetic/congenital condition (40.8%), whereas children with cancer only made up 19.8% of the cohort. The complexity of the care was reflected in 79.6% of children requiring at least one form of long-term medical technology, with 59.6% having a feeding tube of some description (48.5% gastrostomy). The other notable supports were a central venous catheter (22.3%), tracheostomy (10.5%), and 18% having a requirement for assisted respiration.

Similarly, a Malaysian observational analysis by Chong et al. [6] indicated an age spread that was more consistent with general pediatric mortality data, with 44.8% of the 315 children reviewed being one year of age or younger, and 14.6% in the of adolescent age group (13 years to 18 years). The dominant ICD-10 coding identified was similar to the North American study, with 37.1% of children having 'congenital malformations, deformations and chromosomal abnormalities', followed by 'diseases of the nervous system' (24.1%) and 'neoplasms' (19.0%). Again, children with neurological diseases had significantly more physical needs than the other two diagnostic categories (OR = 3.95; 95% CI 1.47 to 10.61, $p < 0.01$).

Case 2. "B" was diagnosed at six months of age with a peroxisomal biogenesis disorder, having been hypotonic and troubled by feeding difficulties since birth. She had had a more recent decline in vision and hearing, as well as gross motor and language development. Her liver function tests had become abnormal, with an increased risk of coagulopathy. There was no known treatment for her condition, and while the prognosis was uncertain, it was expected that she would develop progressive white matter degeneration with increasing disability, and ultimately a shortened life expectancy. A referral was made to the hospital PPC service, which transitioned her care to the community, with respite support arranged.

These findings were reflective of a general trend for children admitted to pediatric hospitals having increasingly complex care needs, with attendant high resource use [7–10]. This data has been further enriched by an elegant, descriptive study [11] of home-based PPC. The most telling finding for these 33 Italian families was the eight hours and 54 minutes per day spent, on average, caring for their child. Feeding was the single most time-consuming activity, at 174 minutes per day, with the additional six hours of care devoted to maintaining an average of five different life-supporting medical appliances. A feeding device was required by 72% of the children, 36% had a tracheostomy, and 55% were on mechanical ventilator support. Care was provided under the duress of tiredness as a result of broken sleep, as caregivers were awake for an average of 67 minutes per night to attend to the child.

3. Integration

The diversity of conditions affecting children that could benefit from palliative care and the medically fragile nature of these children requires a hospital-based PPC service to be an integral part of the pediatric hospital. Very little direction exists on how PPC services can achieve such assimilation, although a review on the early integration of palliative care for children with high-risk cancer [12] suggests a model for cancer that could be translated to non-cancer conditions.

The model addresses three tiers of service delivery within an institution to "function synergistically to maximize early provision". It proposes a broad institutional palliative approach by supporting primary teams through education and policy initiatives to allow the delivery of core elements of PPC from the time of diagnosis. A middle level identifies specific populations, including children, at the end of life so that they may receive palliative care from the child's primary pediatric service by way of standardized guidelines or other such management pathways. This leaves specialist palliative care to be available as the third layer to deal with more complex issues, such as difficult symptom management cases or challenging decision-making issues.

The vignette below provides a glimpse into how the early integration of the PPC service and the palliative approach in the tertiary children's hospital setting can, amongst other things, aid relationship development and parental adjustment, and assist communication and decision-making [13].

Case 2: Integration. "B" developed a series of neurological, respiratory, and gastrointestinal complications over the next four years, including recurrent life-threatening respiratory tract infections and compromised liver function. This required frequent hospital attendances, either as an inpatient or for outpatient consultations with her primary pediatric care provided by the pediatric metabolic service. Several other services were also involved including the pediatric neurology, pediatric gastroenterology, and child liaison psychiatry services. In addition, she had a team of allied health practitioners, including a physiotherapist, occupational therapist, and dietician to help support her developmental, nutritional, and equipment needs. These services were guided by hospital policy for a palliative approach, and through an advance care plan, which the family had previously prepared. The plan was reviewed and modified with the family at times of significant changes in the child's condition. The hospital PPC team maintained contact at outpatient appointments and during admissions, allowing a strong relationship to be established over time, even though the family had moved to another town distant from the pediatric hospital. This allowed the PPC team to address advance care plan reviews, be involved in managing difficult symptoms, and aid communication with the family between services at times of dissonance.

4. Symptom Assessment and Management

The reality is that a hospital-based PPC service will be required to deal with the "relief of suffering by means of early identification and impeccable assessment and treatment of pain and other problems" [14] on a relatively frequent basis. At the beginning of the millennium, the sentinel paper by Wolfe et al. exposed the need for a service with a focus on impeccable symptom management in pediatric hospitals [15].

This exploration of parent perception on the end-of-life care of 102 children dying from cancer indicated that 89% of the children were felt to have suffered "a lot" or "a great deal" from at least one symptom in their last month of life, with this most commonly due to pain, fatigue, or dyspnea. The emphasis for the paper, and arguably the most quoted finding, is that treatment was only successful in 27% of children with pain, and 16% of children with dyspnea. However, as important was the finding that suffering from pain was more likely in children where the physician was not actively involved in providing end-of-life care (OR 2.6; 95% CI 1.0 to 6.7).

The success of having such a program based at a children's hospital was underlined by a prospective study [16] of the symptom burden for 30 children who died as a result of a medical condition in a large, tertiary center. The symptom burden was high, with children having a mean number of symptoms of 11.1 ± 5.6 in the last week of life. Children dying on the ward had significantly more symptoms than those dying in intensive care (14.3 ± 6.1 vs. 9.5 ± 4.7, $p < 0.02$).

Six symptoms, including pain, occurred with a prevalence of 50% or more, and while symptoms were at times distressing, the majority of children were able to be kept "always comfortable" to "usually comfortable" in the last week (64%) and day (76.6%) of life.

Case 2: Symptom Management. "B" was readmitted to hospital after further decline in her vision and the development and onset of distressing severe muscle spasms, intractable irritability, gastrointestinal pseudo-obstruction, and gastric bleeding of unknown cause. The PPC service worked in collaboration with the pediatric metabolic, neurology, and gastroenterology services to modify feeding, bowel care, and coagulopathy management. New medications (baclofen, gabapentin, amitriptyline, clobazam) were introduced and titrated to best effect, while non-pharmacological measures (positioning, gastrostomy venting, distraction, and relaxation techniques for parents to use with "B") were employed to successfully reduce distress, such that her parents were able to contemplate a return home. When she was ready for discharge, several videoconferences were held with the local general pediatric and palliative care teams to ensure a smooth coordinated handover of care. A detailed symptom management plan was drawn up by the palliative care and metabolic teams, and a system for contact was set up so that her parents knew who to call and where to get help.

In 2008, a follow-up study by Wolfe et al. [17] compared the 102 children who died of cancer between 1990–1997 with a follow-up cohort of 119 children who died between 1997–2004 using a similar retrospective parent survey and chart review methodology. The only difference between the two cohorts was the formation of a Pediatric Advanced Care team at the hospital in 1997.

The comparison found no change in the number of children experiencing pain, fatigue, and dyspnea, but reports of "a lot" or "a great deal" of suffering decreased for all of the symptoms in the follow-up group except fatigue. Specifically, parents reporting this level of suffering from pain were down to 47% in the follow-up cohort versus 66% for the baseline cohort (adjusted risk difference 19%, $p = 0.018$), and dyspnea was also lower at 37% versus 58% (adjusted risk difference 21%; $p = 0.02$). Importantly, parents from the follow-up cohort felt "very prepared" for the medical problems experienced by their child at the end of life (56% versus 27%, $p < 0.001$), and for the circumstances at the time of death (49% versus 25%, $p = 0.002$).

The value of a hospital-based PPC service was further reinforced by a retrospective chart review at another major US pediatric hospital, with the analysis of the inpatient deaths of 114 children [18]. This study compared the outcomes of the 25% of children who received a PPC consult with those children who were not seen by the PPC service. The PPC consult group experienced a higher rate of pain assessment during the last 12 to 24 h of admission (adjusted relative risk 1.57; 95% CI 1.16 to 2.10), better documentation around specific actions to manage pain at 12-hourly intervals during the last 72 h of life (adjusted OR 3.14; 95% CI 1.08 to 9.16 to OR 6.51; 95% CI 1.92 to 22.12), and more likely to have a do-not-resuscitate order in place at the time of death (adjusted OR 7.92; 95% CI 2.02 to 31.12).

5. Conclusions

Ultimately, these discoveries strongly suggest that the application of the palliative care paradigm and the presence of a pediatric palliative care service in the pediatric hospital is an important enhancement to the palliative care community. Hospital services can aid in the identification of children and their families who could benefit from palliative care, and by way of system integration and the early involvement of a palliative approach, palliative care can help ensure that palliative and dying children are exposed to the minimum amount of suffering by applying, amongst other things, a more aggressive approach to symptom control.

Conflicts of Interest: The author declares no conflict of interest.

References

1. Feudtner, C.; Womer, J.; Augustin, R.; Remke, S.; Wolfe, J.; Friebert, S.; Weissman, D. Pediatric palliative care programs in children's hospitals: A cross-sectional national survey. *Pediatrics* **2013**, *132*, 1063–1070. [CrossRef] [PubMed]
2. Hain, R.; Devins, M.; Hastings, R.; Noyes, J. Paediatric palliative care: Development and pilot study of a 'Directory' of life-limiting conditions. *BMC Palliat. Care* **2013**, *12*, 43. [CrossRef] [PubMed]
3. Brook, L.; Hain, R. Predicting death in children. *Arch. Dis. Child.* **2008**, *93*, 1067–1070. [CrossRef] [PubMed]
4. Fraser, L.K.; Parslow, R. Children with life-limiting conditions in paediatric intensive care units: A national cohort, data linkage study. *Arch. Dis. Child.* **2017**. [CrossRef] [PubMed]
5. Feudtner, C.; Kang, T.I.; Hexem, K.R.; Friedrichsdorf, S.J.; Osenga, K.; Siden, H.; Friebert, S.E.; Hays, R.M.; Dussel, V.; Wolfe, J. Pediatric palliative care patients: A prospective multicenter cohort study. *Pediatrics* **2011**, *127*, 1094–1101. [CrossRef] [PubMed]
6. Chong, L.A.; Khalid, F.; Khoo, T.B.; Wong, J.J. Clinical spectrum of children receiving palliative care in Malaysian hospitals. *Med. J. Malaysia* **2017**, *72*, 32–36. [PubMed]
7. Simon, T.D.; Berry, J.; Feudtner, C.; Stone, B.L.; Sheng, X.L.; Bratton, S.L.; Dean, J.M.; Srivastava, R. Children with complex chronic conditions in inpatient hospital settings in the United States. *Pediatrics* **2010**, *126*, 647–655. [CrossRef] [PubMed]
8. Berry, J.G.; Hall, D.E.; Kuo, D.Z.; Cohen, E.; Agrawal, R.; Feudtner, C.; Hall, M.; Kueser, J.; Kaplan, W.; Neff, J. Hospital utilization and characteristics of patients experiencing recurrent readmissions within children's hospitals. *JAMA* **2011**, *305*, 682–690. [CrossRef] [PubMed]
9. Cohen, E.; Berry, J.G.; Camacho, X.; Anderson, G.; Wodchis, W.; Guttmann, A. Patterns and costs of health care use of children with medical complexity. *Pediatrics* **2012**, *130*, e1463–e1470. [CrossRef] [PubMed]
10. Davies, D.; Hartfield, D.; Wren, T. Children who 'grow up' in hospital: Inpatient stays of six months or longer. *Pediatr. Child. Health* **2014**, *19*, 533–536. [CrossRef]
11. Lazzarin, P.; Schiavon, B.; Brugnaro, L.; Benini, F. Parents spend an average of nine hours a day providing palliative care for children at home and need to maintain an average of five life-saving devices. *Acta Pediatr.* **2017**. [CrossRef] [PubMed]
12. Kaye, E.C.; Friebert, S.; Baker, J.N. Early integration of palliative care for children with high-risk cancer and their families. *Pediatr. Blood Cancer* **2016**, *63*, 593–597. [CrossRef] [PubMed]
13. Mack, J.W.; Wolfe, J. Early integration of pediatric palliative care: for some children, palliative care starts at diagnosis. *Curr. Opin. Pediatr.* **2006**, *18*, 10–14. [CrossRef] [PubMed]
14. World Health Organisation. *WHO Definition of Palliative Care;* World Health Organisation: Geneva, Switzerland, 2002.
15. Wolfe, J.; Grier, H.E.; Klar, N.; Levin, S.B.; Ellenbogen, J.M.; Salem-Schatz, S.; Emanuel, E.J.; Weeks, J.C. Symptoms and suffering at the end of life in children with cancer. *N. Engl. J. Med.* **2000**, *342*, 326–333. [CrossRef] [PubMed]

16. Drake, R.; Frost, J.; Collins, J.J. The symptoms of dying children. *J. Pain Symptom Manag.* **2003**, *26*, 594–603. [CrossRef]
17. Wolfe, J.; Hammel, J.F.; Edwards, K.E.; Duncan, J.; Comeau, M.; Breyer, J.; Aldridge, S.A.; Grier, H.E.; Berde, C.; Dussel, V.; Weeks, J.C. Easing of suffering in children with cancer at the end of life: Is care changing? *J. Clin. Oncol.* **2008**, *26*, 1717–1723. [CrossRef] [PubMed]
18. Osenga, K.; Postier, A.; Dreyfus, J.; Foster, L.; Teeple, W.; Friedrichsdorf, S.J. A comparison of circumstances at the end of life in a hospital setting for children with palliative care involvement versus those without. *J. Pain Symptom Manag.* **2016**, *52*, 673–680. [CrossRef] [PubMed]

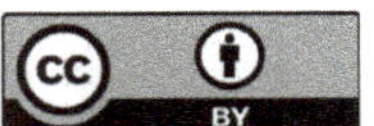

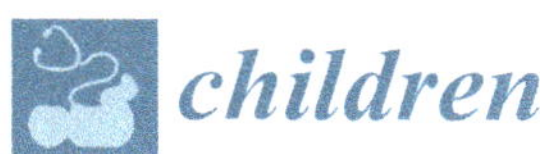
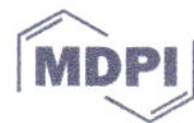

Case Report

From Inpatient to Clinic to Home to Hospice and Back: Using the "Pop Up" Pediatric Palliative Model of Care

Martha F. Mherekumombe

Department of Palliative Care, The Children's Hospital at Westmead, The Sydney Children's Hospitals Network, Westmead, NSW 2145, Australia; martha.mherekumombe@health.nsw.gov.au

Received: 6 March 2018; Accepted: 23 April 2018; Published: 26 April 2018

Abstract: Children and young people with life-limiting illnesses who need palliative care often have complex diverse medical conditions that may involve multiple hospital presentations, medical admissions, care, or transfer to other medical care facilities. In order to provide patients with holistic care in any location, palliative care clinicians need to carefully consider the ways to maintain continuity of care which enhances the child's quality of life. An emerging model of care known as "Pop Up" describes the approaches to supporting children and young people in any facility. A Pop Up is a specific intervention over and above the care that is provided to a child, young person and their family aimed at improving the confidence of local care providers to deliver ongoing care. This paper looks at some of the factors related to care transfer for pediatric palliative patients from one care facility to another, home and the impact of this on the family and medical care.

Keywords: pediatric; palliative; Pop Up; discharge; inpatient; life-limiting; hospice; hospital; goals of care

---

1. Introduction

Children and young people with life-limiting illnesses requiring palliative care spend a variable amount of time in the hospital. They have variable care requirements related to their underlying disease or condition, and at some point of their medical treatment, their care needs may need to continue in another care facility. Whatever the reason for such a transfer, it is important to provide the best support for the child and the caregivers in the preferred or appropriate location of care where possible. Parents and caregivers often prefer being closer to home to maintain some family normality [1–3].

These diverse and often complex care needs should be considered when arranging patient transfer along with an assessment of the local health care's capacity to care for the child and their family. This paper discusses the general factors related to the patient transfer of care, maintaining holistic care, and the impact of the transfer on the child and family.

2. Case Report

Patrick (not his actual name) was an eight-month-old baby with a neurodegenerative disorder. He was the youngest child born to non-consanguineous Caucasian parents Sam and Melissa (not actual names). Melissa had an uncomplicated pregnancy and Patrick was born at term with a normal birth weight at a primary care facility. Around 30 h of age, he was noted to have respiratory distress and hypothermia and was transferred to the neonatal care unit. Shortly after admission, he developed seizures and investigations revealed a deranged pathology suggestive of a severe metabolic disorder, after which he was transferred to a tertiary hospital for specialist treatment.

Over the next few weeks, his stay was complicated by periods of instability. After a month his condition stabilized and he was discharged home. His time at home was very difficult and exhausting for the family. At the age of 5 months, Patrick's parents were given the choice to consider a liver transplant and after much deliberation, his parents made the difficult decision not to proceed and instead opted to maximize his quality of life and a referral to palliative care was made.

Patrick's seizures continued to be a concern and he deteriorated further necessitating a readmission to the tertiary hospital. Patrick's goals of care were determined, and these were to limit life-prolonging interventions that had little benefit and for Patrick to be cared for closer to home.

Patrick was in the hospital for a further month. When his condition stabilized plans were made for a transfer to his local healthcare facility as a step down prior to the final discharge home. A multidisciplinary meeting was convened to review his medical and nursing needs. Changes were made to Patrick's care plan to ensure local services were able to support him closer to home. This included revising his medications and limiting technology such as equipment devices that were unable to be used by the local health providers.

2.1. The Local Healthcare Facility

The transfer was uneventful; unfortunately, after a short period of stability Patrick's clinical condition continued to deteriorate and he was admitted to the local hospital with the care plan that had been put in place. He remained at the facility for three weeks before being discharged home with ongoing support re-initiated by the local community health facility and the community palliative care service.

2.2. Hospital

Patrick enjoyed six weeks at home and was re-presented to the hospital with further deterioration. Though the goals of care were clear, Patrick's parents needed further reassurance that there was no reversible disorder contributing to the deterioration. This admission was different because Patrick was dying. He was transferred to the hospice as per his parents' wishes, where he died peacefully in his mother's arms.

Reflecting back the family reported that being at the local healthcare facility enabled them to spend time away from the tertiary hospital. The goals of care for Patrick as he deteriorated were for him to be cared for at home or as close to home as possible. His advance care plan was to ensure comfort by managing symptoms, offering psychosocial and spiritual support. They were comforted by the knowledge that they did the best they could for their little boy. Being at the hospice for Patrick's death was like a home to them, this meant they could be parents to both the children and feel "normal" for a very short time.

3. Transfer from an Acute Care Facility

The hallmark of pediatric palliative care is providing holistic care. This can be achieved wherever a patient is located, and the care can vary globally. Patients are transferred between care facilities for various reasons [4]. It is important to consider the patient, their family's wishes, and their preferences during a transfer from an acute care facility to ensure that their quality of life is maintained. Goals of care form the framework in which we define what is important for the family by aligning the needs and interests of the child with the goals and wishes of the family [5]. During the planning processes and transfer, these goals of care frame the basis of support.

Goals of care may change during a child's illness and should be re-assessed throughout episodes of a life-threatening condition, clinical deterioration, or transfer of clinical care [6,7]. At the time of clinical diagnosis or referral to palliative care, it is important to establish the family's overarching wishes, to document these, and to inform the relevant agencies.

The process of planning a transfer from an acute facility to a non-acute facility can be multifaceted, involving considerations around care complexity, technology, and equipment support [4]. Other reported pertinent elements include the functional and social aspects of the child and family, including the psychosocial and spiritual domains [8]. Involving key healthcare providers in coordinating the discharge ensures that the patient has the required supports in place, the necessary paperwork such as a current discharge summary, and an acute management plan for deterioration along with advanced care directives [4,9]. Other considerations are finances, insurance, and local governance processes such as policies and procedures related to the transfer or discharge to ensure that there is a continuity of care and to minimize unnecessary transfers [4].

A patient transfer occurs when a child is discharged from one facility to another. There are generally three described processes that are required to initiate discharge of a hospitalized child. These include specifying discharge goals, assessment of discharge healthcare needs, and identifying factors that could affect the child's well-being [10]. Discharge readiness is a concept that signifies the ability to understand and execute the intended discharge care plan in a safe and timely manner [10].

Occasionally, to facilitate care transfer or discharge, the accepting provider may need to be supported to care for the child or young person and this support is given through adopting a model of care known as "Pop Up" [11].

3.1. Pop Up Model of Care

Pop Up model of care is a concept established to enhance access to specialist pediatric palliative care services when needed. The intervention facilitates timely and well-coordinated palliative care by providing in-time training and education to local health providers.

Through a Pop Up intervention, the specialist pediatric palliative care (SPPC) service builds the capacity of the local care providers in response to a clinical or family need. The SPPC team is a team of health professionals with formal training in the provision of pediatric palliative care. A Pop Up intervention occurs when an SPPC service responds to the needs of an individual child, young person, or family and builds capacity with the local community to establish a 'bespoke' pediatric network incorporating the following triad:

1. Family/caregiver.
2. Local health services (such as the family practitioner, community nursing, local hospital services, or local care facility).
3. Specialist pediatric palliative care (PPC) Service [11].

Central to a Pop Up is providing just-in-time training that aims to build capability and capacity for local health providers to continue delivering high-quality palliative care to the child and their family. Pop Up can also be used to support bereavement provision [11]. With this model of care, patients and families can advocate for the appropriate care within their goals of care which was important for Patrick's parents. Patrick's Pop Up was a combination of a face to face meeting and telemedicine which has been reported as an effective tool to provide consultations [12].

In the case study above, discharge planning from hospital commenced in the weeks prior to the transfer when Patrick was stable. The planning meetings helped to identify the level of support that was needed to maintain his quality of life in a non-tertiary setting. A Pop Up was convened closer to discharge and a management plan was outlined considering the local health provider capabilities and resources. Although Patrick's parents wanted him to be cared for in a non-tertiary facility and to be at home, the representations to the hospital were related to their anxiety. This anxiety related to the increased burden of care. Parents and caregivers often experience this when caring for a child with a life-limiting illness as the child or young person's condition deteriorates. Patrick's parents received the appropriate support and counseling to assist them with their grief and the impending loss of their son. Local supports were notified to intensify their support during this time. Children with life-limiting illnesses are reported as having frequent readmissions and are at risk for recurrent hospitalizations, and this needs to be anticipated [13]. In preparing for discharge, care planning to ensure that the necessary supports and an assessment of the family's home is important. The role of palliative care includes helping to decrease hospitalizations and the unmet care needs when the child leaves the hospital [13].

A comprehensive management plan was formulated during Patrick's discharge planning, with the contact details of the main medical providers, pertinent medical and social history, medications, and an emergency medical care plan. The plan was formalized during the Pop Up and it included plans of end-of-life care. The hospice was the family's preferred location for the end-of-life care and all these plans were finalized with all the relevant parties including the receiving team with a predetermined transfer date. In some countries, there are inpatient facilities known as hospices which are care facilities providing support, respite, and end-of-life care for children with life-limiting illnesses and their families. These facilities can also be used when children need to transition to a less acute facility from a hospital, prior to being discharged home. The term hospice in some other countries refers to a model of care providing end-of-life care and is not inferred as such in this section, but rather the former [14–16].

There are reported benefits to Pop Up, which include:

1. Enabling discussions around the current and anticipated medical concerns in a considerate and sensitive manner.
2. Assessing all aspects pertaining to care such as equipment, provisions, or needs.
3. Individualizing the comprehensive care plan to the child's needs with the local services.
4. Providing networking opportunities between the hospital and community health providers.
5. Providing family-centered care and supporting family goals including choices for location of the care.
6. Providing SPPC support to manage the escalating symptoms in a timely manner [11].

3.2. *Challenges Relating to Care Transfer*

There are few challenges in a patient transfer that can occur and these may include the discontinuity of care and changes to treatment including medication regimes and therapies [4]. Discontinuity of care is often an outcome of poor communication related to the swift transfer with inadequate preparation, limited finance, conflict, limited medical staffing, or inexperienced staff at the recipient facility [5]. The transfer processes can be complex, contingent on the healthcare systems and the family working together. Other factors include the inclusion of the appropriate health professionals, completing discharge requirements, having post discharge contingency plans, and providing education to patients and parents [4,9].

Components of hospital discharge have also been examined and aspects such as the medical care team's involvement, addressing clinical needs, contingency plans, and parent readiness rank highly in relative importance among clinicians [4,9]. Pediatric palliative care services and primary care teams need to work collaboratively to provide continuity of care and maintain the patient's and families' well-being [2,17]. Continuity of care is only possible when realistic expectations are in place. It is also helpful to have one contact person such as the pediatrician or a senior nurse. Parents and caregivers need to be prepared for the transfer process as much as possible by providing them with information about the new facility and the relevant updated actions or emergency management plans. The handover processes should occur between physicians and also among the nursing staff. Information pertaining to advanced care planning should also be communicated and this informs the focus of care and helps establish and communicate the care expectations.

Other factors to consider which affect the transfer includes aspects relating to the child's health and safety such as having the appropriate medical insurance, finances, and parent-health care professional communication [10,12].

3.3. *Impact on the Child/Family*

Pediatric palliative care patients including those with rare medical disorders are becoming more challenging because their prognosis has changed with the advancement of medical technology and these children are living longer than they were previously. This uncertainty impacts decision making processes, families, and discharge or transfer plans [5]. The complex care needs of some of these patients are further complicated by having multiple specialties involved in patient care which can result in fragmentation and adversely affect the children [5]. Having a written plan for difficult symptoms is important because poor symptom management impacts negatively on the child and the family [18]. From the limited literature available, we know that the lives of patients can be disrupted during periods of transfer [12,19,20]. Further research on improving the patient experience is needed.

4. Conclusions

Care planning is vital to the success of the transfer of care. Pop Up was used to facilitate the transfer in the case reported. The benefits of this have been reported, however, the processes for patient transfer from the hospital to their home or to another facility require further research. The impact of transfers on children and their families also needs to be explored to determine ways to improve patient care and patient experience. Some pertinent elements required for patient transfer has been discussed and each patient is an individual and needs to be considered on a case by case basis.

Conflicts of Interest: The authors declare no conflicts of interest.

References

1. Hynson, J.L.; Gillis, J.; Collins, J.J.; Irving, H.; Trethewie, S.J. The dying child: How is care different? *Med. J. Aust.* **2003**, *179*, S20. [PubMed]
2. Armitage, N.; Trethewie, S. Paediatric palliative care-the role of the GP. *Aust. Fam. Physician* **2014**, *43*, 176–180. [PubMed]
3. Goldman, A.; Beardsmore, S.; Hunt, J. Palliative care for children with cancer—Home, hospital, or hospice? *Arch. Dis. Child.* **1990**, *65*, 641–643. [CrossRef] [PubMed]
4. Nageswaran, S.; Radulovic, A.; Anania, A. Transitions to and from the acute inpatient care setting for children with life-threatening illness. *Pediatr. Clin.* **2014**, *61*, 761–783. [CrossRef] [PubMed]
5. Himelstein, B.P.; Hilden, J.M.; Boldt, A.M.; Weissman, D. Pediatric palliative care. *N. Engl. J. Med.* **2004**, *350*, 1752–1762. [CrossRef] [PubMed]
6. Liben, S.; Papadatou, D.; Wolfe, J. Paediatric palliative care: Challenges and emerging ideas. *Lancet* **2008**, *371*, 852–864. [CrossRef]
7. Klick, J.C.; Hauer, J. Pediatric palliative care. *Curr. Probl. Pediatr. Adolesc. Health Care* **2010**, *40*, 120–151. [CrossRef] [PubMed]
8. Kane, R.L. Finding the right level of posthospital care: "We didn't realize there was any other option for him". *JAMA* **2011**, *305*, 284–293. [CrossRef] [PubMed]
9. Blaine, K.; Rogers, J.; O'neill, M.R.; McBride, S.; Faerber, J.; Feudtner, C.; Berry, J.G. Clinician Perceptions of the importance of the components of hospital discharge care for children. *J. Healthc. Qual.* **2017**, *40*, 79–88. [CrossRef] [PubMed]
10. Berry, J.G.; Blaine, K.; Rogers, J.; McBride, S.; Schor, E.; Birmingham, J.; Schuster, M.A.; Feudtner, C. A framework of pediatric hospital discharge care informed by legislation, research, and practice. *JAMA Pediatr.* **2014**, *168*, 955–962. [CrossRef] [PubMed]
11. Mherekumombe, M.F.; Frost, J.; Hanson, S.; Shepherd, E.; Collins, J. Pop Up: A new model of paediatric palliative care. *J. Paediatr. Child Health* **2016**, *52*, 979–982. [CrossRef] [PubMed]
12. Bradford, N.K.; Armfield, N.R.; Young, J.; Herbert, A.; Mott, C.; Smith, A.C. Principles of a paediatric palliative care consultation can be achieved with home telemedicine. *J. Telemed. Telecare* **2014**, *20*, 360–364. [CrossRef] [PubMed]
13. Bogetz, J.F.; Ullrich, C.K.; Berry, J.G. Pediatric hospital care for children with life-threatening illness and the role of palliative care. *Pediatr. Clin.* **2014**, *61*, 719–733. [CrossRef] [PubMed]
14. American Academy of Pediatrics. Committee on Bioethics and Committee on Hospital Care. Palliative care for children. *Pediatrics* **2000**, *106*, 351–357.
15. Corr, C.A.; Corr, D.M. Pediatric hospice care. *Pediatrics* **1985**, *76*, 774–780. [PubMed]
16. Armstrong-Dailey, A.; Zarbock, S.F. *Hospice Care for Children*; Oxford University Press: New York, NY, USA, 2001.

17. Moore, D.; Sheetz, J. Pediatric palliative care consultation. *Pediatr. Clin.* **2014**, *61*, 735–747. [CrossRef] [PubMed]
18. Behrman, R.E.; Field, M.J. (Eds.) *When Children Die: Improving Palliative and End-of-Life Care for Children and Their Families*; National Academies Press: Washington, DC, USA, 2003.
19. Dose, A.M.; Rhudy, L.M.; Holland, D.E.; Olson, M.E. The experience of transition from hospital to home hospice: Unexpected disruption. *J. Hosp. Palliat. Nur.* **2011**, *13*, 394–402. [CrossRef]
20. Bluebond-Langner, M.; Beecham, E.; Candy, B.; Langner, R.; Jones, L. Preferred place of death for children and young people with life-limiting and life-threatening conditions: A systematic review of the literature and recommendations for future inquiry and policy. *Palliat. Med.* **2013**, *27*, 705–713. [CrossRef] [PubMed]

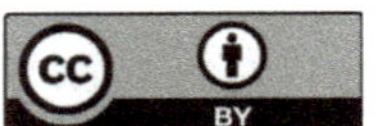

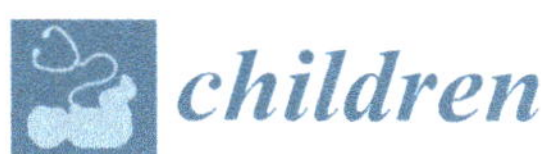 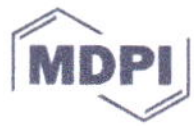

Case Report

Interdisciplinary Pediatric Palliative Care Team Involvement in Compassionate Extubation at Home: From Shared Decision-Making to Bereavement

Andrea Postier [1,*], Kris Catrine [1,2] and Stacy Remke [3]

1 Pain Medicine, Palliative Care and Integrative Medicine Program, Children's Hospitals and Clinics of Minnesota, 2525 Chicago Avenue South, Minneapolis, MN 55404, USA; Kris.catrine@childrensmn.org
2 Department of Pediatrics, University of Minnesota, Minneapolis, MN 55404, USA
3 School of Social Work, University of Minnesota, Saint Paul, MN 55404, USA; remke005@umn.edu
* Correspondence: andrea.postier@childrensmn.org

Received: 19 January 2018; Accepted: 5 March 2018; Published: 7 March 2018

Abstract: Little is known about the role of pediatric palliative care (PPC) programs in providing support for home compassionate extubation (HCE) when families choose to spend their child's end of life at home. Two cases are presented that highlight the ways in which the involvement of PPC teams can help to make the option available, help ensure continuity of family-centered care between hospital and home, and promote the availability of psychosocial support for the child and their entire family, health care team members, and community. Though several challenges to realizing the option of HCE exist, early consultation with a PPC team in the hospital, the development of strategic community partnerships, early referral to home based care resources, and timely discussion of family preferences may help to make this option a realistic one for more families. The cases presented here demonstrate how families' wishes with respect to how and where their child dies can be offered, even in the face of challenges. By joining together when sustaining life support may not be in the child's best interest, PPC teams can pull together hospital and community resources to empower families to make decisions about when and where their child dies.

Keywords: compassionate extubation; psychosocial care; children; palliative care; advance care planning; terminal care; end of life

1. Introduction

Death inevitably involves uncertainty [1]. When the parents of a child are faced with the devastating prospect of a terminal diagnosis, research has shown that being able to plan and make decisions is most important to them, and engaging in shared end-of-life (EOL) decision-making may lead to better parental adjustment [2,3] after the child's death [4–6]. For many parents, this includes planning the location of their child's death when possible.

Between 40–60% of pediatric deaths in the intensive care unit (ICU) setting occur following decisions to end life-sustaining therapies [7]. When a child is being maintained by using artificial ventilation in a neonatal or pediatric intensive care unit (NICU/PICU) setting, the option to die at home is usually possible, but all too often, it may not be offered as professionals may not realize this EOL option exists [8–10]. A recent systematic review reported that, while some parents may feel more comfortable keeping their child in the hospital or hospice facility, many parents in the USA, Western Europe, and Australia prefer the home setting [11]. Choosing death at home requires careful review of options, anticipatory guidance around expectations, and the availability of capable home-based care resources, all of which pediatric palliative care (PPC) teams are uniquely trained to provide or locate in the community. However, many times opportunities to consult with PPC teams while a child is in the ICU are missed. This may be because health care providers are unaware that home compassionate extubation (HCE) is even an option, due to potential resource-related barriers (e.g., time needed to consult with PPC team, lack of staffing needed to support the HCE, lack of information regarding home based care options and resources), or based upon misconceptions about the role of PPC. However, if consultations with PPC teams are incorporated earlier on in the hospital setting, especially as the goals of care are beginning to shift from a life-sustaining focus to a focus on minimizing suffering, they may be able to help facilitate open communication around EOL planning with families and hospital staff.

Everyone involved in caring for the child should play an active role in the discussion; communicating care and engendering trust that the plans being made reflect continued care and not abandonment. Decision-making requires good communication between the child, family, and all of the professionals that are involved in the child's life [12]. Whenever possible, parents should be offered all viable options, as well as adequate time to ask questions and make an informed decision. Comprehensive and early communication that involves the opportunity to plan location of death is in line with palliative care principles, and is associated with more favorable outcomes, such as death in the desired location and lower regret about actual location of death [5].

Pediatric palliative care teams can offer careful navigation of discussions about the option of HCE with families during a time of distress as they face their child's EOL. This is a time when families can be assisted to reclaim more family autonomy and intimacy if well planned. Each of the three domains of PPC apply, from early communication and support for complex decision making, to coordination of emotionally and logistically complex care in the home; through bereavement support and helping families and friends make connections to community support services after the child has died.

In a recent qualitative study of bereaved parents' experiences with transport home from the ICU for compassionate extubation, parents described it as positive, deeply meaningful, and providing a sense of control and comfort to themselves and other family members [13]. Most articles that address the topic of pediatric home extubation have been written from an intensive care perspective [14–16], with emphasis on the development of care pathways [12,15,17,18] and transport logistics [9]. Few peer reviewed articles have been published from a PPC perspective about HCE and the role of PPC teams [19,20]. The critical care-based EOL care guidelines [12,15,17,18] offer suggestions for family-centered planning, pre- and post-transfer, and care during and after the extubation with critical care and community resources. However, these lists of steps do not capture the nuanced aspects of expert communication and coordination that PPC teams are trained to offer around planning, shared decision-making with families and health care teams, the EOL event itself, and the bereavement period. The composure of PPC team members who are familiar with this procedure contributes to an atmosphere of psychological safety and competence instead of crisis.

There is an opportunity for further collaboration between intensive care teams, hospital-based PPC teams, community-based palliative care, and hospice teams when cure is no longer possible and being home is a priority for the family. An interdisciplinary approach is needed in order to ensure success [2,15,21]. Inter-professional teams are an important component of bridging gaps in care, and PPC teams are uniquely positioned to provide care across environments (e.g., hospital, home) and circumstances (e.g., early decision-making, bereavement support). Pediatric palliative care teams are specifically designed to offer services that ensure family preparation and coping before and after the child's death. They are comprised of health care staff that are positioned well and are distinctively experienced in offering the three core PPC task-oriented domains as described by Feudtner et al.: problem-solving/decision-making (e.g., working to define goals and hopes of care with families), interventions (e.g., emotional support, anticipatory guidance, and complex symptom management), and logistics (e.g., coordinating care across environments, from hospital to home) [1].

This paper contains two case reports of children of different ages, medical conditions, and family situations that underwent HCE with direct involvement from a PPC program at a large United States (US) tertiary pediatric hospital system (see Table 1 for a summary). Fictional names have been used and some details changed to protect privacy. These case reports highlight the unique spectrum of services PPC teams play throughout the process, from decision-making through bereavement. Feudtner's [1] core PPC domains serve as a framework for discussion.

Table 1. Patient and Family Characteristics.

Case	Age	Sex	Medical History	Days on Ventilator	PPC Team Involvement	Non-PPC Staff Involvement	Time to Death Following Extubation	Challenges
1	15 years	F	Severe anoxic brain injury secondary to attempted suicide by hanging	2 days	Physician, nurse, MSW, CLS	RT, chaplain	30 min	Portable vent; ambulance transport cost; physician on-call demands; CLS challenges; large and varied family/ community "audience"
2	18 months	M	Spinal muscular atrophy, Type I	8 months	Physician, MSW, nurse, chaplain	Community hospice nurses (adult-focused), pediatric home care nurses, local chaplain	7 days	Inexperienced local hospice; training needs; psychosocial support needs; collaboration with two remote agencies; unanticipated (longer) time to death

2. Case Presentations

2.1. Case 1: Teen with Anoxic Brain Injury and Parental Preference for Death Surrounded by Friends and Family at Home

Jane, a 15 year-old female, was transported to the hospital with severe anoxic brain injury following an attempted suicide by hanging. The PPC team was contacted following intubation in the ICU. The PPC team, physician, and social worker met with Jane's neurologist and ICU attending physician, and arranged a family conference to help the family understand the child's condition and to discuss goals of care. Options that were discussed over the ensuing days were: organ donation after cardiac death, compassionate extubation in the PICU, tracheostomy/vent placement with observation for any neurologic improvement, or home extubation to allow for natural death. The parents chose home extubation, requesting that the child have time at home with family and friends (which included children of all ages) at the bedside. This required access to an ambulance, a portable vent, suctioning equipment, cleaning supplies, multiple IV medications, and adequate medical and psychosocial support staffing on short notice.

The PPC team arranged for involvement of a home hospice nurse, social worker (MSW), child life specialist (CLS), and respiratory therapist (RT) who was not part of the PPC team. Before the day of the transport, the PPC physician prepared medications for home transport while the CLS and MSW spoke with the family, Jane's siblings, and friends to help prepare them and answer questions the day before the transport. That evening, the CLS and MSW met to debrief about any concerns they had after meeting with Jane's family and friends, including an assessment of potential psychosocial challenges that may arise based on their past experiences with HCE. A do not resuscitate (DNR) order was placed in the chart, and all hospice enrollment paperwork was completed. Strategies for managing logistical, financial, and emotional challenges had to be determined quickly (e.g., payment for the ambulance transport and portable vent equipment, which are not covered by insurance).

> *Key Point, Core PPC Domain 1 (Problem-solving and decision-making): This case is an example of how a hospital-based PPC team facilitated medical decision making with the family and medical team & addressed the unique logistical complexities of this case while facing time constraints. The palliative care team gathered an interdisciplinary group of staff members to help facilitate problem-solving and logistical planning by simultaneously drawing upon each team member's skills.*

The care team met together on the morning that Jane was to go home and included PPC, intensive care, and other hospital staff. They jointly reviewed the planned process in a step-wise fashion, which allowed team members to ask questions and identify additional needs or potential issues. Following this, the team met with family briefly to verify the plan and to inquire about any new psychosocial developments. Jane was transported by ambulance along with the hospice nurse in charge of comfort medications and the RT who was responsible for operating the portable ventilator and suctioning equipment. The PPC physician drove the MSW and a physician fellow with her to Jane's home separately. A PPC fellow was in attendance in order to learn, and also to field any pages the PPC physician received to ensure dedicated attention to Jane and her family, while simultaneously attending to any urgent calls from other patients and families.

Jane's family friend drove her parents to their home from the hospital. The CLS was already at the home with family and friends when Jane arrived to provide support and prepare them for what they were likely to witness. Jane was placed in her own bed with continuous monitoring for comfort and suctioning needs. Once in the home, the MSW and CLS addressed Jane's loved ones to explain the process in broad strokes and to offer opportunities to say goodbye for those who did not wish to be present during the actual extubation. Those who remained were educated by the physician and nurse about the physical changes that they were likely to witness, including agonal breathing and temperature change. All present gathered at the bedside, a religious blessing was conducted, medications were provided, and the RT removed the ventilator and the endotracheal tube. The PPC team treated excessive secretions with atropine drops and observed for signs of dyspnea or distress (which were not observed) before the PC physician pronounced death 30 min later.

Key Point, Core PPC Domain 2 (Interventions): The PPC team, experienced and licensed to practice in the home, was able to bring both medical care and psychosocial support to the child's family and friends on short notice. The team's knowledge and experience in providing end-of-life care was critical to being able to orchestrate medical transport, manage symptoms and provide bedside support, thus honoring Jane's family's wishes.

Dark blue blankets, opaque garbage bags, and pressure dressings were used for draping and discretely removing the IV lines and foley catheter so that the secretions and bloodstaining were barely visible. This helped allow family and friends to continue to grieve and console each other without disturbance, and to prevent the potential trauma to the observers. Jane's mother fled the room at the time that death was pronounced and was consoled by a designated relative and additional friend. The MSW checked in with her after a few minutes and she chose to return to the bedside where Jane's sister was crying and being supported by her father. Jane's father addressed everyone that was present, and many of Jane's high school friends remained in the home consoling each other. During this intensely emotional situation, those who were attending to the immediate family members were able to provide the needed support under the guidance of the psychosocial team members. The total time spent at Jane's house following the transport was three hours. The MSW, hospice nurse, and CLS stayed until the funeral home came to remove Jane's body, providing supportive counseling, anticipatory guidance, and acute support. The nurse disposed of the comfort medications, while the PPC physician and RT took the remaining equipment back to the hospital in her car. Bereavement support was arranged including follow-up home visits by the PPC team. The CLS visited Jane's school to assist with communication and offering grief support resources to classmates.

2.2. Case 2: Collaboration with Rural Hospice Agency and Unanticipated Length of Time before Death after Extubation at Home

AJ was an 18 month-old with spinal muscular atrophy (SMA) Type I and respiratory failure. He received a tracheostomy with ventilation at 11 months of age, spending much of his life in the hospital. His family lived in a semi-rural area one hour from the hospital. His family and team recognized he was losing ground to his disease, and his quality of life was deteriorating. They decided that HCE was the best option, but they wanted to be able to spend some time with him at home first. He was referred to the PPC team after this decision had been made at a PICU care conference. After meeting with the family and acknowledging the complex nature of this situation (including the remote geographic location), the PPC team facilitated referrals to a local hospice agency and a home care agency to coordinate support and provide extended hours nursing. The family's local chaplain was also contacted for additional, familiar support. Both of the agencies had limited to no pediatric experience, including how to provide ventilator support in the home. However, they wanted to help the child and his family, who they considered to be part of their community.

Prior to the extubation, the hospital-based PPC team played an integral role in the process by providing the local care team with "just in time" training around pediatric hospice and EOL care. The hospice staff had questions about how to care for a child, and the home-based hospice nurses had questions about how to provide EOL care versus the ICU level of home care they were accustomed to. A PPC team MSW and nurse met with local hospice staff on several occasions to provide consultation and support. As the local team became familiar with the situation and the family, their anxieties lessened, and they felt more capable. The PPC team was available by phone as needed, offering 24/7 consultation. The child's death was planned collaboratively with the family, home nursing agency, and local hospice team. The PPC team sent a hospice nurse, PPC physician, MSW, and chaplain to the family's home to assist the local teams during the extubation.

> *Key Point, Core PPC Domain 3 (Logistics): This case presented logistical challenges up front due to the family's rural home location, lack of a local community home hospice team with pediatric experience, PPC staffing limitations due to the distance, and medical transport and supply challenges. The palliative care team served as a bridge between the family and their community resources to equip both with the necessary education and coordination to enable AJ to be at home in a community without pediatric-specific end of life resources. This case presented an opportunity for PPC teaching and network-building in the community.*

It was expected that AJ would die within minutes to hours of extubation, but he lived for two days. This presented some unanticipated challenges to the family and the trusted PPC team staff when it came to leaving the home when the situation had stabilized. When the MSW planned to leave, the parents expressed their distress, so she stayed a couple of hours longer until the family seemed more confident in the support they had; their needs for intimacy with their family taking precedence. After this additional transition time, the family was much more at ease and was comfortable with additional staff taking leave. Home nursing staff remained in the home overnight to provide extra support. Nurses confronted some unanticipated, emergent needs for more morphine, respiratory toilet supplies, and sudden need for flexibility of staff to cover shifts on short notice. Fast planning under pressure was required, away from the family's view to avoid additional distress for them. While well managed, the unanticipated events resulted in high stress for the team; stress that perhaps would have been lower if some contingency plans had been made. This was an important lesson for the team going forward. AJ ultimately died peacefully with his family surrounding him. The PPC team MSW and nurse held a debriefing meeting with the local care teams. Bereavement support for the family was coordinated through the local hospice agency.

3. Discussion

The two case presentations depict how an interdisciplinary PPC team can play an integral role in making HCE possible and successful, even under very different clinical, patient, and family circumstances. Each case report illustrates the importance of flexibility and teamwork across different types of environments and medical and psychosocial providers. Experiences are subjective and nuanced, diverse, and unique to all of the individuals involved, regardless of the person's role in the process (e.g., staff, family, friends, community members). Success in the context of HCE requires "systems" thinking: noting how the different aspects of the care system interact, where gaps and needs for linkages are surfacing, and how the needs of the child and family can best be addressed. Pediatric palliative care teams routinely focus on complex communication, decision making, creative problem solving, and advocacy for the preferences of patients and their families. We recommend that intensive care staff consider consulting with PPC teams as soon as continued ventilator support is deemed non-beneficial by the family and care team. See Table 2 for a list of key considerations when considering HCE.

The essential steps in the process of HCE presented in the two cases above can be described using Feudtner's [1] three core palliative care domains framework, with particular attention to the unique psychosocial support PPC teams can offer in the home to patients, their families, and health care teams during a time that the child's family will remember for the rest of their lives.

3.1. Problem-Solving/Decision-Making

Pediatric palliative care teams are trained to offer family-centered care and comprehensive communication throughout the decision-making and bereavement process, and across environments of care [1,22]. Communication involves depiction and detection; reframing and re-anchoring. In the context of EOL decisions, each of these dimensions occurs in a situation fraught with complexity, emotion, and high stakes for the family, as well as the whole team of health care providers, including hospital and home based practitioners. For example, when AJ lived longer than anticipated, it was important to reassess and adjust the plan on short notice in order to ensure continued safe care in the face of quickly diminishing resources. Focus was on accessing needed people, plans, and supplies in the background so that the situation did not evolve into an unnecessary crisis for the family. Communication with the family focused on reassurance and offering updates in a reassuring manner. Communication was specific and direct, reducing the potential for additional family distress.

The majority of families prefer a shared decision-making model when faced with critical choices. This has been well established in previous research [23–26]. However, there remain some families who prefer to make decisions autonomously or to defer entirely to their medical teams. The gravity of these choices warrant the expertise of a PPC team trained to assess the specific family's preferences and facilitate decision-making discussions. The importance of this involvement is elevated in situations for which there are additional complicating factors, such as family discord, reluctance to engage in decision-making, lack of alignment between family needs and the child's care team's (e.g., ICU staff) comfort in discussing the issue, and the lack of sufficient time to engage in lengthy discussions. One of the most important aspects of care at this EOL phase is ensuring that the best possible decision-making process occurs in order to minimize the potential for regrets later, and to facilitate future clarification in the event that new questions or concerns arise.

Shared decision-making involves more than simply shared understanding of facts and exchanges of information. It is a process that encompasses emotional, relational, and psychological intensity with "high stakes" implications for the family and their integrity and identity as a family unit going forward [1,27]. All of this unfolds within a context of uncertainty, grief, and the compelling nature of unique situations. Early referral to PPC may enable this process to unfold over time, as complex decisions often require "sitting with facts" and processing emotions as clarity emerges. Trust between the team and the family evolves through this process, underscoring the value of time and patience. Collaboration between the attending team, the PPC team and the family can promote opportunity for successful transfer of the family's trust to future health care teams. Therapeutic relationships with skilled clinicians who possess a thorough understanding of the situation can offer the family a "container" in one sense, and can contribute to establishing psychological safety for the family at a critical time when there is high potential for trauma and unintended, negative outcomes. Skilled clinicians, such as MSWs, must be prepared to anticipate potential events in order to manage them successfully. In the context of HCE, this means minimizing family anxiety and their sense of uncertainty, and also reinforcing a sense of control in the midst of a situation that feels inherently out of control.

Table 2. Key Considerations Prior to Home Compassionate Extubation in Infants and Children with the Possibility of Continued Life at Home.

Topic	Things to Consider
1. Medication supply	✓ Who will provide initial supply and refill or prescribe new medications if needed (e.g., child lives longer than expected)? Where will they be filled? How will they be discarded after death?
2. Transportation	✓ Can the child be taken in private vehicle, or will she require medical transportation? Who will drive? Are there arrangements to transport needed staff and family?
3. Medical equipment	✓ Will suction or a portable vent be needed? How will equipment be returned to the hospital after death?
4. Staffing in the child's home	✓ Anticipate all possible psychosocial support staffing needs in the home before/after HCE (e.g., CLS, MSW, chaplain). ✓ How long will staff (e.g., nurses) be able to remain in the home? If needed, is there a plan for staff relief? ✓ If collaborating with a community home hospice team, is training necessary (e.g., rural hospice team with no pediatric experience)? ✓ Consider communication and collaboration with child's community-based pediatrician as appropriate.
5. Financial and legal	✓ HCE may pose additional legal consequences for some stakeholders and as such should be carefully considered. However, this should not be the overriding concern when the focus is on what is best for the child. Consider an ethics consultation if necessary. ✓ Ensure insurance or private payment is available to cover the cost of ambulance transport, ventilator, home nursing, IV medications, etc.). Check for gaps in insurance coverage if transitioning to a community-based resource. ✓ If child has life insurance plan, death must be designated as due to a disease process rather than as assistance in dying for benefits to be paid. ✓ Provide documentation of anticipated death in a format that meets local legal and community standards for advanced directives. These could include MD letter, POLST or other, and vary by jurisdiction. ✓ If child is in state custody or foster care, check to see if specific regulations apply.
6. Autopsy and organ donation	✓ Ensure family is well informed about organ and tissue donation options and limitations (e.g., cost of autopsy and additional transportation).
7. Anticipatory guidance for the family	✓ Prepare family for what they will witness at end of life (i.e., sights, sounds, smells) [28]. Provide information at the appropriate developmental level and paced to match the emotional needs of family members and friends. ✓ Discuss feeding and hydration with child's family in advance. Consider discontinuation of artificial nutrition and hydration in patients who are unconscious, or if likely to cause burdensome symptoms [29]. Consider feeding/hydration to comfort for those who are wakeful and express hunger or thirst. ✓ Consider referring parents/staff to additional support/educational resources. Examples are videos Choosing Thomas—Inside a family's decision to let their son live, if only for a brief time [30] and Making Every Moment Count [31]; the online support site Courageous Parents Network [32], and Cameron's Arc: Creating a Full Life: Teaching and Resource Guide [33].

Table 2. *Cont.*

Topic		Things to Consider
8. Prognostication	✓	Discuss the likely length of life after extubation, but also prepare for living longer than expected. Confirm family's wishes to continue care at home versus re-hospitalization or transport to a hospice facility.
9. Plan priorities for the child's time at home	✓	Discuss how family wishes to spend their time at home with the child, incorporating any rituals or important practices, and adjusting the medical plan as needed to accommodate. Plan and allow for legacy activities, such as photos, videos, hand/foot prints, locks of hair, as well as storytelling, reminiscing, etc.
10. Comprehensive assessment of the family's emotional, psychological and practical capacity for managing the compassionate extubation event in their home.	✓	In most instances emergency mental health resources will be unfamiliar with this unique sequence of events. Therefore, the PPC team should be prepared to manage unanticipated emotional or psychological crises that may occur. However, in practice we have not observed this to be a significant concern with careful planning.

Real, active involvement of parents in conversations is critical, as is family-centered care with adequate staffing to accommodate it. For example, Jane's family chose to include family and friends at the bedside at the time of the extubation, creating the notable challenges of helping to support many people who are at varying developmental stages, enlisting family and community members to support each other during their own grief experience, and preparing for the potential of emotional crisis in several attendees simultaneously. The CLS and MSW were scheduled on short notice to provide counseling support for anticipatory grief, decision-making, and to offer support to the family and friends of the dying child. This support extended beyond the extubation to being present and ready to manage unanticipated events, while remaining off to the side so that friends and family could console each other. The presence of the PPC team members can also offer families and staff a sense of reassurance that events are unfolding as they should. In Jane's case, the CLS and MSW provided coaching to the health care team and family about how best to respond to the patient, and empowered the family to proactively ask the health care team to address any needs they felt the child had in her last moments of life. This provided an opportunity for family to honor their child's life by gathering with loved ones in a setting and manner consistent with how her previous milestones in life had been honored, and to create a shared memory of the event as a lasting legacy. The family viewed Jane's death as dignified, in part due to the active prevention of suffering and presence of the PPC team in Jane's home setting alongside her community of friends and family.

3.2. Interventions

Depth and breadth of psychosocial services that are available to the patient, parents, siblings, and the family's community (e.g., school) ensures holistic, appropriate care across settings and time. The range of services that families and their children often need include anticipatory guidance, supportive counseling, episodic problem-solving assistance, parent guidance, age appropriate information and education for siblings, friends and neighbors, reinforcement of coping, and crisis management assistance. As indicated in both case examples, unanticipated events and inexperienced people that are involved in providing EOL care required the presence and active guidance by experienced PPC staff. The MSW is charged with attending to the family's well-being, providing supportive counseling, carrying out assessments of emotional and psychological issues that require intervention, and maintaining a systems-oriented perspective on practical management of the entire situation. The CLS provides anticipatory guidance, age appropriate information and preparation, age appropriate activities for children present, legacy-oriented engagement, and emotional support to the patient and any children present. A chaplain can provide religious and/or spiritual support and reassurance at a critical time, often collaborating with community clergy who might not have experienced a child's death before.

In addition to psychosocial support for HCE, medical expertise can be offered by PPC physicians and nurse practitioners (NP), as well as hospice nursing staff. Pediatric palliative care team physicians and NPs have experience anticipating symptoms, titrating comfort medications in proportion to a child's changing symptom burden while reassuring families that symptoms are being continuously managed, can prepare families for likely physical changes around the time of death, and can help dispel myths about hastening death or other ethical concerns that families may have. Experienced PPC nurses can ensure adequate supply and equipment management, anticipate potential issues with the technical aspects of the HCE plan, provide expert symptom assessment, help to minimize the visual impact of needed cares on the family, and help to establish a close and trusting working relationship with the family.

Diverse family situations require sensitive and individualized responses from the care team. The only way to achieve this is through engaging a process that emphasizes nuanced communication and confident clinical practice around EOL care. Attending to a child at the EOL requires a hybrid approach that blends clinical expertise with counseling, education, and support that travels in many directions at once. For example, in AJ's case, care went into providing support not only to the patient and family, but also to staff from the two agencies that were brought in to provide care in the home. Consideration with respect for the feelings of the PICU team that discharged AJ was important, acknowledging the fact that they were very emotionally invested in him and his family through the care they had provided. Their trust in the PPC team in turn inspired the family's ability to trust the PPC team. The PPC team was also aware of the significance that AJ's broader home community network would play in supporting the family in their bereavement over time. Everyone invested in caring for AJ and his family along the way would benefit from psychosocial support.

There is sometimes concern that family may panic and decide not to allow the discontinuation of the ventilator once at home. This requires a MSW readiness assessment in advance, but unexpected reactions may still emerge in the moment. In Jane's case, the large crowd of friends and family of different ages was a factor for the medical team to plan for. What if something went wrong? What if distressing symptoms emerged? Planning for such unanticipated events includes social work, child life, chaplaincy and others (e.g., music therapy, volunteers) as best practice. This support extends beyond the child's immediate family (friends, school, other health care workers) to include their circle of support in the community.

3.3. Logistical Efforts

Collaborating across sites and units for care involves complex steps and processes. We are not just bridging a gap and promoting continuity of EOL care, but when PPC already has an established relationship with the NICU, PICU, and other services, practitioners can link across relationships to promote trust and logistical safety. Finesse involved in managing from behind the scenes without family/friends being aware—bodily fluids; crisis of unexpected time to die and morphine shortage—while managing the complex array of emotions and relationship challenges is required. Active problem solving and intervention around emerging issues is required on the fly. Experience and expertise is essential. Sometimes children live longer than expected after the ventilator is removed [28], like AJ. Parallel planning should take place, as a recent study found one third of children transferred from an intensive care setting to a hospice for EOL survived beyond two weeks [20] and a recent literature review of six case series and reports on pediatric critical care transports from ICU to home for terminal extubation showed that, while the vast majority of infants and children died within hours to days after extubation, one study reported two children living as long as 17 and 40 days [9].

If hospital staff have good experiences collaborating with PPC to help grant parents their wishes, staff will be more likely to engage PPC in conversations in the intensive care setting and feel good about being able to offer a choice—a "good death"—to parents in the future. For example, several months after AJ's death, another pediatric case was referred to the same local hospice. They readily accepted the referral because they felt so gratified by their PPC program. Support meetings were also offered, but the local team felt able to handle the situation with phone consultations as needed, thanks to the relationship formed between the PPC staff and local hospice team during AJ's case.

3.4. *Staffing/Resources*

Compassionate extubation at home requires both physical and staffing resources. Palliative care teams may be helpful in planning for the support systems required. Jane's care brought several resource-related issues to light that can serve to inform the practice of HCE going forward. First, her size and condition required ambulance transportation rather than by private family vehicle. This is not normally an insurance-covered expense and can be cost-prohibitive for many families. Our MSW team has successfully sought assistance through "wish" and charity organizations for some families, but this assistance may not be equally available to all of the children because of their diagnosis. Additionally, some families request the opportunity to spend a prolonged period of time at home before extubation, which requires having a transport ventilator in the home.

Staffing coverage can be an issue, especially on weekends. In Jane's case, the physician was on call the day of the extubation, so she brought a PPC physician fellow along to answer any pages during the event. The logistical issues of being exclusively present for a child and family around the time of extubation can be challenging to navigate when a single physician is on call for many other patients. In Jane's case, the PPC fellow was able to assist with other patient needs, but many PPC services do not have trainees or the availability of backup staffing. Finally, the availability of MSW and CLS support was critical in Jane's case, as a large number of teenage friends were present. Availability of these services can be limited depending upon the day of the week, or dependent on the availability of such resources in a community without a dedicated home-based PPC and hospice program.

It is important to note that the children described in this study were cared for in the US context, where a lack of insurance and financial stability exist, resulting in inability to support a hospice home model [34] that is more commonly available in the UK, Europe, and Canada. Lack of a hospice home option may reduce the likelihood in the US of viewing HCE as a viable option.

4. Summary

With careful planning and collaborative goal-setting, parents can usually be given a choice about where their child dies. There are often great collaborative opportunities for intensive care and PPC teams to make this happen. Ideally, intensivists would contact the PPC team before continued/active treatment has been deemed unhelpful and distressing to the child and family. Early engagement of PPC encourages positive and trusting relationship-building, opportunities for presenting options to the family, and giving families the space they need to actively participate in EOL decision-making for their child. Pediatric palliative care teams are uniquely positioned to bridge resources between the hospital and community as a result of specialized training in dealing with psychosocial issues during the EOL and bereavement periods. We hope that this article encourages timely collaboration between intensive care teams and PPC teams, with the shared goal of involving parents at every stage of the decision-making process in order to successfully grant the wishes of parents in a tragic situation.

Author Contributions: A.P., K.C., and S.R. conceptualized and contributed to all aspects of the manuscript. A.P. drafted the manuscript and compiled the case reports, which were contributed by K.C. and S.R. All authors contributed substantially to the writing. The final version was reviewed and approved by A.P., K.C. and S.R.

Conflicts of Interest: The authors declare no conflicts of interest. No funding was received for this effort.

References

1. Feudtner, C. Collaborative communication in pediatric palliative care: A foundation for problem-solving and decision-making. *Pediatr. Clin. N. Am.* **2007**, *54*, 583–607. [CrossRef] [PubMed]
2. Longden, J.V.; Mayer, A.P. Family involvement in end-of-life care in a paediatric intensive care unit. *Nurs. Crit. Care* **2007**, *12*, 181–187. [CrossRef] [PubMed]
3. Lauer, M.E.; Mulhern, R.K.; Schell, M.J.; Camitta, B.M. Long-term follow-up of parental adjustment following a child's death at home or hospital. *Cancer* **1989**, *63*, 988–994. [CrossRef]
4. Siden, H.; Miller, M.; Straatman, L.; Omesi, L.; Tucker, T.; Collins, J.J. A report on location of death in paediatric palliative care between home, hospice and hospital. *Palliat. Med.* **2008**, *22*, 831–834. [CrossRef] [PubMed]
5. Dussel, V.; Kreicbergs, U.; Hilden, J.M.; Watterson, J.; Moore, C.; Turner, B.G.; Weeks, J.C.; Wolfe, J. Looking beyond where children die: Determinants and effects of planning a child's location of death. *J. Pain Symptom Manage.* **2009**, *37*, 33–43. [CrossRef] [PubMed]
6. Friedrichsdorf, S.J.; Postier, A.; Dreyfus, J.; Osenga, K.; Sencer, S.; Wolfe, J. Improved quality of life at end of life related to home-based palliative care in children with cancer. *J. Palliat. Med.* **2015**, *18*, 143–150. [CrossRef] [PubMed]
7. Burns, J.P.; Rushton, C.H. End-of-life care in the pediatric intensive care unit: Research review and recommendations. *Crit. Care Clin.* **2004**, *20*, 467–485. [CrossRef] [PubMed]
8. Craig, F.; Mancini, A. Can we truly offer a choice of place of death in neonatal palliative care? *Semin. Fetal Neonatal Med.* **2013**, *18*, 93–98. [CrossRef] [PubMed]
9. Noje, C.; Bernier, M.L.; Costabile, P.M.; Klein, B.L.; Kudchadkar, S.R. Pediatric Critical Care Transport as a Conduit to Terminal Extubation at Home: A Case Series. *Pediatr. Crit. Care Med.* **2017**, *18*, e4–e8. [CrossRef] [PubMed]
10. Meert, K.L.; Sarnaik, A.P. Choosing between death at home or in the hospital: Respecting the principle of autonomy. *Pediatr. Crit. Care Med.* **2010**, *11*, 438–439. [CrossRef] [PubMed]
11. Bluebond-Langner, M.; Beecham, E.; Candy, B.; Langner, R.; Jones, L. Preferred place of death for children and young people with life-limiting and life-threatening conditions: A systematic review of the literature and recommendations for future inquiry and policy. *Palliat. Med.* **2013**, *27*, 705–713. [CrossRef] [PubMed]
12. Sine, D.; Sumner, L.; Gracy, D.; von Gunten, C.F. Pediatric extubation: "Pulling the tube". *J. Palliat. Med.* **2001**, *4*, 519–524. [CrossRef] [PubMed]
13. Nelson, H.; Mott, S.; Kleinman, M.E.; Goldstein, R.D. Parents' Experiences of Pediatric Palliative Transports: A Qualitative Case Series. *J. Pain Symptom Manag.* **2015**, *50*, 375–380. [CrossRef] [PubMed]
14. Simpson, E.C.; Penrose, C.V. Compassionate extubation in children at hospice and home. *Int. J. Palliat. Nurs.* **2011**, *17*, 164–169. [CrossRef] [PubMed]
15. Laddie, J.; Craig, F.; Brierley, J.; Kelly, P.; Bluebond-Langner, M. Withdrawal of ventilatory support outside the intensive care unit: Guidance for practice. *Arch. Dis. Child.* **2014**, *99*, 812–816. [CrossRef] [PubMed]
16. Needle, J.S. Home extubation by a pediatric critical care team: Providing a compassionate death outside the pediatric intensive care unit. *Pediatr. Crit. Care Med.* **2010**, *11*, 401–403. [CrossRef] [PubMed]
17. Oppenheim, S.; Bos, C.; Heim, P.; Menkin, E.; Porter, D. Developing guidelines for life-support therapy withdrawal in the home. *J. Palliat. Med.* **2010**, *13*, 491–492. [CrossRef] [PubMed]
18. Cottrell, S.; Edwards, F.; Harrop, E.; Lapwood, S.; McNamara-Goodger, K.; Thompson, A. *A Care Pathway to Support Extubation within a Children's Palliative Care Framework*; Doveton Press: Bristol, UK, 2011.
19. Zwerdling, T.; Hamann, K.C.; Kon, A.A. Home pediatric compassionate extubation: Bridging intensive and palliative care. *Am. J. Hosp. Palliat. Care* **2006**, *23*, 224–228. [CrossRef] [PubMed]
20. Gupta, N.; Harrop, E.; Lapwood, S.; Shefler, A. Journey from pediatric intensive care to palliative care. *J. Palliat. Med.* **2013**, *16*, 397–401. [CrossRef] [PubMed]
21. Hawdon, J.M.; Williams, S.; Weindling, A.M. Withdrawal of neonatal intensive care in the home. *Arch. Dis. Child.* **1994**, *71*, F142–F144. [CrossRef] [PubMed]
22. Jones, B.L.; Contro, N.; Koch, K.D. The duty of the physician to care for the family in pediatric palliative care: Context, communication, and caring. *Pediatrics* **2014**, *133* (Suppl. 1), S8–S15. [CrossRef] [PubMed]
23. Meert, K.L.; Thurston, C.S.; Sarnaik, A.P. End-of-life decision-making and satisfaction with care: Parental perspectives. *Pediatr. Crit. Care Med.* **2000**, *1*, 179–185. [CrossRef] [PubMed]

24. Kon, A.A. Life and death choices in neonatal care: Applying shared decision-making focused on parental values. *Am. J. Bioeth.* **2011**, *11*, 35–36. [CrossRef] [PubMed]
25. Sharman, M.; Meert, K.L.; Sarnaik, A.P. What influences parents' decisions to limit or withdraw life support? *Pediatr. Crit. Care Med.* **2005**, *6*, 513–518. [CrossRef] [PubMed]
26. Lipstein, E.A.; Brinkman, W.B.; Britto, M.T. What Is Known about Parents' Treatment Decisions? A Narrative Review of Pediatric Decision Making. *Med. Decis. Mak.* **2012**, *32*, 246–258. [CrossRef] [PubMed]
27. Browning, D.M.; Solomon, M.Z. Relational learning in pediatric palliative care: Transformative education and the culture of medicine. *Child Adolesc. Psychiatr. Clin. N. Am.* **2006**, *15*, 795–815. [CrossRef] [PubMed]
28. Catlin, A.; Carter, B. Creation of a neonatal end-of-life palliative care protocol. *J. Perinatol.* **2002**, *22*, 184–195. [CrossRef] [PubMed]
29. Hellmann, J.; Williams, C.; Ives-Baine, L.; Shah, P.S. Withdrawal of artificial nutrition and hydration in the neonatal intensive care unit: Parental perspectives. *Arch. Dis. Child. Fetal Neonatal Ed.* **2013**, *98*, F21–F25. [CrossRef] [PubMed]
30. The Dallas Morning News. Choosing Thomas—Inside a Family's Decision to Let Their Son Live, If Only for a Brief Time. Available online: https://www.youtube.com/watch?v=ToNWquoXqJI (accessed on 28 February 2018).
31. National Film Board of Canada. Making Every Moment Count. Available online: http://www.nfb.ca/film/making_every_moment_count/ (accessed on 28 February 2018).
32. Courageous Parents Network. Available online: https://courageousparentsnetwork.org/ (accessed on 28 February 2018).
33. American Academy of Pediatrics. Cameron's Arc: Creating a Full Life; Teaching and Resource Guide. Available online: https://shop.aap.org/camerons-arc-creating-a-full-life/ (accessed on 28 February 2018).
34. National Hospice and Palliative Care Organization (NHPCO). *NHPCO's Facts and Figures: Pediatric Palliative and Hospice Care in America*; NHPCO: Alexandria, VA, USA, 2015.

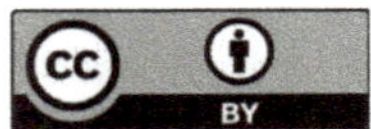

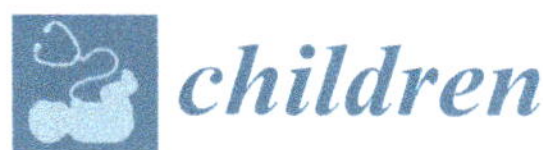

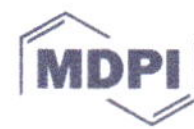

Perspective

Integrative Approaches in Pediatric Palliative Care

Kate Shafto [1], Suzanne Gouda [2], Kris Catrine [3] and Melanie L. Brown [3,4,*]

1 Department of Internal Medicine and Pediatrics, University of Minnesota, Minneapolis, MN 55455, USA; kshafto@umn.edu
2 Department of Pediatrics, University of Chicago, Chicago, IL 60637, USA; suzanne.gouda@uchospitals.edu
3 Department of Pain Medicine, Palliative Care and Integrative Medicine, Children's Hospitals and Clinics of Minnesota, Minneapolis, MN 55404, USA; kris.catrine@childrensmn.org
4 Department of Pediatrics, University of Minnesota, Minneapolis, MN 55455, USA
* Correspondence: melanie.brown@childrensmn.org; Tel.: +1-612-813-7888

Received: 16 April 2018; Accepted: 5 June 2018; Published: 13 June 2018

Abstract: Pediatric palliative care is a field which focuses on caring for and treating the symptoms and distress typically associated with life-limiting illness. Integrative medicine is supported by evidence and aims to heal the whole person, including all aspects of one's lifestyle. Therapies offered by integrative medicine often empower patients and families, allowing for a sense of control. This review addresses the merging of integrative medicine philosophy and modalities with the care given to children with life-limiting illness. We review an introduction to integrative medicine, trends in its incorporation in the healthcare setting, application to patients receiving palliative care and the management of specific symptoms. A case study is offered to illustrate these principles.

Keywords: pediatrics; palliative care; integrative medicine; symptom management; mind-body medicine; pain management; acupuncture; yoga

---

1. Introduction: Integrative Medicine

Integrative medicine is not a new concept, though in recent decades the terminology has become solidified and more widely used. Dating back to early human history, there are writings describing how humans are composed of body, mind and spirit, with healers addressing these realms together when illness occurred [1]. The current definitions of integrative medicine center around a goal of healing, the patient's lifestyle, environment, history, and a patient-provider partnership which considers lifestyle, allopathic diagnosis and treatment, environmental factors, emotional/spiritual factors and the role of other healing systems when caring for the patient. The University of Arizona's Center for Integrative Medicine, USA, a leader in training and research around integrative medicine for several decades, defines integrative medicine as: "healing-oriented medicine that takes account of the whole person, including all aspects of lifestyle. It emphasizes the therapeutic relationship between practitioner and patient, is informed by evidence, and makes use of all appropriate therapies" [2].

Integrative medicine is distinct from complementary and alternative medicine (CAM), which refers to a practice or treatment that differs from the conventional approach, or therapies which complement the conventional model. Integrative medicine, as its name suggests, intentionally integrates too-often separate approaches to healing, with an additional emphasis on empowering the patient with skills for self-care, promotion of wellbeing and self-management (at times with even prevention or reversal) of disease.

2. Integrative Medicine Trends in US Healthcare

Modern western medicine is based on a reductionist approach to the body and disease, dating back to the 1600s, out of which grew the current system of medical specialization and compartmentalization of organs and body systems [1]. This model has come at a great cost financially, and, in many cases, led to disempowerment of patients, a fragmented healthcare system, and patient dependence on healthcare providers for treatment and management of disease. Chronic diseases, due to their multi-organ pathophysiology and high correlation with lifestyle, are often not adequately addressed using a reductionist model. Additionally, the locus of control in an allopathic model is frequently external to the patient, being the healthcare provider and their prescribed treatment. A study examining the health locus of control for youths with chronic illnesses found that those with an external locus of control had poorer health outcomes than those with an internal locus of control [3]. Integrative medicine seeks to leverage a combination between the internal and external, which in turn shifts the locus of control to include a patient's own capacity to influence their health or disease in addition to the provider.

There is clear and rising interest among patients as well as providers in a whole-person care model. Fellowships in integrative medicine are providing evidence-informed knowledge and tools for practice [4]; additionally, a myriad of conferences in integrative medicine [5], restorative medicine [6], lifestyle medicine [7], mind-body medicine [8] and nutrition [9] are offering continuing medical education for clinicians. The internet and social media are making consumers/patients more aware of options in addition to medications and surgeries often offered by traditional allopathic healthcare delivery systems.

In the most recent survey from the National Institutes of Health's Center for Complementary and Integrative Health on the use of complementary health approaches, several trends are evident. This 2012 survey collected information on the use of various approaches, including dietary supplements, chiropractic or osteopathic manipulation, yoga, massage, and mind-body practices such as meditation. Findings from this survey demonstrated about 33% of adults and 11.4% of children use some form of complementary health approaches. The survey also found that roughly 59 million Americans spend money out-of-pocket on complementary health approaches, with total spending around $30.2 billion/year. Pain was one of the main reasons people sought out complementary therapies, and the most utilized mind-body approaches were chiropractic manipulation, meditation, massage and yoga. Interestingly, yoga has become more popular among children as well in the last 15 years: 3.1% of US children practiced yoga in 2012, compared to 2.3% in 2007. These are samples of a large set of data illustrating the increase in interest, use and willingness to pay for integrative (here described as complementary) therapies [10].

The growing demand and value recognition of such therapies and practices has led many healthcare systems to incorporate integrative medicine's modalities, practitioners and practices in service to their patients and families. A 2010 survey by Samueli Institute and the American Hospital Association's Health Forum was conducted to study these trends, entitled Complementary and Alternative Medicine Survey of Hospitals [11]. Out of almost 6000 hospitals receiving the 42-question survey, 714 responded (12%), and 299 of respondents (42%) offered one or more complementary and alternative medicine (CAM) therapies. There was significant regional variation, with the largest number of respondents offering CAM being in the East-North-Central region (23%; Illinois, Indiana, Michigan, Ohio, Wisconsin) and the fewest being in the East-South-Central region (3%; Alabama, Kentucky, Mississippi, Tennessee). Almost half of the respondent institutions offering CAM were academic medical centers, or teaching hospitals, and 72% were urban. The most commonly offered inpatient CAM therapies included pet therapy, massage therapy, music therapy, guided imagery and relaxation training, and Reiki or therapeutic touch. Outpatient modalities were most commonly massage therapy, acupuncture, guided imagery, meditation, relaxation and biofeedback [12].

Despite growing interest and demand for an integrative approach in healthcare, acceptance and adoption of these modalities into mainstream healthcare systems remains limited, and thus inaccessible for many patients and families. Contributing factors to this lack of access include inadequate numbers of trained practitioners, lack of insurance reimbursement for interventions, billing or productivity structures which do not support the time needed to do significant patient counseling and education, and other financial or ideological limitations of healthcare institutions and individual providers alike [13,14]. Medical education at all levels remains limited in training physicians with integrative medicine tools and non-pharmacologic alternatives to symptom management or disease treatment and modification. There are, however, increasing efforts among some medical schools to incorporate lifestyle medicine curricula [15], an integrative medicine elective, or some exposure to CAM therapies in their curriculum. According to the Association of American Medical Colleges, 43% of medical schools offered CAM in their curricula as of 2010. In addition, a survey of University of California medical students' perceptions about CAM, 75% felt that "western medicine would benefit from incorporation of CAM therapies and ideas" [11]. At the Graduate Medical Education level, programs such as Integrative Medicine in Residency (IMR), an online curriculum, is now utilized in 63 residency programs nationally and internationally at the time of this writing [16]. In 2014 the American Board of Physician Specialties began offering a national integrative medicine board exam, for physicians who have completed a two-year fellowship in integrative medicine [17], adding further recognition and standardization to the field of integrative medicine.

One common example of a complex, multi-faceted problem seen from primary care to palliative care is anxiety. Children and teens are experiencing anxiety at unprecedented rates, and according to Kessler et al. in a National Comorbidity Survey of adolescents, the lifetime prevalence of any anxiety disorder was 31.9% between the ages of 13–18 years [18], with females (38%) being affected more than males (26%). Although this does not separate adolescents with comorbidities, it is well known that this population group often suffers from anxiety at higher rates [19,20].

Our understanding of anxiety grows by the week, with more studies detailing the connection between gut health and its role in anxiety [21], depression [22,23], pain, obesity, diabetes [24], autoimmune diseases, and the list goes on. Additionally, a history of adverse childhood experiences (ACEs) such as trauma, neglect or abuse predisposes one to an increased risk of developing anxiety over their lifetime [25]. Social media use, sleep deprivation and social isolation have all been associated with higher rates of anxiety [26]. Genetics, diet [27,28], family history and environmental exposures also have significant bearing on an individual's mental health. Given the numerous etiological influences, and individual variation in life experiences and exposures, it is not reasonable to expect that a single drug or treatment would be adequate for such a multidimensional condition.

Numerous studies, as well as centuries of tradition in eastern medicine, support the efficacy of mind-body techniques for management of anxiety, chronic pain, illness and stress. Examples include various types of meditation [29]; hypnosis and self-hypnosis [30,31], mindfulness-based stress reduction (MBSR) [32], and yoga [33]. Despite the evidence-supported efficacy and cost-savings, providers are not routinely trained in these treatments over a pharmaceutical approach. Integrative medicine interventions carry a low risk of harm, making them an attractive adjunct or when appropriate, alternative to pharmaceuticals, which are not without adverse risks. An additional benefit of integrative therapies is the active participation required by the patient in the regulation of their own nervous system or mind when addressing problems, allowing the patient to feel in control. These approaches are highly empowering and without significant cost once the technique has been adequately taught to the patient and family to employ when desired. Integrative medicine combines all appropriate therapies using an evidence-based approach with consideration to safety, tolerability and efficacy. Studies have shown that combining mind-body techniques with pharmacologic interventions can reduce distress. For example, pediatric leukemia patients undergoing painful procedures in a study comparing a combined intervention (CI) with pharmacologic only (PO) demonstrated significant reduction in distress associated with the procedure in the CI arm, compared to the PO group [34].

This example illustrates how complex and multifaceted many of today's medical issues are, and ways in which integrative medicine can address that complexity using a myriad of tools and modalities suited for a variety of settings and preferences. Many such techniques can be employed in the outpatient, inpatient or community health care setting, with little to no cost and are adaptable to a variety of cultures, backgrounds, ages, disease-states and patient preferences.

3. Overview of Integrative Medicine Modalities

Specific domains in which integrative medicine providers offer care, interventions and education for patients may include nutrition, mind-body techniques, regulation of stress physiology, sleep support, therapeutic movement, Reiki and other energy work techniques, use of herbs and supplements, aromatherapy, mental health support and identification/modification of environmental factors contributing to disease. Knowledge of other healing systems, such as traditional Chinese medicine, Ayurveda, naturopathy, chiropractic and homeopathy, allows integrative medicine providers from an allopathic background to appreciate the role these fields play in healing, and appropriately counsel patients seeking care.

We will briefly describe the following common, well-tolerated integrative modalities that can be used to support patients receiving hospice and palliative care: acupuncture/acupressure, relaxation and stress-physiology regulation techniques, essential oils, botanicals and supplements and reiki.

3.1. *Acupuncture/Acupressure*

Acupuncture is an ancient tradition in which the practitioner inserts thin needles in the body to manipulate specific points. It is a key component of traditional Chinese medicine and is also used for the management of distressing symptoms such as pain and nausea. Acupuncture points can also be stimulated noninvasively with the use of low level lasers or microcurrent. Acupuncture is safe when performed by qualified professionals and is well tolerated by children [35,36]. Acupressure uses firm, steady pressure at these same points. Depending on the location of the acupressure points, and the indications, patients are sometimes able to perform this on themselves. Shonishin is another needleless acupuncture technique that uses pressure and massage along the meridians to influence the flow of energy.

3.2. *Relaxation Techniques and Stress-Physiology Regulation*

The ancient practices of meditation, yoga, tai chi and qi gong are making their way into western culture, as well as being utilized to address a range of present day health problems. In each of these practices, the activation of the parasympathetic nervous system, through intentional, regulated breathing, has been shown to improve autonomic nervous system balance, heart-rate variability, chronic pain, fibromyalgia, anxiety, depression, post-traumatic stress disorder and promote overall well-being [37–40]. The activation of the parasympathetic nervous system in what has been termed the "relaxation response", as described above, counters the often overactive sympathetic nervous system stress response, triggered by numerous stimuli that occurs during illness, pain and threatening circumstances. The ability for a person to regulate the stress response and elicit the relaxation response is empowering, and often shifts the locus of control for patients during illness, anxiety, pain and especially at the end-of-life. The use of these physiologic principles in healthcare settings includes modalities such as breathing practices, guided imagery, self-hypnosis and progressive muscle relaxation (PMR). All of these practices have the potential to elicit the relaxation response and can be tailored to individual preferences, functional limitations, age, experiences and culture [41].

3.3. *Essential Oils*

Aromatherapy is the use of aerosolized or inhaled essential oils, the potent extracts of roots, plants or herbs, for therapeutic purposes. Topical application of essential oils diluted in a carrier oil, with or without massage, is also a route by which therapeutic effects may be obtained. The parts of the plant used, the species, and the quality of the extract all bear on the quality of the essential oil and thus its therapeutic effect [42].

Essential oils have been used for centuries in many cultures and have also made their way into western healing practices and alongside allopathic medicine in many places. Examples of these uses will follow, related to specific symptoms commonly encountered in patients who are receiving palliative care services.

3.4. Botanicals and Supplements

For some patients, due to the burden of polypharmacy, additional supplements are not desired. In others, taking supplements may improve symptoms and allow them to feel a greater sense of self-management over their treatment. Supplements can be taken orally, sublingually or absorbed through the skin. It is critical that any health care provider ask patients about their use of supplements and botanicals, with consideration to any possible side effects as well as drug interactions. An extensive treatment of this topic is beyond the scope of this paper; several specific supplements are covered below in the section on symptom management.

3.5. Reiki

Reiki is an ancient healing art which involves the gentle laying on of hands with the intent to connect the universal life-force energy with the person's own innate power to heal. This treatment is individualized, can be empowering to the patient, and generally has no adverse effects or harm.

4. Integrative Medicine for Distressing Symptoms in Critical Illness and Palliative Care

Below we discuss the integrative approach to several common distressing symptoms to those receiving palliative care: nausea and vomiting, pain and neuropathic pain, stress, and dyspnea.

4.1. Nausea and Vomiting

Nausea and/or vomiting are common symptoms that develop in serious illness related to a wide range of disorders and/or the treatments used to address them. Traditional pharmacologic treatments, such as ondansetron and metoclopramide, do not come without side effects and limitations. Integrative therapies have been shown to provide significant relief as both primary and adjunct therapies in the management of nausea/vomiting with few side effects or adverse reactions. Herbal supplements, such as oral ginger, have long been regarded as a natural antiemetic, but its demonstrated effectiveness in scientific studies remains inconclusive. Currently, ginger has been used to address nausea/vomiting related to motion sickness, pregnancy, post-surgical and chemotherapy [43–45]. In a systematic review of randomized control trials studying the efficacy of ginger for post-operative nausea and vomiting, Ernst et al. concluded that ginger was superior to placebo and demonstrated equal effectiveness compared to metoclopramide [46]. There are few trials related to chemotherapy induced nausea and vomiting, a common problem plaguing many pediatric palliative care patients with cancer. Although the availability of literature yields mixed results, some studies have shown statistically significant benefit. One of the largest randomized control trials to date involved 576 patients undergoing chemotherapy cycles demonstrated a significant decrease in nausea when using ginger compared with placebo [47].

Acupuncture and acupressure have also been utilized to address nausea and vomiting. Specific to pediatrics, there is a rising popularity of acupuncture, with now over one-third of pediatric pain treatment programs offering services [48]. Studies have demonstrated many significant benefits for a myriad of systems, with the strongest evidence demonstrated in the post-operative period. For example, a 2015 systematic review of randomized trials utilizing wrist acupuncture for postoperative nausea and vomiting in both children and adults found a significant reduction in symptoms and need for rescue antiemetics compared to sham treatment [49]. Studies involving exclusively pediatric patients remain limited, although a meta-analysis of clinical studies investigating acupuncture for postoperative nausea/vomiting in children following tonsillectomy further supported these findings [50]. Of note, acupuncture has proven to be well tolerated and safe in the pediatric population. One systematic review involving over 140 randomized clinical trials and 12,000 pediatric patients found acupuncture to be safe for when performed by trained practitioners, with over 90% of adverse events being mild [51].

Aromatherapy, via direct application or inhalation, may also provide benefit in the management of nausea and vomiting. For example, the use of peppermint oil has been recognized as an effective treatment for controlling nausea [52]. Other products, such as ginger oil, have also been utilized in aromatherapy application, with the most updated Cochrane review concluding that participants who received aromatherapy may require less antiemetic medications, although the strength of this evidence was lacking [52]. It is important to state that direct application of peppermint oil, specifically products diluted with methanol, to the nares or chest of infants is not recommended due to the documented risk of apnea, laryngeal and bronchial spasms, and acute respiratory distress [53,54].

4.2. Pain

In chronic disease, throughout the continuum of care and at the end-of-life, many patients struggle with uncontrolled pain. The balance between comfort and over sedation can be difficult for caretakers and families. The most common pharmacologic approach to pain management currently relies heavily on opioid medications, which may have unintended side effects. The Support study, which included more than 4000 hospitalized patients at the end-of-life, demonstrated that over 50% of patients suffered from moderate to severe pain in the days before their death [55]. Integrative modalities can be an effective adjunct to traditional pharmacologic approaches to pain.

In recent years, various relaxation techniques in the management of pain have been studied. These include progressive muscle relaxation, guided imagery, and autogenic training, with the goal of inducing one's own natural relaxation response, described above. For example, a meta-analysis of randomized clinical trials utilizing guided imagery for pain control demonstrated a significant reduction in non-musculoskeletal pain in 11 out of 15 trials reviewed [56]. Studies involving pediatric patients remain limited, but the same principles can be extended to this population with adjustments for age and developmental capabilities.

Acupuncture has become increasingly recognized in western medicine for the management of both acute and chronic pain, making it a viable adjunct for patients suffering with pain at the end-of-life. One Cochrane review concluded that acupuncture demonstrated effectiveness as a treatment for pain associated with migraines, headaches, neck pain, arthritis, and low back pain, all of which often plague those in the end-of-life [57]. A majority of research specific to the field of hospice and palliative medicine focuses on cancer patients, with many positive results shown with the use of acupuncture not only in pain relief, but also decreased use of traditional analgesics [58–60]. For example, one case series of 29 cancer patients at the end-of-life with severe pain demonstrated significant relief and discontinuation of injection analgesics (i.e., morphine, hydromorphone, fentanyl) in 62% of patients, and decreased use in an additional 27% [61].

As one of its many benefits, aromatherapy has been used for pain relief, especially when combined with therapeutic massage, and is another modality to be considered in the management of pain, as well as anxiety and stress. A meta-analysis of literature examining the effectiveness of aromatherapy in treating multiple types of pain found a significant positive effect in reducing pain, typically reported on a visual analog scale [62]. Specific to the pediatric population, one study demonstrated a 40% reduction of acetaminophen usage in children recovering from tonsillectomy who were treated with lavender aromatherapy [63]. Although there are no known studies in the pediatric palliative population, given proven benefits in other population groups, further research of the use of aromatherapy should be pursued.

4.3. Neuropathic Pain

Neuropathic pain can be a significant cause of discomfort and distress to those receiving palliative care and at the end-of-life. Neuropathy can result from multiple etiologies, but the mechanism of pain remains the same, with nerve damage and resultant hyperexcitability of peripheral nerves. Traditional therapy modalities for neuropathic pain, such as neuroleptic drugs, antidepressants, and opioids, have variable success and frequent unwanted side effects. Topical capsaicin is a treatment modality that may be considered for neuropathic pain. Produced from chili peppers, capsaicin binds nociceptors in the skin, leading to initial stimulation and release of substance P. Research has shown that repeat applications of capsaicin can deplete substance P, ultimately resulting in nerve desensitization [64]. Several studies have demonstrated symptom relief in comparison to placebo with the use of topical capsaicin, including Mason et al.'s review of randomized, controlled trials examining the use of capsaicin for chronic neuropathic and musculoskeletal pain in adults [65]. In addition, a recent Cochrane review examined the use of high concentration capsaicin (8% capsaicin patch) for treatment of neuropathic pain, finding moderate to substantial pain relief in patients with several types of neuropathic pain. Additional improvements in sleep, fatigue, depression, and quality of life were also demonstrated. The most common adverse effect to be noted is initial burning at the application site, which decreases with continued use [66].

4.4. Stress Response Regulation, Depression, Anxiety and Insomnia

Any clinician caring for a patient who is receiving palliative care must be prepared to address the psychological symptoms common at the end-of-life in addition to the physical ones. Furthermore, the psychological and the physical are physiologically interconnected. Depression and anxiety may plague patients and non-pharmacologic treatments have long been utilized in the management of depression and anxiety.

Mind-body and relaxation techniques, previously detailed for pain relief, have been shown to provide significant relief of depression, anxiety, and stress. A Cochrane meta-analysis of 15 randomized controlled studies of relaxation techniques with patients diagnosed with depression showed improvement compared to no or minimal traditional treatment. It is important to note, the most significant positive outcome was demonstrated when combined with psychological therapies, such as cognitive behavioral therapy [67]. Furthermore, mindfulness meditation has been demonstrated to provide significant improvements in overall mood and well-being, including stress-reduction, anxiety reduction, alleviating depression, and improved sleep cycles [68]. Specific to pediatrics, one study of 13 adolescents suffering from cancer underwent eight weekly meditation sessions (8 of the 13 enrolled). After completion of the course, investigators analyzed differences in overall mood, depression, sleep, and quality-of-life compared to pre-trial participant responses via questionnaire. Those in the treatment group compared to the control group showed a significant improvement in all areas [69].

As noted, aromatherapy and/or massage have also demonstrated benefit in overall well-being, mood, and sleep patterns. A randomized control trial of aromatherapy massage in the hospice setting found statistically significant improvements in sleep scores and depression reduction [70].

Reiki has been shown to have benefits of relaxation, decreased pain perception, anxiety reduction, overall sense of well-being, and quality-of-life in the palliative patient population [71]. Similar to reiki, therapeutic touch has also demonstrated significant benefits [72].

4.5. Dyspnea

Patients often experience shortness of breath, or dyspnea, related to their underlying disease process and this can worsen during the last six months of life and at the end-of-life. Beyond the physical discomfort, dyspnea can also be anxiety-provoking for many patients and caregivers who have to watch their loved ones suffer. Although the most effective management is to modify the underlying etiology, often in the terminally ill this is not possible. Traditional therapies such as opioids, steroids, nebulizers, and supplemental oxygen can be effective, but not always sufficient [73]. Complementary methods and therapies can provide significant relief as an adjunct therapy. For example, Acupuncture and acupressure have proven beneficial in the chronic-obstructive pulmonary disease (COPD) and asthma patient populations. Jobst et al. conducted a single-blind randomized control trial of 24 COPD patients with disabling shortness of breath who underwent 13 sessions of acupuncture over a three-week period compared to sham acupuncture. Patients in the treatment group reported less subjective breathlessness [74]. Although studies remain limited, and more research is needed in the pediatric population, these benefits could be extended to the palliative care population in pediatrics as well.

Below we provide a case illustration to demonstrate how integrative medicine can be used in practice to improve quality of life.

5. Case Illustration

Janey was a 16-year-old who presented to her general practitioner with complaints of abdominal pain and was found to have angiosarcoma of the spleen with metastasis to the liver, spine and portal venous system. She was being raised by her grandparents due to parental substance abuse. Following the diagnosis, she underwent first line therapy with chemotherapy and radiation. Unfortunately, the social disconnection from her peers created by her medical therapies and the psychological distress of her diagnoses led to a mental health crisis that resulted in a suicide attempt by overdose. While Janey recovered medically in the hospital, the Integrative Medicine team was consulted in the hopes that they might offer a more holistic approach to the impacts of cancer on Janey's life.

The integrative medicine practitioner worked intensively with Janey around the use of guided imagery to relieve anxiety and fears related to her diagnosis and uncertain future. Specifically, they chose to focus on scenes in which Janey traveled to Bora Bora, which she had seen in a travel magazine and viewed as the most relaxing location she could imagine. This technique combined with diaphragmatic breathing and aromatherapy was particularly helpful during times of heightened anxiety when waiting for results of imaging studies to evaluate the effectiveness of her ongoing treatment.

Computed tomography (CT) scans early in the second year of her treatment showed progression of the hepatic portion of her cancer. Discussions about the possibility that she may not be cured became more frequent with her medical team. While she proceeded with a new chemotherapy regimen, she also began planning a Make-A-Wish trip to Bora Bora. Planning her trip motivated her to intensify her practice of integrative strategies and she began a daily meditation practice and engaged in biofeedback. With minimal medications, she had excellent symptom management and was able to enjoy the trip and add more depth to her subsequent imagery work.

By the third year of her cancer journey, her tumor was again growing more quickly, and Janey struggled with progressive abdominal pain. She was very reluctant to use opioid pain medications due to fears about addiction raised by her parents' substance abuse histories. She was motivated to maintain as normal a life as possible despite her medical condition and prioritized having a job babysitting for the neighbors' children each afternoon. Her palliative care physician and integrative medicine practitioner worked with her to design a plan involving long- and short-acting pain medications, as well as mind-body practices, to enable her to maintain function, acceptable pain control and still attend to her responsibilities and relationships.

This plan was quite effective for many months before the cancer progressed. At that time, she had processed many of her fears about addiction with psychology support and was able to accept increased medication for pain control when integrative techniques alone could not manage her symptoms. Janey was aware that she was approaching the end of her life and worked with a child life specialist to participate in legacy activities.

Janey spent many weeks planning for a wedding to her longtime boyfriend and utilized her arsenal of imagery, breathing, aromatherapy and techniques learned in biofeedback to minimize medications used during the ceremony and reception. As her liver failure progressed, nausea became a prominent symptom and she sought new strategies for treatment. She found a combination of lorazepam and acupressure wrist bands with peppermint aromatherapy and imagery to be most effective. Near the end of her life, she became minimally wakeful and less able to utilize strategies herself. However, her husband and grandparents were able to perform massage with her lavender essential oil and use home music therapy provided through hospice to keep her relaxed as she died.

Family participation in integrative strategies made loved ones feel empowered to help Janey through the last stage of her life and has provided crucial legacy memories to help them through their grief.

This case illustrates the numerous ways that integrative medicine modalities were employed alongside, and at times in place of, pharmaceutical and conventional treatments, equipping Janey and her family to manage her disease and symptoms. The shared locus of control (both internal and external) concept is also demonstrated in the combination of integrative therapies as well as medication management, which provided Janey with the ability to live out her life in meaningful ways.

6. Summary

Integrative medicine is the multimodal approach to improved quality of life and patient care that respects and builds upon the strengths of the patient in combination with appropriate medical management. In the setting of palliative and end-of-life care an integrative approach can serve to reduce symptom burden and empower patients and their families.

Author Contributions: M.L.B., S.G. and K.S. are primarily responsible for the conception and design of this article. S.G. and K.S. are co- first authors and share the first author position equally. M.L.B. is the senior author. M.L.B., K.S., S.G., and K.C. drafted the text. All authors provided evaluation and revision of the manuscript and have given final approval of the manuscript.

Funding: This research received no external funding.

Acknowledgments: Thank you to Janey (name has been changed for patient privacy) and her family for giving permission for her story to be shared as a part of her legacy project.

Conflicts of Interest: In the past 5 years, M.L.B. has been supported in part by the Coleman Foundation, the Oberweiler Foundation and the Patient-Centered Outcomes Research Institute. The founding sponsors had no role in the design of the study; in the collection, analyses, or interpretation of data; in the writing of the manuscript, and in the decision to publish the results.

References

1. Rakel, D. *Integrative Medicine*, 4th ed.; Elsevier: Philadelphia, PA, USA, 2017.
2. Arizona Center for Integrative Medicine. What is IM/IH? Available online: https://integrativemedicine.arizona.edu/about/definition.html (accessed on 3 March 2018).
3. Nazareth, M.; Richards, J.; Javalkar, K.; Haberman, C.; Zhong, Y.; Rak, E.; Jain, N.; Ferris, M.; van Tilburg, M.A. Relating health locus of control to health care use, adherence, and transition readiness among youths with chronic conditions, North Carolina, 2015. *Prev. Chronic Dis.* **2016**, *13*. [CrossRef] [PubMed]
4. Arizona Center for Integrative Medicine. Fellowship in Integrative Medicine. Available online: https://integrativemedicine.arizona.edu/education/fellowship/index.html (accessed on 3 March 2018).
5. Upcoming Integrative Medicine & Health Events. Available online: https://www.imconsortium.org/events/upcoming-conferences/conferences.cfm (accessed on 3 March 2018).
6. AARM. 2018 Annual Conference. Available online: https://restorativemedicine.org/conferences/2018-annual-conference/ (accessed on 3 March 2018).
7. American Collage of Lifestyle Medicine. Bringing Together Medical Professionals Committed to Lifestyle Medicine As a First Treatment Option. Available online: https://www.lifestylemedicine.org/Lifestyle-Medicine-Conference (accessed on 3 March 2018).
8. The Center for Mind-Body Medicine. Teaching Thousands to Heal Millions. Available online: https://cmbm.org/ (accessed on 3 March 2018).
9. Nutrition & Health. Available online: https://nutritionandhealthconf.org/ (accessed on 3 March 2018).
10. National Center for Complementary and Integrative Health. Use of Complementary Health Approaches in the U.S. Available online: https://nccih.nih.gov/research/statistics/NHIS/2012/key-findings (accessed on 25 March 2018).
11. 2010 Survey of Complementary and Alternative Medicine in Hospitals: Summary of Results. Available online: http://www.samueliinstitute.org/File%20Library/Our%20Research/OHE/CAM_Survey_2010_oct6.pdf (accessed on 25 March 2018).

12. Barnes, P.M.; Bloom, B.; Nahin, R.L. Complementary and alternative medicine use among adults and children: United States, 2007. *CDC Natl. Health Stat. Report.* **2008**, *10*, 1–23.
13. Ross, C.L. Integral healthcare: The benefits and challenges of integrating complementary and alternative medicine with a conventional healthcare practice. *Integr. Med. Insights* **2009**, *4*, 13–20. [CrossRef] [PubMed]
14. Willison, K. Integrating complementary and alternative medicine into primary health care in Canada: Barriers and opportunities. *J. Cancer Integr. Med.* **2005**, *3*, 71–74. [CrossRef]
15. The Institute of Lifestyle Medicine. Medical School Education. Available online: http://www.instituteoflifestylemedicine.org/education-2/medical-school-education/ (accessed on 3 March 2018).
16. Integrative Medicine in Residency. Available online: https://integrativemedicine.arizona.edu/education/imr.html#Sites (accessed on 3 March 2018).
17. American Board of Integrative Medicine. Available online: http://www.abpsus.org/integrative-medicine (accessed on 25 March 2018).
18. Kessler, R.C.; Chiu, W.T.; Demler, O.; Merikangas, K.R.; Walters, E.E. Prevalence, severity, and comorbidity of 12-month DSM-IV disorders in the National Comorbidity Survey Replication. *Arch. Gen. Psychiatr.* **2005**, *62*, 617–627. [CrossRef] [PubMed]
19. Angold, A.; Costello, E.J.; Erkanli, A. Comorbidity. *J. Child Psychol. Psychiatr.* **1999**, *40*, 57–87. [CrossRef]
20. Thapar, P.A.; Collishaw, S.; Pine, D.S.; Thapar, A.K. Depression in adolescence. *Lancet* **2012**, *379*, 1056–1067. [CrossRef]
21. Cryan, J.P.; O'Mahoney, S. The microbiome-gut-brain axis: From bowel to behavior. *Neurogastroenterol. Motil.* **2011**, *23*, 187–192. [CrossRef] [PubMed]
22. Deans, E. Microbiome and mental health in the modern environment. *J. Physiol. Anthropol.* **2017**, *36*, 1–4. [CrossRef] [PubMed]
23. Rogers, G.B.; Keating, D.J.; Young, R.L.; Wong, M.L.; Licinio, J.; Wesselingh, S. From gut dysbiosis to altered brain function and mental illness: Mechanisms and pathways. *Mol. Psychiatr.* **2016**, *21*, 738–748. [CrossRef] [PubMed]
24. Cani, P.D.; Osto, M.; Geurts, L.; Everard, A. Involvement of gut microbiota in the development of low-grade inflammation and type 2 diabetes associated with obesity. *Gut Microbes* **2012**, *3*, 279–288. [CrossRef] [PubMed]
25. Karatekin, C. Adverse Childhood Experiences (ACEs), stress and mental health in college students. *Stress Health* **2018**, *34*, 36–45. [CrossRef] [PubMed]
26. O'Keeffe, G.S.; Clarke-Pearson, K.; Council on Communications and Media. The impact of social media on children, adolescents, and families. *Pediatrics* **2011**, *127*, 800–804.
27. Rahe, C.; Unrath, M.; Berger, K. Dietary patterns and the risk of depression in adults: A systematic review of observational studies. *Eur. J. Nutr.* **2014**, *53*, 997–1013. [CrossRef] [PubMed]
28. O'Neil, A.; Quirk, S.E.; Housden, S.; Brennan, S.L.; Williams, L.J.; Pasco, J.A.; Berk, M.; Jacka, F.N. Relationship between diet and mental health in children and adolescents: A systematic review. *Am. J. Public Health* **2014**, *104*, e31–e42. [CrossRef] [PubMed]
29. Goyal, M.; Singh, S.; Sibinga, E.M.S.; Gould, N.F.; Rowland-Seymour, A.; Sharma, R.; Berger, Z.; Sleicher, D.; Maron, D.D.; Shihab, H.M.; et al. Meditation programs for psychological stress and well-being: A systematic review and meta-analysis. *JAMA Intern. Med.* **2014**, *174*, 357–368. [CrossRef] [PubMed]
30. Liossi, C.; Hatira, P. Clinical hypnosis versus cognitive behavioral training for pain management with pediatric cancer patients undergoing bone marrow aspirations. *Int. J. Clin. Exp. Hypn.* **1999**, *47*, 104–116. [CrossRef] [PubMed]
31. Deng, G.; Cassileth, B.R. Integrative oncology: Complementary therapies for pain, anxiety, and mood disturbance. *CA Cancer J. Clin.* **2005**, *55*, 109–116. [CrossRef] [PubMed]
32. Reibel, D.K.; Greeson, J.M.; Brainard, G.C.; Rosenzweig, S. Mindfulness-based stress reduction and health-related quality of life in a heterogeneous patient population. *Gen. Hosp. Psychiatr.* **2001**, *23*, 183–192. [CrossRef]
33. Tilbrook, H.E.; Cox, H.; Hewitt, C.E.; Kang'ombe, A.R.; Chuang, L.; Jayakody, S.; Aplin, J.D.; Semlyen, A.; Trewhela, A.; Watt, I.; et al. Yoga for chronic low back pain: A randomized trial. *Ann. Intern. Med.* **2011**, *155*, 569–578. [CrossRef] [PubMed]
34. Kazak, A.; Penati, B.; Brophy, P.; Himelstein, B. Pharmacologic and psychologic interventions for procedural pain. *Pediatrics* **1998**, *102*, 59–66. [CrossRef] [PubMed]

35. Brown, M.L.; Rojas, E.; Gouda, S. A mind–body approach to pediatric pain management. *Children* **2017**, *4*, 50. [CrossRef] [PubMed]
36. Jindal, V.; Ge, A.; Mansky, P.J. Safety and efficacy of acupuncture in children a review of the evidence. *J. Pediatr. Hematol. Oncol.* **2008**, *30*, 431–442. [CrossRef] [PubMed]
37. Vohra, S.; McClafferty, H.; Becker, D.; Bethell, C.; Culbert, T.; King-Jones, S.; Rosen, L.; Sibinga, E.; Bailey, M.; Weydert, J.; et al. Mind-body therapies in children and youth. *Pediatrics* **2016**, *138*, 1896. [CrossRef]
38. Pittig, A.; Arch, J.J.; Lam, C.W.; Craske, M.G. Heart rate and heart rate variability in panic, social anxiety, obsessive-compulsive, and generalized anxiety disorders at baseline and in response to relaxation and hyperventilation. *Int. J. Psychophysiol.* **2013**, *87*, 19–27. [CrossRef] [PubMed]
39. Hassett, A.L.; Radvanski, D.C.; Vaschillo, E.G.; Vaschillo, B.; Sigal, L.H.; Karavidas, M.K.; Buyske, S.; Lehrer, P.M. A pilot study of the efficacy of heart rate variability (HRV) biofeedback in patients with fibromyalgia. *Appl. Psychophysiol. Biofeedback* **2007**, *32*, 1–10. [CrossRef] [PubMed]
40. Karavidas, M.K.; Lehrer, P.M.; Vaschillo, E.; Vaschillo, B.; Marin, H.; Buyske, S.; Malinovsky, I.; Radvanski, D.; Hassett, A. Preliminary results of an open label study of heart rate variability biofeedback for the treatment of major depression. *Appl. Psychophysiol. Biofeedback* **2007**, *32*, 19–30. [CrossRef] [PubMed]
41. Lazar, S.W.; Bush, G.; Gollub, R.L.; Fricchione, G.L.; Khalsa, G.; Benson, H. Functional brain mapping of the relaxation response and meditation. *Neuroreport* **2000**, *11*, 1581–1585. [CrossRef] [PubMed]
42. American Cancer Society Aromatherapy. *American Cancer Society Complete Guide to Complementary and Alternative Cancer Therapies*, 2nd ed.; American Cancer Society: Atlanta, GA, USA, 2009; pp. 57–60. ISBN 978-0-944235-71-3.
43. Bode, A.M.; Dong, Z. The amazing and mighty ginger. In *Herbal Medicine: Biomolecular and Clinical Aspects*, 2nd ed.; Benzie, I.F.F., Wachtel-Galor, S., Eds.; CRC Press/Taylor & Francis: Boca Raton, FL, USA, 2011.
44. Dupuis, L.L.; Nathan, P.C. Options for the prevention and management of acute chemotherapy-induced nausea and vomiting in children. *Paediatric Drugs* **2003**, *5*, 597–613. [CrossRef] [PubMed]
45. Quimby, E.L. The use of herbal therapies in pediatric oncology patients: Treating symptoms of cancer and side effects of standard therapies. *J. Pediatr. Oncol. Nurs.* **2007**, *24*, 35–40. [CrossRef] [PubMed]
46. Ernst, E.; Pittler, M.H. Efficacy of ginger for nausea and vomiting: A systematic review of randomized clinical trials. *Br. J. Anaesth.* **2000**, *84*, 367–371. [CrossRef] [PubMed]
47. Ryan, L.J.; Heckler, C.E.; Roscoe, J.A.; Dakhil, S.R.; Kirshner, J.; Flynn, P.J.; Hickok, J.T.; Morrow, G.R. Ginger (*Zingiber officinale*) Reduces Acute Chemotherapy-Induced Nausea: A URCC CCOP Study of 576 Patients. *Support. Care Cancer* **2012**, *20*, 1479–1489. [CrossRef] [PubMed]
48. Lin, Y.C.; Lee, A.C.; Kemper, K.J.; Berde, C.B. Use of complementary and alternative medicine in pediatric pain management service: A survey. *Pain Med.* **2005**, *6*, 452–458. [CrossRef] [PubMed]
49. Lee, A.; Chan, S.K.; Fan, L.T. Stimulation of the wrist acupuncture point PC6 for preventing postoperative nausea and vomiting. *Cochrane Database Syst. Rev.* **2015**, *2*, CD003281. [CrossRef] [PubMed]
50. Shin, H.C.; Kim, J.S.; Lee, S.K.; Kwon, S.H.; Kim, M.S.; Lee, E.J.; Yoon, Y.J. The effect of acupuncture on postoperative nausea and vomiting after pediatric tonsillectomy: A meta-analysis and systematic review. *Laryngoscope* **2016**, *126*, 1761–1767. [CrossRef] [PubMed]
51. Adams, D.; Cheng, F.; Jou, H.; Aung, S.; Yasui, Y.; Vohra, S. The safety of pediatric acupuncture: A systematic review. *Pediatrics* **2011**, *128*, e1575–e1587. [CrossRef] [PubMed]
52. Hines, S.; Steels, E.; Chang, A.; Gibbons, K. Aromatherapy for treatment of postoperative nausea and vomiting. *Cochrane Database Syst. Rev.* **2012**, *18*. [CrossRef] [PubMed]
53. Javorka, K.; Tomori, Z.; Zavarska, L. Protective and defensive airway reflexes in premature infants. *Physiol. Bohemoslov.* **1980**, *29*, 29–35. [PubMed]
54. Blake, K.D.; Fertleman, C.R.; Meates, M.A. Dangers of common cold treatments in children. *Lancet* **1993**, *341*. [CrossRef]
55. A controlled trial to improve care for seriously ill hospitalized patients. The study to understand prognoses and preferences for outcomes and risks of treatments (SUPPORT). The SUPPORT principal investigators. *JAMA* **1995**, *274*, 1591–1598.
56. Paul, P.; Lewandowski, W.; Terry, R.; Ernst, E.; Stearns, A. Guided imagery for non-musculoskeletal pain: A systematic review of randomized clinical trials. *J. Pain Symp. Manag.* **2012**, *44*, 95–104.
57. Lee, M.S.; Emst, E. Acupuncture for pain: An overview of Cochrane reviews. *Chin. J. Integr. Med.* **2011**, *17*, 187–189. [CrossRef] [PubMed]

58. Gadsby, J.G.; Franks, A.; Jarvis, P.; Dewhurst, F. Acupuncture like transcutaneous electrical nerve stimulation within palliative care: A pilot study. *Complement. Ther. Med.* **1997**, *5*, 13–18. [CrossRef]
59. Avellanosa, A.M.; West, C.R. Experience with transcutaneous electrical nerve stimulation for relief of intractable pain in cancer patients. *J. Med.* **1982**, *13*, 203–213. [CrossRef]
60. Ostrowski, M.J. Pain control in advanced malignant disease using transcutaneous nerve stimulation. *Br. J. Clin. Pract.* **1979**, *33*, 157–162. [PubMed]
61. Wen, H.L. Cancer pain treated with acupuncture and electrical stimulation. *Mod. Med. Asia* **1977**, *13*, 12–16.
62. Lakhan, E.S.; Sheafer, H.; Tepper, D. The effectiveness of aromatherapy in reducing pain: A systematic review and meta-analysis. *Pain Res. Treat.* **2016**. [CrossRef] [PubMed]
63. Rasool, S.; Soheilipour, S.; Hajhashemi, V.; Asghari, G.; Bagheri, M.; Molavi, M. Evaluation of the effect of aromatherapy with lavender essential oil on post-tonsillectomy pain in pediatric patients: A randomized controlled trial. *Int. J. Pediatr. Otorhinolaryngol.* **2013**, *77*, 1579–1581.
64. Rains, C.; Bryson, H.M. Topical capsaicin. A review of its pharmacological properties and therapeutic potential in post-herpetic neuralgia, diabetic neuropathy and osteoarthritis. *Drugs Aging* **1995**, *7*, 317–328. [CrossRef] [PubMed]
65. Mason, L.; Moore, R.A.; Derry, S.; Edwards, J.E.; McQuay, H.J. Systematic review of topical capsaicin for the treatment of chronic pain. *BMJ* **2004**, *328*. [CrossRef] [PubMed]
66. Derry, S.; Sven-Rice, A.; Cole, P.; Tan, T.; Moore, R.A. Topical capsaicin (high concentration) for chronic neuropathic pain in adults. *Cochrane Database Syst. Rev.* **2013**, *28*. [CrossRef]
67. Jorm, F.A.; Morgan, A.J.; Hetrick, S.E. Relaxation for depression. *Cochrane Database Syst. Rev.* **2008**, *4*. [CrossRef] [PubMed]
68. Latorraca, C.O.C.; Martimbianco, A.L.C.; Pachito, D.V.; Pacheco, R.L.; Riera, R. Mindfulness for palliative care patients. Systematic review. *Int. J. Clin. Pract.* **2017**, *71*. [CrossRef] [PubMed]
69. Malboeuf-Hurtubise, C.; Achille, M.; Muise, L.; Beauregard-Lacroix, R.; Vadnais, M.; Lacourse, É. A mindfulness-based meditation pilot study: Lessons learned on acceptability and feasibility in adolescents with cancer. *J. Child Fam. Stud.* **2015**, *25*, 1168–1177. [CrossRef]
70. Soden, K.; Vincent, K.; Craske, S.; Lucas, C.; Ashley, S. A randomized controlled trial of aromatherapy massage in a hospice setting. *Palliat. Med.* **2004**, *18*, 87–92. [CrossRef] [PubMed]
71. Burden, B.; Herron-Marx, S.; Clifford, C. The increasing use of reiki as a complementary therapy in specialist palliative care. *Int. J. Palliat. Nurs.* **2005**, *11*, 248–253. [CrossRef] [PubMed]
72. Tabatabaee, A.; Tafreshi, M.Z.; Rassouli, M.; Aledavood, S.A.; AlaviMajd, H.; Farahmand, S.K. Effect of therapeutic touch in patients with cancer: A literature review. *Med. Arch.* **2016**, *70*. [CrossRef] [PubMed]
73. Rome, R.B.; Hillary, H.L.; Deborah, A.B.; Christopher, M.B. The role of palliative care at the end of life. *Ochsner J.* **2011**, *11*, 348–352. [PubMed]
74. Jobst, K.; Chen, J.H.; McPherson, K.; Arrowsmith, J.; Brown, V.; Efthimiou, J.; Fletcher, H.J.; Maciocia, G.; Mole, P.; Shifrin, K.; et al. Controlled trial of acupuncture for disabling breathlessness. *Lancet* **1986**, *2*, 1416–1419. [CrossRef]

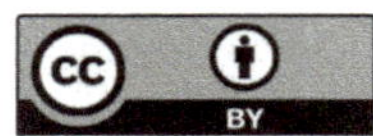

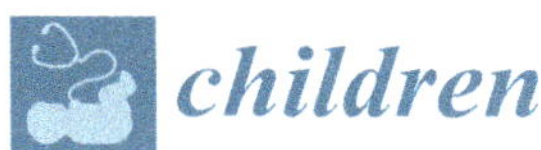

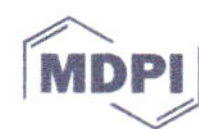

Review

Communicating Effectively in Pediatric Cancer Care: Translating Evidence into Practice

Lindsay J. Blazin [1], Cherilyn Cecchini [2], Catherine Habashy [2], Erica C. Kaye [1] and Justin N. Baker [1,*]

[1] Department of Oncology, Division of Quality of Life and Palliative Care, St. Jude Children's Research Hospital, Memphis, TN 38105, USA; lindsay.blazin@stjude.org (L.J.B.); erica.kaye@stjude.org (E.C.K.)

[2] Department of Pediatrics, Children's National Medical Center, Washington, DC 20010, USA; ccecchin@childrensnational.org (C.C); chabashy@childrensnational.org (C.H.)

* Correspondence: justin.baker@stjude.org; Tel.: +1-901-595-4446

Received: 19 December 2017; Accepted: 6 March 2018; Published: 11 March 2018

Abstract: Effective communication is essential to the practice of pediatric oncology. Clear and empathic delivery of diagnostic and prognostic information positively impacts the ways in which patients and families cope. Honest, compassionate discussions regarding goals of care and hopes for patients approaching end of life can provide healing when other therapies have failed. Effective communication and the positive relationships it fosters also can provide comfort to families grieving the loss of a child. A robust body of evidence demonstrates the benefits of optimal communication for patients, families, and healthcare providers. This review aims to identify key communication skills that healthcare providers can employ throughout the illness journey to provide information, encourage shared decision-making, promote therapeutic alliance, and empathically address end-of-life concerns. By reviewing the relevant evidence and providing practical tips for skill development, we strive to help healthcare providers understand the value of effective communication and master these critical skills.

Keywords: pediatric oncology; pediatric cancer; pediatric palliative care; communication

---

1. Introduction

Approximately 16,000 cases of cancer are diagnosed each year in children in the United States [1]. Although advances in treatment have led to remarkable gains in survival over the past century, an estimated 20% of children with cancer still die of their disease [1]. The field of pediatric palliative oncology (PPO) has emerged in response to the burden of suffering experienced by children with cancer and their families [2]. A core tenet of PPO is the use of effective communication to enhance therapeutic alliance and align the provision of medical interventions with the goals of care of the patient and family. Optimal communication in the context of pediatric oncology should begin at the time of diagnosis [3] and continue throughout the illness trajectory to enhance the therapeutic relationship, explore the hopes and goals of patients and families, and deliver care that maximizes quality of life and minimizes decisional regret.

Studies have demonstrated that patients with cancer desire effective communication with their healthcare providers (HCPs) [4,5]. Here, we will use the term healthcare providers to reference all members of a patient's interdisciplinary team, a critical functional unit of care delivery that will be discussed in greater detail below. In this context, the National Cancer Institute and the American Society of Clinical Oncology have called for improvements in patient–provider communication [6]. Effective communication is associated with improved quality of life [7] and is essential for promoting and facilitating shared decision-making between HCPs, patients, and families [8]. Even for patients for whom no curative treatments exist, open and empathic conversations with trusted HCPs can offer hope and healing [9]. For these reasons, HCPs who strive to provide optimal care for pediatric oncology patients should prioritize high-quality communication.

Effective communication is one of the primary means through which therapeutic relationships are established and developed. Six core functions of patient–provider communication were previously identified by Epstein and Street (Table 1) [6]. This conceptual framework can aid providers in understanding the importance of patient-centered communication and gaining critical skills. A recent review article on communication in pediatric oncology is framed in part around this model and provides an overview of recent research in this field [5].

Table 1. Six core functions of patient–provider communication.

Functions	Communication Methods
Responding to emotions	Evaluate and appraise distress Offer validation, empathy, and support
Exchanging information	Identify depth of information the patient or caregiver desires Acknowledge the abundance of information available online Consider findings presented without seeming dismissive
Making decisions	Partner with patient and family to identify goals of care Align treatment plan with stated goals
Fostering healing relationships	Develop mutual trust, understanding, and commitment Clarify roles and expectations of patient and provider
Enabling self-management	Encourage active engagement in all aspects of care Invite discussion and questions from patients and families
Managing uncertainty	Recognize limitations in knowledge Name uncertainties and address associated fears

2. Communicating Diagnosis to Families in Distress

For many HCPs, the first opportunity for effective and empathic communication with a patient and family comes at the time of diagnostic disclosure. Here, we discuss strategies for approaching this difficult task.

The period of illness preceding cancer diagnosis is fraught with considerable psychosocial distress. Communicating diagnoses to patients and families living under such a strain can be challenging. The manner in which this information is delivered can affect patient and family adjustment to the diagnosis, both positively and negatively [10]. Because of the importance of what we say and how we say it, much thought has gone into developing communication guides for diagnostic disclosure.

One such guideline has been provided by Mack and Grier in "The Day One Talk" [3]. In this report, the authors describe the steps that HCPs can take to optimize the communication of difficult information to a family in distress (summarized in Table 2) [3].

By clearly naming the diagnosis, outlining the treatment plan, and correcting misinformation about causation, HCPs can use communication around diagnostic disclosure to foster a lasting therapeutic alliance. Although no family ever wishes to receive a cancer diagnosis, some may find relief from learning the cause of their child's symptoms. A known diagnosis, defined treatment plan, and trusted HCP can help patients and families feel empowered to engage in treatment and prepare for the coming cancer journey.

Much of pediatric oncology is practiced in tertiary care medical centers with diverse patient populations. Excellent communicators must cultivate an awareness of and respect for the unique cultural experiences of each patient and family and work to develop a shared understanding of the essential health information. Alternative explanatory models of disease and treatment should be elicited and explored to allow the patient, family, and HCPs to develop partnerships and move toward shared decision-making. While this is a valuable topic, a full review of cross-cultural communication is beyond the scope of this article.

Table 2. A structured approach to diagnosis disclosure.

Components	Key Steps	Examples
Prepare the setting	Quiet location	
	All desired parties present and seated	
	Minimize interruptions	
Elicit understanding	One HCP takes the lead, asks family to describe their current understanding	"What have you heard so far about what is going on?"
Provide "warning shot"		"I'm afraid we have difficult news to discuss." "Unfortunately, the scans didn't show what we hoped."
Give the diagnosis	Use clear language Avoid euphemisms Use the word cancer	"Your child has leukemia, which is a kind of cancer."
Pause	Stop speaking	
	Allow the family to process information	
	Elicit questions	
Discuss treatment	Discuss expected location and duration of treatment	"We will use a combination of surgery followed by medicines called chemotherapy to treat the cancer. Most of the chemotherapy will be given during inpatient hospitalizations lasting 3–5 days. Overall, treatment will last for about 6 months."
	Explain different modalities	
	Provide alternative options	
Pause	Stop speaking	
	Allow the family to process information	
	Elicit questions	
Define goals of therapy	Provide clear, honest communication regarding curative intent	"The goal of therapy is to cure your child's cancer."
		"Unfortunately, there is no cure for this cancer at this time. The goal of treatment will be to minimize symptoms, improve quality of life, and prolong life."
Pause	Stop speaking	
	Allow the family to process information	
	Elicit questions	
Address causation	If accurate, clearly state that cancer was not preventable	"We don't know what causes this kind of cancer, but we know that there is nothing that you or your child did to cause it. You did the right thing by bringing your child in when you did."
	Dispel concerns that cancer resulted from something child or family did or did not do	
Summarize key points	Restate the diagnosis, goals of therapy, and discussion of causation	"For today, what I want you to understand is that your child has cancer. We plan to treat with chemotherapy and the goal of treatment is cure. There is nothing you or your child could have done to prevent this and this is not your fault."
Conclude conversation	Offer reassurance that information will be discussed again at future visits	"We will discuss all of this information again, so don't worry if you can't remember everything. I will see you in clinic again tomorrow afternoon. If you have any concerns before then, you can always call the clinic at..."
	Plan for next visit	
	Provide contact information for urgent issues	

3. Prognostic Communication and the Importance of Hope

After sharing the diagnosis, HCPs should address the ways in which the disease may impact the child, including likelihood of cure and expected complications. Prognostic disclosure often provokes anxiety for HCPs and may be greeted with similar apprehension by patients and families [11]. HCPs fear that communication about prognosis may erode hope and cause distress in families who are already overwhelmed [12]. Despite these concerns, research suggests that prognostic disclosure provided by trusted HCPs in an appropriate setting confers a range of benefits to patients and families, irrespective of the nature of the information provided [12,13].

Parents of children with cancer almost unanimously wish to receive prognostic information, and most prefer to hear as much detail as is available [14]. The period following a cancer diagnosis is one of uncertainty and anxiety for patients and families. By addressing this uncertainty through clear prognostic communication, HCPs have an opportunity to help decrease anxiety around fear of the unknown. Providing accurate information may help empower families to engage in medical treatment and optimize quality of life [2].

Additionally, hope is identified as an essential part of the treatment journey by patients with cancer [15]. Although HCPs may avoid disclosing accurate prognostic information for fear of extinguishing hope [16], a growing body of evidence suggests that maintenance of hope and prognostic awareness are not mutually exclusive. A study of parents of children with cancer found that parents who receive more prognostic information experience higher communication-related hope, even when the prognosis is poor [12]. A qualitative study in a similar population found that parents view prognostic communication as difficult but necessary. Prognostic understanding may empower parents to reframe their hopes and goals [17], offering an opportunity for families to maximize quality time with their children [9]. Furthermore, parents who receive high-quality information, including detailed prognosis, self-report less decisional regret than do parents who receive less information [18].

Given that most parents desire prognostic awareness, HCPs must consider how best to communicate highly stressful and upsetting prognostic information. As with most critical conversations, HCPs should carefully plan the setting with the goal of maximizing privacy and minimizing interruptions. At the start of a conversation, patients and families should be asked about their current prognostic understanding and what additional information they wish to learn. Ask-tell-ask is a conversational technique in which HCPs elicit the specific information that a patient and family desire to know, deliver that information, and then ask the family to share what they have heard and understood. Employing this technique allows providers to gain insight into a family's current understanding while also demonstrating a willingness to listen [19]. Simple questions such as "What have you been told?" and "What would you like to know?" can enable HCPs to tailor a conversation to the needs of a patient and family [11]. With regards to prognostic disclosure, some patients and families may wish to know numeric survival rates, while others may seek a general sense of likelihood of cure. For patients with no curative options, prognostic disclosure may center on estimations of survival length with anticipatory guidance about expected disease trajectory. Prognosis also may comprise discussions about what the disease means for a child's future, irrespective of survival. By understanding the family's informational needs, the HCP can be prepared to answer questions and empathically disclose additional information that may be both helpful and difficult to hear.

Despite clear communication of prognostic information, patients and families may demonstrate a nonlinear evolution of prognostic awareness. HCPs may feel frustrated when patients and families discuss future goals that do not align with a child's realistic projected survival. However, research suggests that parents of children with cancer are able to report accurately on their child's prognosis while simultaneously maintaining a wide range of hopes, including hope for cure [16]. HCPs should help patients and families identify and reframe new and different hopes by frequently asking the paired questions, "What are you hoping for?" and "What else are you hoping for?" By exploring these additional hopes, HCPs can broach conversation about realistic goals and encourage meaningful choices to optimize quality time for patients approaching the end of life.

Patients and families may further benefit from serial discussions about prognosis over time. HCPs may consider a longitudinal approach to prognostic disclosure in which providers facilitate prognostic awareness throughout the illness journey [20]. This approach may be particularly relevant for patients with progressive refractory disease, as they and their families struggle to reconcile their hopes for cure with the reality of incurable illness. (Table 3) [20].

Table 3. Cultivating prognostic awareness over time.

Step 1. Assess understanding of disease and prognosis	
• What have you been told about your/your child's disease/prognosis? • What is your sense of what the future holds? • How worried are you? What has you the most worried?	
Step 2. Facilitate development of prognostic awareness by imagining poorer health	
• Have you ever thought about what it might be like if you/your child got sicker? • It might be good to think about what might happen if you/your child got sicker. It is good to be prepared in case that does happen.	
Step 3. Assess response and consider urgency of need to deliver prognostic information	
If the patient is ambivalent about prognostic discussion and disease is stable:	• Delay giving prognostic information • Repeat steps 1–3 over time to cultivate prognostic awareness
If the patient is ambivalent about prognosis discussion but disease is worsening:	• Align with the patient • Name the dilemma: "It seems like it is hard for you to talk about the possibility that you/your child might get sicker."
If the patient is ready to discuss prognosis, regardless of disease state:	• Deliver prognostic information • Ask-tell-ask: Find out what the patient wants to know, deliver information, then ask what they make of it • Pair hope and worry: "I hope you will feel good for a long time, but I am worried because your scans look much worse."

Adapted with permission from [20].

In summary, effective prognostic communication is a difficult but essential task for HCPs to practice and prioritize. Patients and families who understand prognosis are empowered to make informed decisions that align with their stated goals of care. Although an engaged approach to decision-making is important for every patient, it is particularly critical for patients with no further curative options. Further communication strategies for these patients are discussed in additional detail below.

4. Communication with Families at the End of Life and During Bereavement

In addition to assisting patients and families with end-of-life decision-making, HCPs must also provide anticipatory guidance about the dying process. End-of-life physiology can be highly distressing for family members, particularly if inadequately explained. Expected levels of responsiveness, grimacing, agonal breathing, and other common end-of-life symptoms should be discussed in clear and specific terms prior to the onset of anticipated changes. Such explanations may help provide reassurance to parents who often feel ill-equipped to care for their children during the final stage of illness.

A critical aspect of communication around anticipatory guidance at the end of life includes discussion with families about symptom management plans and the availability of staff to ensure the highest possible level of comfort. Providing a comfortable death to children with cancer is paramount and has been identified by the National Quality Forum as a critical measure of quality care [21]. Specific symptom management plans, including contingency plans for new symptoms, should be developed in partnership with patients and parents. HCPs should be available in person or by phone to troubleshoot additional issues that may arise.

Parents of children who died of cancer strongly advocate for children to continue to receive the same level of care as they approach end of life, and many parents express fears of abandonment by HCPs when goals of care shift from cure to comfort [22]. HCPs should make every effort to assuage such fears through clear communication and actions. Evidence suggests that families who observed professionalism in the interactions between HCPs and the dying patient and who were reassured that the patient was comfortable were more satisfied with care [23]. Additionally, families that were coached on how to care for the patient were allowed adequate time to grieve after death, and those who could not overhear medical conversations outside the patient's room reported lower levels of distress at time of patient death [23].

HCPs also can support patients and families by offering updates on clinical status. Although the timing of death can be difficult to predict, an experienced HCP should attempt to provide information regarding anticipated timeline as the patient's end of life approaches. Providing a diagnosis of hours, days, or weeks allows families to prepare, both emotionally and pragmatically, in terms of making funeral arrangements and ensuring that loved ones can be present at the time of death. A bereavement plan of care should be developed in collaboration with the patient (when developmentally appropriate) and family during earlier advance-care planning conversations and implemented by the HCP after the patient's death.

Following a child's death, the role of the HCP changes yet remains highly important. The death of a child is a devastating event, and the grieving process is often intense and prolonged [24] and may include feelings of helplessness and guilt [25]. Many factors that affect parental grief are immutable, including the timing and manner of death. Some variables, however, can be moderated by HCPs in ways that influence the bereavement experience. Parents who perceive an uncaring or "too busy" attitude among staff as their child was dying report higher levels of grief near time of death. Similarly, parents who thought HCPs were being evasive were less effectively able to manage their grief. Parents who felt adequately informed and were satisfied with their child's end of life care experienced lower levels of early grief [26].

In addition to the death of their child, many parents grieve the loss of their hospital community. Research suggests that feelings of abandonment can complicate parental grief [27]. Understandably, many bereaved parents wish to remain connected with their child's care teams [28]. Parents of children who died of cancer specifically desire to continue relationships with the HCPs involved in their child's care, and they identify communication with their child's prior HCPs as an important part of their grieving process. Additionally, connecting with bereaved families may benefit HCPs by providing closure and healing. Although bereavement resources are limited in many institutions, a brief phone call to a family can be multiply beneficial by screening for complicated grief, connecting families with local resources, and, importantly, reminding the family that their child was important and is not forgotten [29].

Caring for a dying child and his/her family is a trying experience for HCPs. By optimizing comfort through effective symptom management, providing up-to-date clinical and prognostic information, and delivering empathic, patient-centered care, HCPs can support patients and families through this devastating event.

5. Cultivating Therapeutic Alliance in the Patient–Provider Relationship

Therapeutic alliance encompasses the personal bond and shared therapeutic goals among the patient, family, and HCP [30]. Establishment of a therapeutic alliance begins at the first meeting and further develops over time. Optimal communication strengthens the therapeutic alliance, providing HCPs with necessary credibility when difficult decisions must be made.

Stronger therapeutic alliance between patients and physicians is associated with improvements in patient and family psychosocial outcomes, including illness coping, quality of life, and treatment satisfaction [31]. Additionally, a strong alliance is associated with increases in perceived social support, decreased illness-related grief among adolescents and young adults with cancer, and improvements in treatment adherence [31]. The latter finding is particularly salient to note, as rates of nonadherence in adolescents with cancer approach 60% and are associated with poor clinical outcomes.

Relationships between patients and families and the care team become increasingly important in the context of refractory, progressive, or relapsed disease. Although HCPs may worry that frank discussions about prognosis may weaken or damage the patient–provider relationship [12], open conversations about end-of-life care do not adversely impact therapeutic alliance [32]. On the contrary, a strong therapeutic alliance is associated with greater emotional acceptance of incurable illness in patients with cancer [32]. By devoting time and effort towards establishing and developing therapeutic alliance, HCPs can help empower patients and families to confront their cancer diagnoses and reframe their hopes and goals for the future.

Furthermore, the benefits of a strong therapeutic alliance extend beyond the patient. Caregivers of patients with cancer who perceive a supportive alliance between the patient and HCP self-report decreased role limitation, enhanced social function, and improved physical and psychological health [33]. Importantly, caregiver benefits persist after the death of the patient [33].

Given the myriad of benefits for patients and families, establishing a therapeutic alliance should be a priority for HCPs. Many of the skills detailed above can serve to develop and strengthen the therapeutic alliance. The International Society for Paediatric Oncology (SIOP) developed guidelines to assist HCPs in developing a therapeutic alliance with families (Table 4) [34].

Establishment of a strong therapeutic alliance with HCPs benefits patients and families. Effective, empathic communication is one of the primary means by which this alliance is forged. Over time, the strength of the therapeutic bond with a family allows HCPs to discuss more difficult topics. If done well, these challenging conversations serve to further deepen the therapeutic alliance and create space for future discussions. Effective communication deepens the therapeutic alliance, which, in turn, allows for more open communication. In this way, these two concepts are mutually reinforcing and foster greater connections between patients, families, and HCPs over time (Figure 1).

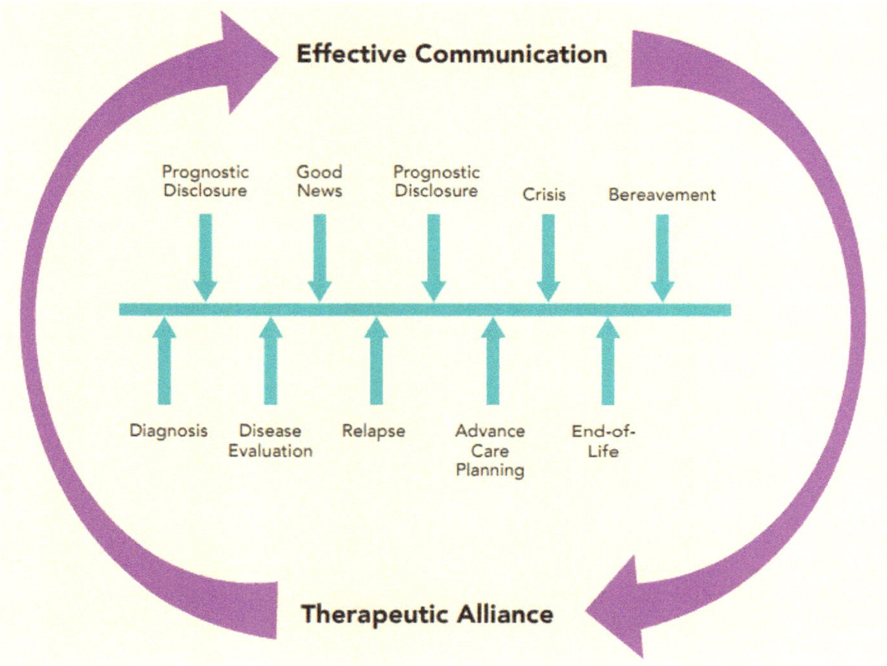

Figure 1. Diagram of the cyclic, reinforcing relationship between effective communication and therapeutic alliance throughout illness trajectory.

Table 4. Guidelines for developing therapeutic alliance with patients and families.

- Treat all members of the interdisciplinary team with professionalism and respect for their expertise
- Invite patients and families to be members of the medical team and recognize their unique skills and contributions
- Elicit needs and preferences from patients and families; avoid assumptions
- Provide education about diagnosis and treatment; ensure understanding
- Recognize the burdens associated with diagnosis; empathize with frustrations related to medical bureaucracy
- Meet regularly with the interdisciplinary team to discuss the psychosocial wellbeing of patients and families and strategize approaches to improve this wellbeing
- Support pediatric patients' needs for autonomy and encourage them to take control of appropriate aspects of care

6. Involving the Child

Determining how and when to involve pediatric patients in medical conversations is a critical skill for pediatric oncology HCPs to master. Most childhood cancer survivors and their families believe that a cancer diagnosis should be discussed with a child early in the disease course [35]. Effectively including children in medical conversations requires excellent communication skills, strong alliance with parents, and a thorough grasp of developmentally-appropriate communication strategies (Table 5) [36]. Though challenging, it is important that HCPs engage children in conversations about their health to ensure that their unique questions, fears, and uncertainties are addressed [37].

Table 5. Communication goals by patient age.

Age	Communication Goals
Infants	• Soothe and relieve distress • Show care through gentle touch
Toddlers	• *Includes prior goals for infants* • Elicit bothersome symptoms • Validate emotional experiences
School-Aged Children	• *Includes prior goals for infants and toddlers* • Obtain information needed to diagnose and treat • Encourage cooperation and adherence with recommendations • Educate about disease • Demonstrate respect for individual choice and voice
Adolescents	• *Includes prior goals for infants, toddlers, and school-aged children* • Recruit for discussions about goals of care and medical decision-making • Elicit hopes, worries, fears

Any plan to involve a child in medical conversations should be developed with parents. Out of a desire to protect their child, some parents are hesitant to disclose illness information. In these circumstances, HCPs should broach conversations by asking parents to share what they believe their child already knows. Even young patients can understand serious illness and participate in medical decisions as long as conversations are led in an age-appropriate manner [38]. Furthermore, children often perceive the seriousness of their illness prior to hearing formal disclosure by family or HCPs.

By helping parents recognize the level of their child's illness awareness, HCPs can empower parents to explore difficult topics with their child.

A majority of chronically ill adolescents wish to be involved in their medical decision-making [39]. The degree of engagement varies, with many adolescents preferring to play an active role in their medical decision-making [40]. Even those that prefer less active roles still desire to be informed about their health [40]. HCPs should make every effort to involve adolescent patients in medical conversations, to the level that is desired by the adolescent and family. Even participation in relatively minor care conversations may allow adolescent patients to regain control and build trust with HCPs [40].

The literature also supports the involvement of adolescent patients in advance care planning. Family-centered advance care planning (ACP) elicits input from adolescent patients and their parents and is associated with improved congruence of end-of-life care with the stated goals of patients and families [41]. Patients and families who participate in family-centered ACP find the conversations to be difficult but worthwhile [42], report a greater understanding of end-of-life wishes, and are more likely to receive early palliative care [43]. Importantly, all of these studies used structured conversation guides to facilitate discussions. Evidence-based conversation guides, such as Voicing My CHOICES (available from Aging With Dignity [44]), are available to assist HCPs who wish to enter into these difficult but necessary discussions with patients facing life-limiting illnesses.

The benefits of engaging patients in medical conversations persist even when there is no longer chance for cure. Parents who involve their children in discussions about prognosis and impending death generally do not regret doing so [45,46]. Disclosing to a family that there are no further curative options for their child's disease is challenging. HCPs facilitating these conversations should be mindful of the language they choose and avoid terminology that may seem dismissive or offensive (Table 6) [47]. Other team members including child life specialists and spiritual care providers may be particularly helpful for navigating these challenging discussions.

Table 6. Communication in the context of progressive or refractory disease.

Potential Pitfalls	Phrases to Avoid	Alternative Phrases
Placing burden of understanding on the family	"Do you understand what I've told you?"	"Does this make sense?""Tell me what you've been hearing from the team."
Appearing to give up	"There is nothing more we can do."	"I wish we had a treatment to cure this disease. We will continue to do everything in our power to care for (child's name)."
Claiming understanding	"I understand how you feel."	"I can't imagine how you must be feeling. I wish we had better news. What might be helpful for you right now?"
Using clichés, emphasizing the positives	"This will make you a better/stronger person."	"May I just sit with you for a while?"

In summary, facilitating patient involvement in their own care is one of the essential functions of HCPs. While challenging, there is a growing body of evidence that suggests involving pediatric patients in medical conversation in age-appropriate ways has benefits for both patients and families.

7. Communicating with Siblings and the Extended Family

In addition to interacting directly with patients and parents, HCPs also play an important role in facilitating communication within the larger family unit [48]. In particular, HCP communication with siblings of children with cancer can considerably affect how a family adjusts to the diagnosis [49]. The families of children who die from cancer are also impacted by their interactions with HCPs. Bereaved parents appreciate HCPs who engage the family in conversations about care decisions [24].

Siblings who receive adequate communication at the end of their sibling's life have lower levels of long-term maladjustment. Importantly, the inverse is also true: siblings who did not perceive satisfactory communication around their sibling's death subsequently report higher levels of anxiety later in life [50].

In communication with the family unit, HCPs must remain mindful of parent and sibling preferences as well as relevant spiritual and cultural beliefs or practices. HCPs can encourage parents to openly discuss a patient's illness with his/her siblings while respecting parental wishes and beliefs related to information sharing. Families who choose to discuss a patient's illness with siblings and other family members may require support from trusted HCPs. It may be beneficial for HCPs to meet with parents before discussions with the extended family to answer questions and develop strategies for sharing medical information. Some families may benefit from having the HCP available during the conversation to answer questions.

HCPs and parents can employ several strategies when conveying truths about a patient's disease with the extended family. HCPs should state that they are available to assist parents with these conversations and will respect their decisions regarding what information to disclose and to whom. HCPs should either be present during the conversation or be available at a set time to answer questions from the extended family. Remind parents that, though they can be difficult to say, words like "death," "dying," and "cancer" should be used to make sure family members understand the clinical situation. Parents may be worried about responding to emotions or about their own emotional reactions. HCPs can reassure that a wide range of emotional responses to this kind of information is normal. Parents may find phrases like "Mommy is crying because she is sad that (child's name) is sick" helpful in these situations. For parents discussing a cancer diagnosis with the patient's siblings, additional effort should be made to ensure information is discussed in a developmentally appropriate way.

In summary, a cancer diagnosis in one child affects the entire family. By facilitating communication with and among all family members, HCPs can help family members adjust to their new roles, process their emotions, interact appropriately with the patient, and cope with the aftermath of the death of a child.

8. An Interdisciplinary Team Approach to Communication

To best support the physical, emotional, and spiritual needs of patients and families, pediatric palliative oncology care should be provided through an interdisciplinary team (IDT) [51]. This team may be composed of physicians, nurses, advance practice clinicians, social workers, chaplains, child life specialists, and other psychosocial support staff. IDT members must communicate effectively with one another and with the patient and family in order to ensure provision of optimal medical, psychosocial, and spiritual care.

Individual members of the IDT should meet with the patient and family to provide targeted support of their physical, emotional, and spiritual needs. The IDT should meet at regular intervals so that insights gleaned from individual conversations can be shared with the entire team [52]. The primary goal of the IDT is to integrate the clinical perspectives and expertise of a diverse group of providers to develop a holistic care plan that supports the expressed and perceived needs of the patient and family.

Clinicians who participate in the IDT meeting should be cognizant of the common phenomenon in which patients' biomedical needs are reviewed in detail with relatively little attention given to spiritual and emotional needs [52]. HCPs should guard against the biomedical bias by conducting IDT meetings with a structured format that ensures an appropriate balance of physical, emotional, and spiritual issues. Ideally, one designated clinician should lead the meeting to facilitate efficient discussion and transitions. This clinician should share a one-line medical summary for the patient then invite other interdisciplinary colleagues to provide salient information to enhance the team's collective understanding and facilitate improved care coordination/planning for the patient and family.

Often, information discussed during an IDT meeting needs to be shared with patients and families. Typically, this transfer of information is best facilitated through a family conference. Figure 2 depicts the typical clinical progression from individual HCP conversations to IDT meeting to family conference [53].

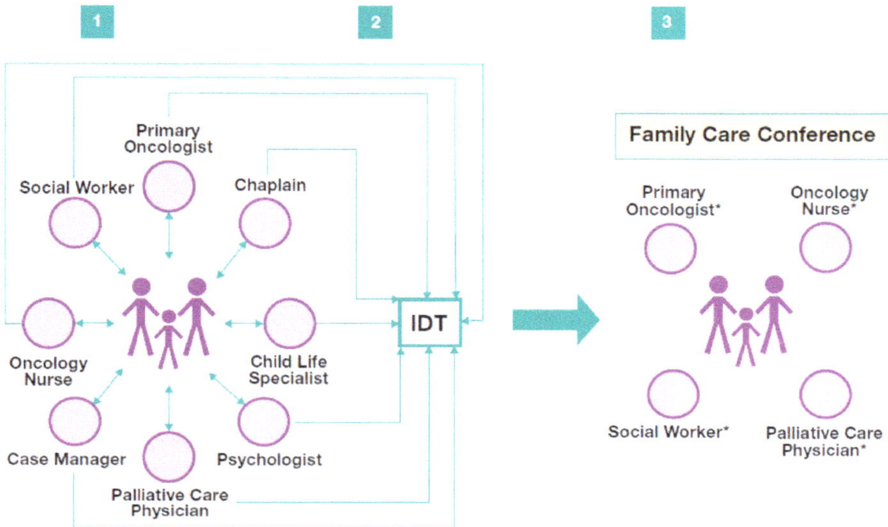

Figure 2. Flowchart demonstrating ideal collaborative efforts to promote effective communication of comprehensive care plans. Panel **1** illustrates individual interdisciplinary team (IDT) members meeting with patient and family; Panel **2** illustrates the IDT meeting; and Panel **3** illustrates the family care conference conducted based on recommendations from the IDT meeting. IDT members will be chosen to participate in the family conference based on the information to be discussed and the needs of the patient and family.

A family conference can be loosely defined to include any planned meeting between IDT members, patients, and family members in which discussions of the patient's clinical status, illness trajectory, treatment plan, prognosis, goals of care, or disposition planning occur [54]. HCPs may identify the need for a family conference in the setting of a change in clinical status, in anticipation of future decision making, prior to an upcoming transition, in the context of fragmented or ineffective communication, or in response to moral distress or ethical concerns raised by the care team or family [55].

While the objectives of individual family conferences vary based on the clinical circumstances and key stakeholders unique to each case, the primary goal underpinning the agenda for all family conferences should be to ensure that the patient, family, and HCPs have a shared understanding of the illness trajectory, appropriate treatment plan, and overall goals of care. Prior to initiating a family conference, the IDT should discuss and identify what information should be conveyed to the patient and family. Based on this, the team then may elect certain representatives to lead and attend the family conference.

The optimal time to schedule a family conference is when the patient's clinical condition is reasonably stable and the patient and/or family are already aware of the illness and its implications [56]. However, often family conferences occur in circumstances of extremis, in which the patient is acutely ill or worsening and/or families are unaware of the gravity of the situation. HCPs should strive to coordinate family conferences prior to catastrophic events, yet they should not shy away from scheduling conferences even during times of extreme stress.

An effective family conference requires preparation, particularly from the HCP that will be leading the conference. It is critical that HCPs have a comprehensive understanding of the patient's medical condition, realistic treatment options, and goals of care. The patient and family should be given adequate notice regarding the timing of the conference and a time and location should be chosen that accommodates the family and all key team members. In advance of the meeting, patients and families should be encouraged to create an agenda or question list to be addressed during the meeting.

It is also important for HCPs to ask the patient and family who would be most helpful to have in attendance at the conference, including members of the IDT, other members of the medical team, and family members. The patient may or may not attend the conference, depending on age/developmental stage, clinical status, and personal or family preferences. If the patient does not attend, arrangements should be made in advance for an appropriate family member or clinician (e.g., a child life specialist, music therapist, or other known and trusted HCP) to remain with the patient if desired by the child or family.

Although family conferences occur frequently within the pediatric oncology setting, the majority of HCPs do not receive formal training on how to effectively lead or communicate in these conferences [57,58]. The following discussion outlines general recommendations for facilitating a family conference, including guidance regarding language options for HCPs to use.

At the specified time, all attendees should gather and be seated. The HCP designated to lead the conference should facilitate introductions of all team members and family members in attendance. The conference leader should then review the agenda for the meeting and ensure concurrence between family and providers. Prior to sharing medical information, the conference leader should ask the patient and family a few open-ended questions to elicit their understanding of the clinical situation. This may include statements like, "Tell me what you've heard the doctors say" or "What have you been told about how (the patient) is doing?" The responses of the patient and family to these questions should shape the structure and content of the remainder of the conference.

The meeting leader should provide a concise summary of the relevant medical facts and an overview of therapeutic options, if relevant, taking care to only include plans considered reasonable and feasible for the patient [55]. The leader should also facilitate the sharing of information from subspecialized experts in attendance, encouraging each clinician to provide information and then summarizing and integrating the input into the larger clinical picture. Depending on case-specific factors, the conference leader's role may focus more on facilitating the transfer of information between other experts and the family, as opposed to delivering information directly. An important responsibility of the conference leader is to make statements related to the most likely disease trajectory and outcome, providing anticipatory guidance even in the context of prognostic uncertainty.

During each phase of a family conference, HCPs must strive to provide clear information devoid of medical jargon, using language that accurately and frankly describes the patient's current status and most likely anticipated outcome. Questions from the patient and family must be answered honestly and concisely, ideally in 2–3 sentences, followed by a significant pause to allow the family to process the information. Regardless of the prognosis or treatment options offered, it is imperative to provide reassurance that the patient will continue receiving excellent, attentive care. Statements that affirm that the IDT will remain highly engaged in the patient's management and strive to provide care that aligns with the goals of the patient and family can be helpful, and positive language that emphasizes what CAN and WILL be done is preferable to language that describes what cannot or will not be done. For example, saying, "We will continue to do everything possible to ensure that (the patient) lives as well as possible for as long as possible" or "We will continue to fight to do everything we can so that (the patient) is as comfortable as possible" can help the patient and family know that their team continues to prioritize their needs and will not abandon them in the face of progressive illness.

Additionally, HCPs should strive to maintain a respectful environment wherein all conference attendees are able to offer insights and interruptions are minimized [56]. Patients and family members should be encouraged throughout the conference to share their hopes, fears, and concerns so that these may be addressed as specifically as possible by the IDT members in attendance. Questions such as "What are you most worried about?" also offer helpful ways for HCPs to transition into conversations about prognosis and goals of care. Sitting in silence can be another effective way to elicit difficult emotions and concerns; HCPs should be reminded before the conference of the value of sitting quietly and not filling the silence, but rather deferring to the patient, family, and meeting leader to determine the duration of pauses.

Lastly, at the conclusion of a conference, patients and families should be provided with clear and specific information about the next time they will meet and how to reach the team if new questions or concerns arise in the interim. Within 24 h after the conference, at least one member of the IDT should follow up with the family to help them process the information and address any lingering questions or concerns. An overview of the conference should also be documented systematically and clearly in the patient's medical record, with copies sent to all IDT members to ensure that the team moves forward collaboratively and communicates with the patient and family in ways that align with the information shared during the family conference.

In summary, comprehensive care of pediatric oncology patients and their families in the modern health care system extends beyond the capabilities of any one clinician. The complexity of patient medical needs is mirrored by multifaceted and overlapping communication lines between the patient and family and all participating HCPs. IDT meetings and family conferences are two ways in which HCPs can coordinate the efforts of a variety of providers and collaborate with patients and families to optimize the provision of holistic, goal-concordant care.

9. Conclusions

Effective communication is an essential skill in the practice of PPO. Mastery of effective communication enables HCPs to expertly disclose diagnoses, facilitate the development of prognostic awareness, navigate advance care planning discussions, identify goals of care, provide comfort at the end of life, and support bereaved families during the difficult grief journey. Improving skills with regards to development of therapeutic alliance, involving pediatric patients in medical discussions, communicating with the whole family unit, and collaborative dialogue in the context of an IDT approach allows HCPs to provide optimal care to patients and families. A large body of evidence demonstrates the benefits of effective communication on patient and family experiences and outcomes. HCPs who strive to provide excellent, whole-person care must devote time and attention to the development of these critical communication skills.

Acknowledgments: The authors received no funding for this work. The authors would like to acknowledge Nisha Badders for her work on formatting the manuscript and Jessica Anderson for creation of the included figures.

Author Contributions: Catherine Habashy and Cherilyn Cecchini conducted extensive reviews of the literature and drafted large sections of the manuscript. Lindsay J. Blazin determined the overall structure and content of the paper and drafted the final manuscript, incorporating the work of the other authors. Justin N. Baker provided oversight of concept development and provided editorial feedback related to content, structure, and style. Erica C. Kaye provided critical feedback related to the tone and structure of the text and provided additional literature review.

Conflicts of Interest: The authors have no conflict of interest to declare.

References

1. Ward, E.; DeSantis, C.; Robbins, A.; Kohler, B.; Jemal, A. Childhood and adolescent cancer statistics, 2014. *CA Cancer J. Clin.* **2014**, *64*, 83–103. [CrossRef] [PubMed]
2. Wolfe, J.; Klar, N.; Grier, H.E.; Duncan, J.; Salem-Schatz, S.; Emanuel, E.J.; Weeks, J.C. Understanding of prognosis among parents of children who died of cancer. *JAMA* **2000**, *284*, 2469–2475. [CrossRef] [PubMed]
3. Mack, J.W.; Grier, H.E. The Day One Talk. *J. Clin. Oncol.* **2004**, *22*, 563–566. [CrossRef] [PubMed]
4. Hagerty, R.G.; Butow, P.N.; Ellis, P.M.; Dimitry, S.; Tattersall, M.H.N. Communicating prognosis in cancer care: A systematic review of the literature. *Ann. Oncol.* **2005**, *16*, 1005–1053. [CrossRef] [PubMed]

5. Sisk, B.A.; Mack, J.W.; Ashworth, R.; DuBois, J. Communication in pediatric oncology: State of the field and research agenda. *Pediatr. Blood Cancer* **2018**, *65*, e26727. [CrossRef] [PubMed]
6. Epstein, R.M.; Street, R.L., Jr. *Patient-Centered Communication in Cancer Care: Promoting Healing and Reducing Suffering*; NIH Publication No. 07-6225; National Cancer Institute: Bethesda, MD, USA, 2007.
7. Hays, R.M.; Valentine, J.; Haynes, G.; Geyer, J.R.; Villareale, N.; Mckinstry, B.; Varni, J.W.; Churchill, S.S. The seattle pediatric palliative care project: Effects on family satisfaction and health-related quality of life. *J. Palliat. Med.* **2006**, *9*, 716–728. [CrossRef] [PubMed]
8. Mack, J.W.; Weeks, J.C.; Wright, A.A.; Block, S.D.; Prigerson, H.G. End-of-life discussions, goal attainment, and distress at the end of life: Predictors and outcomes of receipt of care consistent with preferences. *J. Clin. Oncol.* **2010**, *28*, 1203–1208. [CrossRef] [PubMed]
9. Nyborn, J.A.; Olcese, M.; Nickerson, T.; Mack, J.W. "Don't try to cover the sky with your hands": Parents' experiences with prognosis communication about their children with advanced cancer. *J. Palliat. Med.* **2016**, *19*, 626–631. [CrossRef] [PubMed]
10. Ptacek, J.T.; Ptacek, J.J. Patients' perceptions of receiving bad news about cancer. *J. Clin. Oncol.* **2001**, *19*, 4160–4164. [CrossRef] [PubMed]
11. Mack, J.W.; Smith, T.J. Reasons why physicians do not have discussions about poor prognosis, why it matters, and what can be improved. *J. Clin. Oncol.* **2012**, *30*, 2715–2717. [CrossRef] [PubMed]
12. Mack, J.W.; Wolfe, J.; Cook, E.F.; Grier, H.E.; Cleary, P.D.; Weeks, J.C. Hope and prognostic disclosure. *J. Clin. Oncol.* **2007**, *25*, 5636–5642. [CrossRef] [PubMed]
13. Mack, J.W.; Cook, E.F.; Wolfe, J.; Grier, H.E.; Cleary, P.D.; Weeks, J.C. Understanding of prognosis among parents of children with cancer: Parental optimism and the parent-physician interaction. *J. Clin. Oncol.* **2007**, *25*, 1357–1362. [CrossRef] [PubMed]
14. Mack, J.W.; Wolfe, J.; Grier, H.E.; Cleary, P.D.; Weeks, J.C. Communication about prognosis between parents and physicians of children with cancer: Parent preferences and the impact of prognostic information. *J. Clin. Oncol.* **2006**, *24*, 5265–5270. [CrossRef] [PubMed]
15. Thorne, S.; Oglov, V.; Armstrong, E.-A.; Hislop, T.G. Prognosticating futures and the human experience of hope. *Palliat. Support. Care* **2007**, *5*, 227–239. [CrossRef] [PubMed]
16. Kamihara, J.; Nyborn, J.A.; Olcese, M.E.; Nickerson, T.; Mack, J.W. Parental Hope for Children with Advanced Cancer. *Pediatrics* **2015**, *135*, 868–874. [CrossRef] [PubMed]
17. Feudtner, C. Collaborative Communication in Pediatric Palliative Care: A Foundation for Problem-Solving and Decision-Making. *Pediatr. Clin. N. Am.* **2007**, *54*, 583–607. [CrossRef] [PubMed]
18. Mack, J.W.; Cronin, A.M.; Kang, T.I. Decisional regret among parents of children with cancer. *J. Clin. Oncol.* **2016**, *34*, 4023–4029. [CrossRef] [PubMed]
19. Back, A.L.; Arnold, R.M.; Baile, W.F.; Tulsky, J.A.; Fryer-Edwards, K. Approaching difficult communication tasks in oncology. *CA Cancer J. Clin.* **2005**, *55*, 164–177. [CrossRef] [PubMed]
20. Jackson, V.A.; Jacobsen, J.; Greer, J.A.; Pirl, W.F.; Temel, J.S.; Back, A.L. The cultivation of prognostic awareness through the provision of early palliative care in the ambulatory setting: A communication guide. *J. Palliat. Med.* **2013**, *16*, 894–900. [CrossRef] [PubMed]
21. National Quality Forum. *National Voluntary Consensus Standards for Nursing-Sensitive Care: A Consensus Report*; National Quality Forum: Washington, DC, USA, 2004.
22. Maurer, S.H.; Hinds, P.S.; Spunt, S.L.; Furman, W.L.; Kane, J.R.; Baker, J.N. Decision making by parents of children with incurable cancer who opt for enrollment on a phase I trial compared with choosing a do not resuscitate/terminal care option. *J. Clin. Oncol.* **2010**, *28*, 3292–3298. [CrossRef] [PubMed]
23. Shinjo, T.; Morita, T.; Hirai, K.; Miyashita, M.; Sato, K.; Tsuneto, S.; Shima, Y. Care for imminently dying cancer patients: Family members' experiences and recommendations. *J. Clin. Oncol.* **2010**, *28*, 142–148. [CrossRef] [PubMed]
24. Michon, B.; Balkou, S.; Hivon, R.; Cyr, C. Death of a child: Parental perception of grief intensity—End-of-life and bereavement care. *Paediatr. Child Health* **2003**, *8*, 363–366. [CrossRef] [PubMed]
25. Higgs, E.J.; McClaren, B.J.; Sahhar, M.A.R.; Ryan, M.M.; Forbes, R. "A short time but a lovely little short time": Bereaved parents' experiences of having a child with spinal muscular atrophy type 1. *J. Paediatr. Child Health* **2016**, *52*, 40–46. [CrossRef] [PubMed]
26. Meert, K.L.; Thurston, C.S.; Thomas, R. Parental coping and bereavement outcome after the death of a child in the pediatric intensive care unit. *Pediatr. Crit. Care Med.* **2001**, *2*, 324–328. [CrossRef] [PubMed]

27. Contro, N.; Larson, J.; Scofield, S.; Sourkes, B.; Cohen, H. Family perspectives on the quality of pediatric palliative care. *JAMA* **2002**, *156*, 14–19. [CrossRef]
28. Snaman, J.M.; Kaye, E.C.; Torres, C.; Gibson, D.V.; Baker, J.N. Helping parents live with the hole in their heart: The role of health care providers and institutions in the bereaved parents' grief journeys. *Cancer* **2016**, *122*, 2757–2765. [CrossRef] [PubMed]
29. Jankovic, M.; Masera, G.; Uderzo, C.; Conter, V.; Adamoli, L.; Spinetta, J.J. Meetings with parents after the death of their child from leukemia. *Pediatr. Hematol. Oncol.* **1989**, *6*, 155–160. [CrossRef] [PubMed]
30. Mead, N.; Bower, P. Patient-centredness: A conceptual framework and review of the empirical literature. *Soc. Sci. Med.* **2000**, *51*, 1087–1110. [CrossRef]
31. Trevino, K.M.; Fasciano, K.; Prigerson, H.G. Patient-oncologist alliance, psychosocial well-being, and treatment adherence among young adults with advanced cancer. *J. Clin. Oncol.* **2013**, *31*, 1683–1689. [CrossRef] [PubMed]
32. Mack, J.W.; Block, S.D.; Nilsson, M.; Wright, A.; Trice, E.; Friedlander, R.; Paulk, E.; Prigerson, H.G. Measuring therapeutic alliance between oncologists and patients with advanced cancer: The human connection scale. *Cancer* **2009**, *115*, 3302–3311. [CrossRef] [PubMed]
33. Trevino, K.M.; Maciejewski, P.K.; Epstein, A.S.; Prigerson, H.G. The lasting impact of the therapeutic alliance: Patient-oncologist alliance as a predictor of caregiver bereavement adjustment. *Cancer* **2015**, *121*, 3534–3542. [CrossRef] [PubMed]
34. Masera, G.; Spinetta, J.J.; Jankovic, M.; Ablin, A.R.; Buchwall, I.; Van Dongen-Melman, J.; Eden, T.; Epelman, C.; Green, D.M.; Kosmidis, H.V.; et al. Guidelines for a therapeutic alliance between families and staff: A report of the SIOP Working Committee on Psychosocial Issues in Pediatric Oncology. *Med. Pediatr. Oncol.* **1998**, *30*, 183–186. [CrossRef]
35. Slavin, L.A.; O'Malley, J.E.; Koocher, G.P.; Foster, D.J. Communication of the cancer diagnosis to pediatric patients: Impact on long-term adjustment. *Am. J. Psychiatry* **1982**, *139*, 179–183. [CrossRef] [PubMed]
36. Palazzi, D.L.; Lorin, M.I.; Turner, T.L.; Ward, M.A.; Cabrera, A.G. *Communicating with Pediatric Patients and Their Families: The Texas Children's Hospital Guide for Physicians, Nurses and Other Healthcare Professionals*; Texas Children's Hospital: Houston, TX, USA, 2015.
37. Levine, D.; Lam, C.G.; Cunningham, M.J.; Remke, S.; Chrastek, J.; Klick, J.; Macauley, R.; Baker, J.N. Best practices for pediatric palliative cancer care: A primer for clinical providers. *J. Support. Oncol.* **2013**, *11*, 114–125. [CrossRef] [PubMed]
38. Nitschke, R.; Caldwell, S.; Jay, S. Therapeutic choices in end-stage cancer. *J. Pediatr.* **1986**, *108*, 330–331. [CrossRef]
39. Lyon, M.E.; McCabe, M.A.; Patel, K.M.; D'angelo, L.J. What do adolescents want? An exploratory study regarding end-of-life decision-making. *J. Adolesc. Health* **2004**, *35*, 529.e1–529.e6. [CrossRef] [PubMed]
40. Weaver, M.S.; Baker, J.N.; Gattuso, J.S.; Gibson, D.V.; Sykes, A.D.; Hinds, P.S. Adolescents' preferences for treatment decisional involvement during their cancer. *Cancer* **2015**, *121*, 4416–4424. [CrossRef] [PubMed]
41. Lyon, M.E.; Garvie, P.A.; McCarter, R.; Briggs, L.; He, J.; D'Angelo, L.J. Who will speak for me? Improving end-of-life decision-making for adolescents with HIV and their families. *Pediatrics* **2009**, *123*, e199–e206. [CrossRef] [PubMed]
42. Dallas, R.H.; Kimmel, A.; Wilkins, M.L.; Rana, S.; Garcia, A.; Cheng, Y.I.; Wang, J.; Lyon, M.E. Acceptability of family-centered advanced care planning for adolescents with HIV. *Pediatrics* **2016**, *138*, e20161854. [CrossRef] [PubMed]
43. Madrigal, V.N.; McCabe, B.; Cecchini, C.L.M.E. The respecting choices interview: Qualitative assessment. In Proceedings of the Pediatric Academic Societies Meeting, San Francisco, CA, USA, 6–9 May 2017.
44. Aging with Dignity. Available online: https://www.agingwithdignity.org/shop/product-details/voicing-my-choices (accessed on 8 March 2018).
45. Van der Geest, I.M.M.; van den Heuvel-Eibrink, M.M.; van Vliet, L.M.; Pluijm, S.M.F.; Streng, I.C.; Michiels, E.M.C.; Pieters, R.; Darlington, A.-S.E. Talking about death with children with incurable cancer: Perspectives from parents. *J. Pediatr.* **2015**, *167*, 1320–1326. [CrossRef] [PubMed]
46. Kreicbergs, U.; Valdimarsdóttir, U.; Onelöv, E.; Henter, J.-I.; Steineck, G. Talking about death with children who have severe malignant disease. *N. Engl. J. Med.* **2004**, *351*, 1175–1186. [CrossRef] [PubMed]

47. Kaye, E.C.; Snaman, J.M.; Johnson, L.; Levine, D.; Powell, B.; Love, A.; Smith, J.; Ehrentraut, J.H.; Lyman, J.; Cunningham, M.; et al. Communication with children with cancer and their families throughout the illness journey and at the end-of-life. In *Palliative Care in Pediatric Oncology*; Wolfe, J., Jones, B.L., Kreicbergs, U., Jankovic, M., Eds.; Springer: Berlin, Germany, 2017.
48. Levetown, M. Communicating with children and families: From everyday interactions to skill in conveying distressing information. *Pediatrics* **2008**, *121*, e1441–e1460. [CrossRef] [PubMed]
49. Gaab, E.M.; Owens, G.R.; MacLeod, R.D. Siblings caring for and about pediatric palliative care patients. *J. Palliat. Med.* **2014**, *17*, 62–67. [CrossRef] [PubMed]
50. Eilertsen, M.-E.B.; Eilegård, A.; Steineck, G.; Nyberg, T.; Kreicbergs, U. Impact of social support on bereaved siblings' anxiety. *J. Pediatr. Oncol. Nurs.* **2013**, *30*, 301–310. [CrossRef] [PubMed]
51. Dahlin, C. (Ed.) *Clinical Practice Guidelines for Quality Palliative Care*, 3rd ed.; National Concensus Project for quality palliative care; Hospice and Palliative nurses Association: Pittsburgh, PA, USA, 2013.
52. Moore, A.R.; Bastian, R.G.; Apenteng, B.A. Communication within hospice interdisciplinary teams: A narrative review. *Am. J. Hosp. Palliat. Med.* **2016**, *33*, 996–1012. [CrossRef] [PubMed]
53. Linz, A. *Interdisciplinary Care Team Development for Pediatric Oncology Palliative Treatment*; The University of Oklahoma Health Sciences Center: Oklahoma City, OK, USA, 2016.
54. Fineberg, I.C. Preparing professionals for family conferences in palliative care: Evaluation results of an interdisciplinary approach. *J. Palliat. Med.* **2005**, *8*, 857–866. [CrossRef] [PubMed]
55. Powazki, R.D.; Walsh, D. The Family conference in palliative medicine: A practical approach. *Am. J. Hosp. Palliat. Med.* **2014**, *31*, 678–684. [CrossRef] [PubMed]
56. Powazki, R.D. The family conference in oncology: Benefits for the patient, family, and physician. *Semin. Oncol.* **2011**, *38*, 407–412. [CrossRef] [PubMed]
57. Roth, M.; Wang, D.; Kim, M.; Moody, K. An assessment of the current state of palliative care education in pediatric hematology/oncology fellowship training. *Pediatr. Blood Cancer* **2009**, *53*, 647–651. [CrossRef] [PubMed]
58. Kushner, K.; Meyer, D. Family physicians' perceptions of the family conference. *J. Fam. Pract.* **1989**, *28*, 65–68. [PubMed]

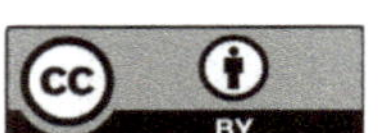

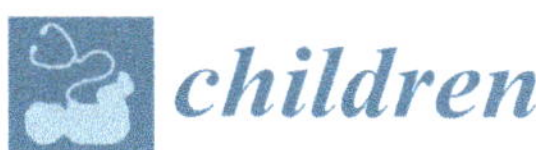

MDPI

Article

Supporting Parent Caregivers of Children with Life-Limiting Illness

Kendra D. Koch * and Barbara L. Jones

Steve Hicks School of Social Work, University of Texas at Austin, 1925 San Jacinto Blvd., D3500, Austin, TX 78712, USA; barbarajones@mail.utexas.edu
* Correspondence: kdkoch@utexas.edu; Tel.: +1-512-475-9367

Received: 6 June 2018; Accepted: 20 June 2018; Published: 26 June 2018

Abstract: The well-being of parents is essential to the well-being of children with life-limiting illness. Parents are vulnerable to a range of negative financial, physical, and psychosocial issues due to caregiving tasks and other stressors related to the illness of their child. Pediatric palliative care practitioners provide good care to children by supporting their parents in decision-making and difficult conversations, by managing pain and other symptoms in the ill child, and by addressing parent and family needs for care coordination, respite, bereavement, and social and emotional support. No matter the design or setting of a pediatric palliative care team, practitioners can seek to provide for parent needs by referral or intervention by the care team.

Keywords: palliative care; special needs; parent; respite; life-limiting illness; caregiver; pediatric; psychosocial; stress; medically complex

---

1. Introduction: Available and Needed Pediatric Palliative Care Services

Pediatric palliative care (PPC) programs typically help children and families with decision-making, communication, psychosocial support, pain and symptom management, and bereavement care [1]. However, as the population of children and families receiving pediatric palliative care services has grown to include those who have life-limiting, complex illnesses, recent research suggests that parents and families may need an expansion of these domains to include care coordination, respite, and education and support for medical complexity [2].

As developments in treatment and technology have led to prolonged life-spans for children with life-threatening, complex, chronic conditions, patients and families have expressed a need for support in the broadest definition of palliative care beyond end-of-life care [2–5]. Pediatric palliative care research and practice has begun to change the emphasis of palliative care articles from end-of-life topics to include more comprehensive topics that cover the span of a child's life, from diagnosis to death, and all the life in between [2,6,7].

The American Academy of Pediatrics (AAP) recommends that patient- and family-centered care is an essential component of good pediatric palliative care practice [8]. Additionally, the International Meeting for Palliative Care in Children, Trento (IMPaCCT) standards developed by the 2006 consensus meeting of health professionals from Europe, Canada, the United States, and Lebanon adopted the stance of the World Health Organization (WHO) that "Palliative care for children is the active total care of the child's body, mind and spirit, and also involves giving support to the family" [9]. In 2015, the professional consensus, "Standards for the Psychosocial Care of Children With Cancer and Their Families" [10] identified pediatric palliative care with an emphasis on care for the family, as one of its 15 essential standards of psychosocial care for children with cancer [11].

Despite consensus, and although increasing in number and scope, Pediatric Palliative Care (PPC) services internationally still do not meet the needs of many pediatric patients. International reviews of palliative care services find that even in countries with the most developed PPC programs, the vast number of children who might benefit never have access to PPC services [12–15].

While all countries have barriers to implementing adequate PPC services, lower- and middle-income countries are disproportionately challenged by lack of medical and financial resources, problems of access, lack of awareness of what PPC services offer, and lack of trained health care and social workers. Proponents of PPC have developed a framework to overcome barriers which includes, (1) working at all levels from health centers to governments to increase advocacy and awareness; (2) educating health care and social work professionals at different levels of expertise from a general approach to a specialist level of pediatric palliative care; (3) continuing to address disparity issues regarding access to medications; (4) implementing and evaluating a range of pediatric palliative care service models to meet differing resource, geographic, cultural, and disease-specific need; and (5) prioritizing pragmatic and translational research that acknowledges the need for culturally- and regionally-specific studies to provide medical and social best practices for providers [12].

Even in more integrated programs, referrals may be more likely to be made at the end-of-life and consider end-of-life concerns from the healthcare provider. Providers using a lifespan philosophy of palliative care would offer more holistic care that is closer to the time of a child's diagnosis of a life-threatening illness [15]. This particular barrier to PPC underscores the need for healthcare providers to not only understand PPC best practices and philosophy, but also to continue to implement and refer to services that are holistic, comprehensive, and timely. Screening instruments may also be used by providers to standardize referrals, increasing the likelihood that patients and families will have the benefit of palliative care support [16].

Depending on the model of the pediatric palliative care service, healthcare professionals may not be able to directly provide needed services for families, however, PPC teams should be prepared to intervene or offer referrals for issues that further stress families, even if they do not seem to be covered by the umbrella of what PPC might typically address. In addition to more typical PPC services, the intent of PPC to prevent and relieve suffering can be best achieved when primary stressors for parent caregivers are addressed, including: (1) care coordination; (2) respite care; (3) peer and emotional support; (4) insurance and employment benefits; and (5) health and related supports [17]. Research outcomes for these five areas support (1) streamlining services and (2) minimizing the effects of caregiving burden. In addition, intervention research emphasizes healthy and intentional collaborations between healthcare professionals and families [17].

2. Parents as Caregivers

Understanding the types of caregiving that parents offer their children may help to guide the types of support a PPC professional might offer. Caregiving can be divided into five basic types of support: instrumental, personal, informational, medical, and emotional [18]. Instrumental, personal, and informational support are social supports. Instrumental caregiving, also known as instrumental activities of daily living (IADL) are those supports that allow a person (in this case a child) to live and engage in community. For example, going to school, driving (or being transported), communication with peers or teachers, or caring for a family pet. Instrumental activities are important to the social well-being of the child. Personal caregiving or personal activities of daily living (also known as habilitation) include those tasks of caregiving that are personal to the child: feeding, personal hygiene, managing incontinence, and dressing are in this category. Informational caregiving is generally managing information, medical or otherwise, for issues that need to be addressed by the person for whom the caregiver is caring. Although, this generally applies to geriatric populations. Medical decision-making, information on diagnosis, care coordination, and other information-specific exchanges might be the pediatric equivalent of this caregiving type. Emotional caregiving is what it seems—it is the care provided to the child to address emotional needs. In the world of children who receive PPC services, emotional care may reflect more specifically a parent's need to address emotions associated with illness, such as sadness, hope, hopelessness, or fear. Finally, Medical supports are fulfilling those tasks associated with medical care, for example: changing a g-tube, tube feeding, suctioning, administering nebulizer treatments, managing a tracheostomy, adhering to a medicine regimen, positioning a child, or monitoring seizure activity [18]. Often overlooked is self-care. Self-care is a factor in caregiving because it promotes that caregivers also prioritize their own care. For many caregivers, this domain is the easiest to overlook. Primary caregivers may react with amusement or anger to suggestions that they care for themselves, because for them the word "care" implies not an affective state, but another task to be wedged in to a regimen of care that may already be full.

Parent caregivers of children with life-limiting illness are expected to assume many roles that extend across physical, emotional, social, and spiritual domains, including, everyday instrumental care provider, medical and financial decision-maker, advocate in education, patient advocate, nurse, relationship manager, care coordinator, communicator, transport service, insurance and financial support manager, and "typical parent" [19,20]. The level at which a care provider gives instrumental care may depend on the course or severity of the child's disease, minimizing or increasing the need for help with tasks like hygiene, dressing, feeding, lifting, and transport [2,19]. A recent Italian study of 33 families who cared for children with life-limiting diseases showed parents spent an average of nine hours a day meeting medical needs [21].

Some tasks are more constant, requiring unaccounted for hours of mental time from caregivers. One of these—medical decision-making—begins at the point of birth and continues throughout the course of the child's illness. The parent is the surrogate decision maker deciding on what treatments the child is to have, what medicines they will take, and which specialists they will see. This is the case whether the child is born healthy developing illness later, as in cancer or some neurodegenerative diseases, or if the child is born with congenital illness. Many parents express that decision-making adds to the burden of care for the child, but that it is an essential role of parenting [22,23]. In addition, complicated family dynamics or familial struggles, sleeplessness, financial or other stress, and pre-existing needs such as poverty may complicate care and decision-making [24]. The medical caregiving role is in addition to and sometimes at odds with the typical parental caregiving for the child because medical caregiving asks the parent to subject their child to difficult and sometimes painful procedures and experiences while the typical parental role is to protect the child from pain and discomfort [25].

Parent caregivers of children with life-limiting illness are vulnerable to negative social, psychological, physical, relational, individual, and financial sequelae. They are more likely to have depressive symptoms [26,27] and more likely to be fatigued, lack vitality, and have problems with sleep than are caregivers of typical children [19,28]. Parents of children with life-limiting illness suffer from social isolation due to caregiving tasks, threat of their child being exposed to pathogens, lack of respite care, and frequent hospitalizations [29]. They are also more likely than parents of typical children to encounter financial problems from healthcare costs and the need to reduce work to meet caregiving demands [19,26,30].

Each family constructs care for their ill child in a way that is unique to their family structure, strengths, and challenges. Caregiving may be both indirect and direct (instrumental), and parents who offer more direct care to the child are at higher risk of personal negative outcomes [26]. Because 90% of primary caregivers of children with chronic or complex needs are mothers [26], it makes sense that mothers of these children, more than fathers, are more often affected by anxiety, depression, pain, and physical health symptoms [31–33]. Pediatric Palliative Care (PPC) standards include caring for both the ill child and their family [1].

Care for the parent in pediatric palliative care has been justified by the ethical imperative of caring for the whole family in pediatric palliative care [34,35]. Although the impact of a child's life-limiting illness on parents is well articulated in the literature [36], providing services that are supportive of parents is sometimes still not well executed, perhaps in practice still being treated as an ancillary or optional part of pediatric palliative care practice [3]. As the child's primary caregivers, parents are a direct and highly influential factor in child wellness and health outcomes, and caring for the parents is essential to caring for the child [1,35].

Ethics and professionally agreed upon consensus statements have provided compelling reasons for professionals to care for families, including parent caregivers. To reinforce this foundation, in addition to offering practical direction for healthcare professionals to provide the best support to parents, this article will articulate how care for the parent directly impacts the ill child. By offering a brief overview of supportive research, this article underscores that caring for the parents of children with life-limiting illness is more than preferred, it is evidence-based and essential and ultimately leads to better outcomes for the ill child.

3. Care for the Parent Directly Impacts the Child

The most pragmatic justification for directly assessing and addressing parental need is in the understanding of the parent-child connection, which is a continual interaction of cognitive, behavioral, and emotional factors designed to protect the child [37]. Because of this connection, children with life-limiting illness may be directly affected by the psychological well-being of their parents. For example, a parent's response to their child's pain may affect the child's experience of that pain [38]. In one study, children whose parents were oriented toward their pain and distress, without being self-oriented (responding out of self-protection to the distress that the child's pain may have caused in the parent) had less observable pain and distress and a more positive disposition during cancer treatments [39]. Similarly, in children with chronic pain, parents who engaged in catastrophic thinking about pain, had children who engaged in greater catastrophizing of pain [40].

Evidence suggests that parents facing consistent and premorbid stressors may experience a neurologic process dominated by the limbic distress response, instead of a more cognitive response of adaptive coping. This means that parents who are already under strain will become more behaviorally distressed in crisis situations, instead of accessing more adaptive and resilient responses [38,41]. As shown previously, this distress response may increase a mirrored response in the child, affecting both emotional and physical outcomes for children with life-limiting illness. Research also suggests that depression among caregivers may lead to difficulty communicating with providers and less satisfaction with medical care [42,43]. It is not only poor mental health that affects children, parent well-being is also associated with increased well-being in siblings of ill children. Studies of posttraumatic growth (positive changes experienced in the face of adversity) show that higher maternal posttraumatic growth levels are associated with fewer behavior problems in siblings [44].

Given the evidence of such strong associations between parent well-being and child well-being, healthcare providers should offer care to parents, not only because it is compassionate, not only because parents have an ethical claim to care, not only to involve parents in decision making and medical education, and not only because including parents in the care schema acknowledges the context in which the child lives, but also because the well-being of parents, who often provide the most instrumental, daily care for the ill child [32,45], directly affects outcomes for the ill child [32,45].

4. What Providers Can Do

4.1. Assessing Parents

The importance of adequate and ongoing assessment that includes assessing the psychosocial needs of the child and their parent caregivers has been established by the Institute of Medicine, the American Cancer Society, the National Comprehensive Cancer Network, the Psychosocial Standards of Care Project for Childhood Cancer (PSCPCC), and the Association of Pediatric Oncology Social Workers [10,36,46–49]. Initial consensus and literature on the topic of parent caregiver assessment (or screening, which is a less comprehensive approach to identifying problems or needs) began in pediatric cancer [36]. More recently, healthcare providers and researchers have observed the increasing number of medically complex children outside of cancer and more typically progressive diseases, and have suggested that both practice and research focus on increasing assessment and evidence-based practice in that population of children and families as well [2,17].

However, although healthcare professionals are aware of the increased physical, emotional, personal, financial, and relational impact on parent caregivers, assessing their distress in these areas is still not standard practice [45]. Four common barriers to professional assessment of parent needs include: (1) inadequate staff funding that leads to lack of time to address clinical needs; (2) staff inexperience with parent/adult engagement, coupled with lack of training on parent engagement; (3) pediatric institutions having an unwillingness to accept parents, who are seen as "adult patients"; and (4) lack of understanding as to how to bill and document parent experience/treatment in the context of pediatric specialist practice [11]. These barriers create large gaps in care, evidenced by a recent study of Children's Oncology Group Institutions, which reported that a meager 9% of institutions used empirically supported psychosocial evaluations, and further, that only 50% of parents received assessments or psychosocial support within the first 30 days of their child's diagnosis [50]. In some cases, there is a need for increased social work and other psychosocial support staffing to meet the needs of both the child and parent.

While some assessment instruments do exist in the domains of caregiver burden, satisfaction with healthcare delivery, caregiver needs, caregiver quality of life, and caregiver distress [45], they are not always specific to parental distress. Additionally, it is difficult for providers to know if instruments are intended for clinical or research purposes [45]. In a recent review of instruments, researchers found 59 instruments that might be useful for assessment of parents of children with chronic or complex illness, however, of those, only 12 were found to be reliable, valid, self-reported, and minimally burdensome (having fewer than 20 items) [45]. Further, research suggests that even when assessments occur, often the interventions that follow may not be evidence-based. In the multi-site study referenced previously, only 11% of the subsequent interventions (post-assessment), were empirically supported [50].

While parental distress may be assessed in pediatric life-limiting illness, that assessment is still not systematic [10,36]. To ameliorate symptoms and support coping, ideally, parental distress screening and assessment would be routine in all pediatric palliative care settings, but this would require adequate staffing, specific and tailored measures, as well as an increased understanding of the direct impact on the child of parental distress and appropriate interventions to effectively lessen that impact [27,36,51].

4.2. Pain and Physical Distress

Parents report that witnessing physical distress and pain in their children is extremely troubling. Parental well-being is closely tied to the needs and suffering of the ill child [52]. Managing pain and physical distress in the child is the most direct way to meet immediate needs for the child and for their parent. Easing symptoms of physical distress and pain in the patient may have the added benefit of reducing psychological distress in the patient and vice versa [38]. Parents often cite pain management as being the aspect of pediatric palliative care that is most important to them [53,54]. Each disease process presents different physical challenges to pediatric palliative care professionals, who broadly assess for symptoms of physical distress including pain, respiratory symptoms of dyspnea or "air hunger," fatigue, spasticity, gastrointestinal problems including constipation and motility issues, issues of positioning, and chronic irritability, especially in neurologically impaired children [55,56].

4.3. Communication

Second only to pain and symptom control, parents express that good communication is the most highly prioritized aspect of pediatric palliative care [57–59]. Compassionate and effective communication has the potential to foster trusting relationships, provide anticipatory guidance, offer information, support emotions, manage uncertainty, assist in decision-making, and enable patient and family self-management [35,55,60,61].

Throughout their child's life, parents of children with life-threatening illness are asked to understand masses of information, assimilate difficult news, and make decisions based on communication with their child's healthcare team. Parents want to be able to hear information in a manner that allows them to trust the content that they are receiving from their child's team. Parental trust is increased when information and discussion is presented in ways that are accessible and helpful to parents. Communication is made of content (*what* is being communicated) and manner (*how* the content is being communicated). The manner of communication includes the tone, language, style, and cultural sensitivity with which the content is conveyed [61]. Professionals may attend to both the what and the how by focusing on these areas: timeliness (of test results, labs), language (using credentialed interpreters if needed), style (i.e., directive versus non-directive), and intricacies in communication like respect (calling an infant by name), or cultural humility (avoiding the use of culturally-bound metaphors and acknowledging cultural norms of patient and family) [61].

Each family will have specific preferences for the style of communication and amount of information they would prefer to receive. Some parents want limited information, finding certain types of information upsetting or reducing hopefulness. However, most parents express that they want more medical information [62] about their child's illness, not less [63,64]. For these parents, information may help them to cope and regain a sense of control, reducing the uncertainty of the situation. Still, it is important to work with the family to understand their preferred communication style and timing. Healthcare professionals can ask parents, "How would you like information shared? All at once? A little at a time?" "Who needs to be here when we communicate?" "How should we talk with your child?" [55,61,65].

Anticipatory guidance relies on communication to describe future symptoms or conditions that may develop as part of the child's illness. Depending on the illness and its trajectory, the content of each guiding conversation is different. For instance, parents of a non-ambulatory child with static encephalopathy who is at far greater risk of developing recurrent aspiration pneumonia will require different anticipatory guidance than parents whose child has cancer with a poor prognosis [66]. Information regarding potential risks, probable outcome, and choices for treatment are all areas to be explored. In the instance of a child with static encephalopathy, the parents might be told that their child is at risk of recurrent infection from aspiration, opening the discussion to the parents' wishes for future use of medical technology and their values and goals [61]. PPC practitioners understand that communication is often not one conversation, but many. As with all of pediatric palliative care, anticipatory guidance is more than a medical issue, it encompasses social-emotional and spiritual domains of care as well; acknowledging this, Klick and Hauer (2010) offer brief phrases that help PPC to assess for needs and guide discussions with parents and patients, "Who do you use for support?" "Are you able to do the things that you enjoy doing?" "What are the challenges getting through each day?" and, "Do you have a faith or spiritual belief that brings you support?" [67].

Practitioner attunement to the child and family is a critical component of PPC and can enhance delivery of PPC services. Davies et al. recommend that healthcare practitioners attune to the patient and family's situation using six techniques: (1) *orienting* to all of the observable factors present in a conversation, from the state of mind of the practitioner, to the situation of the patient and family; (2) *seeking parents' perspectives* by providing space and asking questions such as, "What do you understand about the illness?" "What supports do you have?" or "What is the thing that you are most afraid of?" (3) *discerning* by observing and listening to parent responses and nonverbal cues to determine how best to approach the conversation and what is most important to them; (4) *shaping* a thoughtful response that considers the parents' states of mind and takes the most salient concerns of the parents to plan direct care activities; (5) *checking* by evaluating the effectiveness of an intervention, or by following up on promises to check back later or find out more information for parents; and (6) *reflecting* by purposefully and objectively considering their interactions with patients and families, their responses, attitudes, worldview, and behavior, noting opportunities to better attune and to find meaning in their experiences [68].

Communication must remain an ongoing and dialogical process that acknowledges that a parents' way of thinking about their child's care may change over time. End-of-life and care transition conversations especially are directly related to the child's health status, symptoms, and quality of life, thus requiring healthcare professionals to reassess the health status of their patient, the needs of the family, and the type of communication needed to address each. Although different in content, each of these conversations require that the PPC clinician uses a team approach, enlisting interdisciplinary expertise to exchange information, promote anticipatory guidance, respond to child- and- family emotions, make decisions (including managing uncertainty and decisional regret), and enable patient and family self-management.

4.4. Decision Making

Decision-making support is the backbone of pediatric palliative care services. Historically, PPC has focused on end-of-life decision-making. Although this trend is changing, often research about parent decision-making for children with life-limiting illness is still overwhelmingly focused on end-of-life. As the field continues to grow and children with life-limiting illness continue to live longer, healthcare professionals can acknowledge the need for continued assessment, treatment, and referral to address the needs of parents of patients who may have illnesses that span decades. These parents engage with decision-making (DM) that often includes considering mundane, everyday questions not related to end-of-life conversations or processing a new illness status or diagnosis.

Practitioners may support parental decision making by considering these factors when guiding parents: (1) the complex and different roles that clinicians and parents have in the decision making process; (2) the parent's changing understanding of the child as someone with a future and on whom now-unmet expectations have been placed; (3) that diagnosis of a life-limiting or life-threatening condition is an assault on the life of the family; (4) that for the sake of the family and preserving and maintaining normalcy, parents tend to push against the intrusion of the disease in everyday life; (5) that an individual's and parent's view of illness changes over time; (6) that parents use information in ways that clinician's may not expect; and (7) that parent's and clinicians may view the child differently [69].

Parents generally desire to be involved in decision-making for their children [63,70–77]. This is not changed by a parents' experiencing decisional regret or guilt, in fact, parents may experience both whether they were the primary decision-maker or not [72,78]. There are, of course, exceptions to this—rarely, parents prefer that the physician or medical team be the decision-makers [78–80].

Parents view their child-focused decision making as part of "being a good parent" [63,81]. Their self-concept as expert, advocate, and protector for the child make their involvement in DM imperative [76,82]. Despite developments in decision-making ethic that promotes patient and parent autonomy as the primary concepts in decision-making practice, parents report barriers to implementation of decision-making that values their choices. Findings suggest that healthcare professionals (especially, physicians) hold values and goals for the ill child that may be at odds or discordant to those held by parents [62,83]. Further, parents sometimes felt that they had not been involved in even life-and-death decisions at all [78–80,82]. In some circumstances, parents felt like they were involved, but given such limited information or choice, that they had only one choice, or the decision was all-but-made for them [22,78,79,84]. Although, at least in principle, medical ethic and discourse have embraced autonomous choice, most parents actually prefer some level of shared or collaborative decision making. They want to be able to talk with healthcare providers and make a decision with them [71,72,85–88].

Whatever the information conveyed from the PPC practitioner, parents need and want information that allows them to make the decisions they feel will be best for the child [63]. Even if it is unpleasant, parents prefer the truth. Parents want the truth presented in ways that they can understand and that "leave room" for hope [64,89,90]. Truth telling is not only the preference of parents, it is a moral imperative. At times when telling the truth is difficult, PPC practitioners can consult with team members for support and remember that telling parents the truth gives them the information that they need to make the best decisions they can for their ill child [64,89]. Practitioners should also remember that they are part of a team and draw on the strengths of the team to support themselves and the family, conveying to parents that, "no matter what comes next, we will be here for you and your child" [35].

Healthcare professionals and families alike may find decision-making (DM) tools (or "Decision Aids," DA) such as the "Ottawa Family Decision Guide" [91] or the "Caring for Health: Child Tracheostomy Decision Guide" [92] to be helpful when making a decision that can be aided by a benefits and burdens paradigm. These DM tools may allow parents and their healthcare team to consider questions in a systematic way that leads to a broader and richer discussion between the PPC team and parents.

4.5. Care Coordination

Although most often associated with primary care or medical home models, care coordination should exist wherever pediatric patients receive care. The vulnerability of children, their "developmental trajectory, dependency on adults, differential epidemiology of chronic disease, demographic patterns of poverty and diversity, and overall dollars" heightens their need for well-coordinated care [93]. A recent study of 735 parents with medically complex children ranked care coordination as one of the top two most challenging areas for parent caregivers [94]. The greatest challenges to care coordination in complex pediatric populations is in poor communication between services and providers [95].

Because PPC teams differ in processes, roles represented, and settings, it is difficult to prescribe one particular method to address care coordination in practice. However, Klick and Hauer suggest that the primary objectives for PPC practitioners addressing care coordination might be (1) collaborating with specialists; (2) identifying resources and partnering with community programs; (3) identifying financial resources and payment mechanisms; and (4) partnering with school programs [67]. The second and third items assume that adequate screening and assessment have been completed to inform the practitioner of the needs and challenges faced by the patient and family [36]. Care coordination is as unique to each family as communication and other palliative care tasks. It should not be limited to providing the same list of generic referrals or general suggestions to every family.

The care coordinator within a PPC team may be filled successfully by any number disciplines, although social worker, nurse, or nurse practitioner are the most commonly represented [96–98]. PPC teams may review resources by considering what types of patients need the most care coordination, and at what times. PPC teams may anticipate care coordination needs by reviewing the characteristics of their population of patients with the understanding that different populations of patients often have different types of needs. One study found shorter but more intensive needs for patients with malignant disease, when compared to patients with non-malignant disease who needed more hours of management and coordination overall, but spread over a much longer period of time [99]. Whatever their discipline, the presence of care coordinators is a particular support to parent caregivers and has been associated with reduced parental stress and increased caregiver satisfaction [94,100,101].

4.6. Respite Care

Parents of children with life-threatening illness need occasional respite from caregiving [26]. Even if it is only a few hours at a time, breaks from direct (instrumental) care help increase parents' quality of life (QOL) and stem burnout, including symptoms of fatigue, psychological adjustment, depression, and anxiety in parent caregivers [102,103]. Children with PPC needs suffer from a range of diagnoses which present varied trajectories of illness, even within the same diagnosis. The unpredictability of these trajectories means that parent caregivers need consistent respite care on which they can rely. Access to respite varies with family resources. Some government programs pay for respite services, some do not. Some families have larger groups of family or friends from which to pull. Some diagnoses are easier to manage without nursing care or medical knowledge. Parents do report that often it is difficult to find trustworthy respite workers and that having respite at the cost of not knowing or fully trusting the worker who is with your ill child is worse than having no respite at all [104].

PPC professionals should ask about parental needs for respite, before parents show signs of burnout, exhaustion, or fatigue. Small and consistent doses of rest throughout the trajectory of illness allow parents to process and adjust in small increments, instead of trying to recover from physical and emotional exhaustion. If parents are open to finding respite resources, PPC teams should have resources and referral information ready to give to parents and should help parents access resources, if needed [105].

4.7. Social and Emotional Support

Parents of children with life-threatening illness have a range of social and emotional needs stemming from an array of feelings, emotional overwhelm, and high levels of stress. The emotional outcomes found in research literature include anxiety and depressive symptoms, guilt, stress, fear, varying degrees of uncertainty and disbelief, denial, powerlessness, anger, sadness, and anticipatory and realized grief [11,21,105].

Psychological interventions aimed at parental distress in PPC cancer settings are still emerging, with studies that are limited by small numbers and lack of appropriate controls [11]. However, among reviewed interventions, several do stand out as offering hopeful outcomes: Problem Solving Skills Training (PSST) has been shown to be effective in reducing negative affect in mothers of children newly diagnosed with cancer [11]. Progressive Muscle Relaxation and Guided Imagery Techniques have both been shown to reduce anxiety and improve mood in parents of children with cancer [106]. When it is available, families are open to information that helps them lessen their own psychological and emotional concerns [107]. Interventions that offer psychoeducation and promote the well-being of the caregiver have some protective effect in limiting increases in distress [17]. These interventions included both face-to-face check-ins as well as interventions that used phone calls, with no face-to-face engagement [17].

Because a lack of social support has been associated with higher levels of distress, psychological morbidity, and post-traumatic stress disorder (PTSD) [108,109], and because increased community and peer social support have been shown to ameliorate distress in parents, it may be beneficial for PPC practitioners to facilitate channels of personal and systems engagement between parents of ill children and community organizations or peer support [108].

Research shows that caregivers' growth in relationships with others during difficult times is likely to have effects on family members, the ill child, and on the caregiver [44,110]. Relationship-focused coping strategies may be helpful to maintain and build relationships during periods of stress. Using these strategies, parents can be encouraged to consider the responses of others involved in care, while being given the reassurance that both similar and dissimilar (complementary) coping styles may exist and be helpful in parent dyads [111]. Relationship-focused coping includes activities such as, putting yourself "in someone else's shoes," active listening, trying to understand how someone else feels, finding equitable solutions, displays of positive feelings, and promoting empathy in relationships. These activities allow caregivers to nurture and sustain relationships, while reducing threat and defensiveness in stressful times [112]. Because of pre-existing socio-ecological issues, PPC services alone may be unable to address the social and emotional needs of parents [108]. However, it has been suggested that it is not necessarily an "intervention" that decreases distress for caregivers, but the practice of good pediatric palliative care that includes the previously-mentioned treatment of symptoms (in the patient), good communication, care coordination, and decision-making support that affect psychological outcomes for parents in PPC settings [108]. By practicing optimal PPC, practitioners help to decrease the likelihood of further deterioration in the parent and decrease the likelihood of further parental stress from poor communication, uncertainty or regret in decision-making, or distress from witnessing the suffering of a child.

5. Modeling Self Care through Reflective Practice

In order to offer the most compassionate care to parental caregivers, healthcare practitioners must engage in reflective practice, acknowledge that providing care to children with life-limiting conditions and their families is emotionally taxing, and practice intentional self-care and self-compassion.

Caring for children who are suffering and their families can naturally lead to a sense of personal struggle and distress often referred to as burnout, compassion fatigue, or secondary traumatic stress [113]. Moral distress can occur for practitioners when they witness patient suffering and when they cannot alleviate that suffering. Moral distress is more common for practitioners delivering direct patient care in acute situations and can be a leading cause of burnout and staff turnover [114].

While it is commonly understood that caring for those who are suffering can lead to distress, how to prevent this is less studied [113]. Self-care and self-compassion are critical skills for the pediatric palliative care practitioner. Strategies that can assist include focusing on work-life balance, identifying a sense of meaning, and developing personal skills that help manage the stress [113]. It is expected that pediatric palliative care practitioners will experience struggle, but the key to managing this is to first engage in reflective practice. This self-reflection and self-care is not only preventative for the practitioners but can serve as a model for family caregivers about the critical importance of self-compassion and care. Institutional solutions in pediatric palliative care that can alleviate suffering include education about compassion fatigue and moral distress, on-site support, debriefing and support groups, mentorship, high functioning interdisciplinary teams, adequate staffing, bereavement, and memorials [113,115]. A recent study found that it can be helpful when pediatric palliative care teams are able to offer each other respect, nonjudgmental validation, and open communication [116]. Reflective practice is important not only to PPC providers, but also to parents. By watching PPC practitioners take time and space for themselves, parents may be inspired to seek out opportunities that promote wellness and caring for self, as well.

6. Bereavement

Sometimes bereavement is confused with grief. Grief is "primarily the emotional (affective) reaction to the loss of a loved one through death. It is a normal, natural reaction to loss" [117], while bereavement is a "broad term that encompasses the entire experience of family members and friends in the anticipation, death and subsequent adjustment to living following the death of a loved one" [118]. Parents who have lost their child to death experience a number of symptoms that, although negative, may be normal parts of bereavement, including: depression, anxiety, grief, guilt, and/or existential or spiritual distress [119,120]. These symptoms may persist over long periods of time [119], and affected mothers are at risk for poorer bereavement outcomes [121].

PPC professionals understand the need for services that address the psychosocial and emotional domains of bereavement, but PPC professionals should remember that bereavement also includes "the adjustment to living" after the death of a loved one. This adjustment may also include changes in health, relationships, and finances [122–126]. After a simple screening, PPC professionals should be prepared to advise and refer parents to appropriate services to receive further assessment and to address needs in these areas [127]. Instruments such as the Bereavement Risk Index or the Prolonged Grief Inventory may be used to assess for grieving that may need intervention or referral from the PPC team to more appropriate, long-term professional help.

Parents and other bereaved family members may grieve for years without complication, but for a subset of parents and other family members the grief can be unrelenting and problematic. Signs of post-traumatic stress disorder (PTSD) (i.e., intrusive memories, avoidance of reminders, negative alterations in cognitions and mood, and marked alterations in arousal and reactivity) [128], or grief that does not subside in intensity and focus over time should alert healthcare professionals that mental health intervention is needed [129,130].

In general, parents indicate that they want and appreciate follow-up by their child's healthcare team during bereavement [131]. The "Standards for the Psychosocial Care of Children with Cancer and Their Families" proposes that "A member of the healthcare team should contact the family after a child's death to assess family needs, to identify those at risk for negative psychosocial sequelae, to continue care, and to provide resources for bereavement support" [131].

There is very little research currently available demonstrating effectiveness of intervention measures for bereaved parents and siblings. A recent review found of 129 studies retrieved for full screening, only eight were rigorous and comparative studies. More well-designed randomized controlled trials are needed to present practitioners with effective interventions for bereaved parents [132].

7. Conclusions

Optimal pediatric palliative care includes care for both the child and the family. The well-being of children depends in large part on their parents' well-being. The presence and involvement of parents in every aspect of their child's care is essential to good care. The role of parents as primary caregivers to the ill child means that parents and practitioners are partners in decisions of care, and that information about the ill child should be provided for the parents and for the ill child. Therefore, care for parents can reduce the distress of both the parental caregiver and the child with life limiting illness. Even if it is in referral, PPC should meet the needs of its expanding complex chronic illness population by more broadly assessing for/meeting family needs. Parents are a critical component of a child's well-being and the PPC interdisciplinary team should strive to provide routine psychosocial assessment, evidence-based interventions, shared decision-making, organized respite, and attention to distress for all parental caregivers. In so doing, PPC meets its goals of caring for the child in their primary context—in their family.

Author Contributions: K.D.K. and B.L.J. have each contributed substantially to the conception, literature review, writing, citing, and editing of this work.

Funding: This research received no external funding.

Conflicts of Interest: The authors declare no conflict of interest.

References

1. Weaver, M.; Heinze, K.; Bell, C. Establishing psychosocial palliative care standards for children and adolescents with cancer and their families: An integrative review. *Palliat. Med.* **2016**, *30*, 212–223. [CrossRef] [PubMed]
2. Cohen, E.; Kuo, D.; Agrawal, R.; Berry, J.G.; Bhagat, S.K.M.; Simon, T.D.; Srivastava, R. Children with medical complexity: An emerging population for clinical research initiatives. *Pediatrics* **2011**, *127*, 529–538. [CrossRef] [PubMed]
3. De Clercq, E.; Rost, M.; Pacurari, N.; Elger, B.S.; Wangmo, T. Aligning guidelines and medical practice: Literature review on pediatric palliative care guidelines. *Palliat. Support. Care* **2017**, *15*, 474–489. [CrossRef] [PubMed]
4. Msall, M.; Tremont, M. Measuring functional outcomes after prematurity: Developmental impact of very low birth weight and extremely low birth weight status on childhood disability. *Ment. Retard. Dev. Disabil. Res. Rev.* **2002**, *8*, 258–272. [CrossRef] [PubMed]
5. Tennant, P.; Pearce, M.; Bythell, M.; Rankin, J. 20-Year survival of children born with congenital anomalies: A population-based study. *Lancet* **2010**, *375*, 649–656. [CrossRef]
6. DeCourcey, D.D.; Silverman, M.; Oladunjoye, A.; Balkin, E.M.; Wolfe, J. Patterns of Care at the End of Life for Children and Young Adults with Life-Threatening Complex Chronic Conditions. *J. Pediatr.* **2018**, *193*, 196.e2–203.e2. [CrossRef] [PubMed]
7. Hunt, A.; Coad, J.; West, E.; Hex, N.; Staniszewska, S.; Hacking, S.; Farman, M.; Brown, E.; Owens, C.; Ashley, N.; et al. *The BiG Study for Life-Limited Children and Their Families*; Kelly, K., Woodhead, S., Eds.; Together for Short Lives: Bristol, UK, 2013; Available online: http://clok.uclan.ac.uk/8951/2/TfSL_The_Big_Study_Final_Research_Report__WEB_.pdf (accessed on 4 June 2018).
8. American Academy of Pediatrics (AAP). Pediatric palliative care and hospice care commitments, guidelines, and recommendations. *Pediatrics* **2013**, *132*, 966–972.
9. Craig, F.; Abu-Saad Huijer, H.; Benini, F.; Kuttner, L.; Wood, C.; Feraris, P.C.; Zernikow, B. IMPaCCT: Standards of paediatric palliative care. *Schmerz* **2008**, *22*, 401–408. [CrossRef] [PubMed]

10. Wiener, L.; Kazak, A.E.; Noll, R.B.; Patenaude, A.F.; Kupst, M.J. Standards for the Psychosocial Care of Children with Cancer and Their Families: An Introduction to the Special Issue: Pediatric Psychosocial Standards of Care. *Pediatr. Blood Cancer* **2015**, *62* (Suppl. 5), S419–S424. [CrossRef] [PubMed]
11. Kearney, J.A.; Salley, C.G.; Muriel, A.C. Standards of Psychosocial Care for Parents of Children with Cancer. *Pediatr. Blood Cancer* **2015**, *62* (Suppl. 5), S632–S683. [CrossRef] [PubMed]
12. Downing, J.; Boucher, S.; Daniels, A.; Nkosi, B. Paediatric Palliative Care in Resource-Poor Countries. *Children* **2018**, *5*, 27. [CrossRef] [PubMed]
13. Knapp, C.; Woodworth, L.; Wright, M.; Downing, J.; Drake, R.; Fowler-Kerry, S.; Hain, R.; Marston, J. Pediatric palliative care provision around the world: A systematic review. *Pediatr. Blood Cancer* **2011**, *57*, 361–368. [CrossRef] [PubMed]
14. Knapp, C.; Sberna-Hinojosa, M.; Baron-Lee, J.; Curtis, C.; Huang, I.C. Does decisional conflict differ across race and ethnicity groups? A study of parents whose children have a life-threatening illness. *J. Palliat. Med.* **2014**, *17*, 559–567. [CrossRef] [PubMed]
15. Twamley, K.; Craig, F.; Kelly, P.; Hollowell, D.R.; Mendoza, P.; Bluebond-Langner, M. Underlying barriers to referral to paediatric palliative care services: Knowledge and attitudes of health care professionals in a paediatric tertiary care centre in the United Kingdom. *J. Child Health Care* **2014**, *18*, 19–30. [CrossRef] [PubMed]
16. Bergstraesser, E.; Hain, R.D.; Pereira, J.L. The development of an instrument that can identify children with palliative care needs: The Paediatric Palliative Screening Scale (PaPaS Scale): A qualitative study approach. *BMC Palliat. Care* **2013**, *12*, 20. [CrossRef] [PubMed]
17. Edelstein, H.; Schippke, J.; Sheffe, S.; Kingsnorth, S. Children with medical complexity: A scoping review of interventions to support caregiver stress. *Child Care Health Dev.* **2017**, *43*, 323–333. [CrossRef] [PubMed]
18. Seeman, T. Support & Social Conflict: Section One-Social Support. MacArthur SES & Health Network. Available online: http://www.macses.ucsf.edu/research/psychosocial/socsupp.php (accessed on 4 June 2018).
19. Caicedo, C. Families with Special Needs Children: Family Health, Functioning, and Care Burden. *J. Am. Psychiatr. Nurses Assoc.* **2014**, *20*, 398–407. [CrossRef] [PubMed]
20. National Cancer Institute (NCI). Family Caregivers in Cancer: Roles and Challenges (PDQ®)-Health Professional Version. 2017. Available online: https://www.cancer.gov/about-cancer/coping/family-friends/family-caregivers-hp-pdq (accessed on 8 March 2018).
21. Lazzarin, P.; Schiavon, B.; Brugnaro, L.; Benini, F. Parents spend an average of nine hours a day providing palliative care for children at home and need to maintain an average of five life-saving devices. *Acta Paediatr.* **2018**, *107*, 289–293. [CrossRef] [PubMed]
22. Brotherton, A.; Abbott, J. Mothers' process of decision making for gastrostomy placement. *Qual. Health Res.* **2012**, *22*, 587–594. [CrossRef] [PubMed]
23. Hellmann, J.; Williams, C.; Ives-Baine, L.; Shah, P.S. Withdrawal of artificial nutrition and hydration in the neonatal intensive care unit: Parental perspectives. *Arch. Dis. Child. Fetal Neonatal Ed.* **2013**, *98*, F21–F25. [CrossRef] [PubMed]
24. Siminoff, L.A.; Rose, J.H.; Zhang, A.; Zyzanski, S.J. Measuring discord in treatment decision-making; Progress toward development of a cancer communication and decision-making assessment tool. *Psycho-Oncology* **2006**, *15*, 528–540. [CrossRef] [PubMed]
25. Jones, B.L. The challenge of quality care for family caregivers in pediatric cancer care. *Semin. Oncol. Nurs.* **2012**, *28*, 213–220. [CrossRef] [PubMed]
26. Brehaut, J.C.; Garner, R.E.; Miller, A.R.; Lach, L.M.; Klassen, A.F.; Rosenbaum, P.L.; Kohen, D.E. Changes over time in the health of caregivers of children with health problems: Growth-curve findings from a 10-year Canadian population-based study. *Am. J. Public Health* **2011**, *101*, 2308–2316. [CrossRef] [PubMed]
27. Steele, A.C.; Mullins, L.L.; Mullins, A.J.; Muriel, A.C. Psychosocial Interventions and Therapeutic Support as a Standard of Care in Pediatric Oncology: Psychosocial Interventions and Therapeutic Support. *Pediatr. Blood Cancer* **2015**, *62* (Suppl. 5), S585–S618. [CrossRef] [PubMed]
28. Hatzmann, J.; Heymans, H.S.; Ferrer-I-Carbonell, A.; Van Praag, B.M.; Grootenhuis, M.A. Hidden Consequences of Success in Pediatrics: Parental Health-Related Quality of Life—Results from the Care Project. *Pediatrics* **2008**, *122*, e1030–e1038. [CrossRef] [PubMed]

29. Collins, A.; Hennessy-Anderson, N.; Hosking, S.; Hynson, J.; Remedios, C.; Thomas, K. Lived experiences of parents caring for a child with a life-limiting condition in Australia: A qualitative study. *Palliat. Med.* **2016**, *30*, 950–959. [CrossRef] [PubMed]
30. Bona, K.; Dussel, V.; Orellana, L.; Kang, T.; Geyer, R.; Feudtner, C.; Wolfe, J. Economic Impact of Advanced Pediatric Cancer on Families. *J. Pain Symptom Manag.* **2014**, *47*, 594–603. [CrossRef] [PubMed]
31. Brehaut, J.C.; Kohen, D.E.; Raina, P.; Walter, S.D.; Russell, D.J.; Swinton, M.; O'Donnell, M.; Rosenbaum, P. The health of primary caregivers of children with cerebral palsy: How does it compare with other Canadian caregivers. *Pediatrics* **2004**, *114*, e182–e191. [CrossRef] [PubMed]
32. Brehaut, J.C.; Kohen, D.E.; Garner, R.E.; Miller, A.R.; Lach, L.M.; Klassen, A.F.; Rosenbaum, P.L. Health Among Caregivers of Children with Health Problems: Findings from a Canadian Population-Based Study. *Am. J. Public Health* **2009**, *99*, 1254–1262. [CrossRef] [PubMed]
33. Clarke, N.E.; McCarthy, M.C.; Downie, P.; Ashley, D.M.; Anderson, V.A. Gender differences in the psychosocial experience of parents of children with cancer: A review of the literature. *Psycho-Oncology* **2009**, *18*, 907–915. [CrossRef] [PubMed]
34. Field, M.; Behrman, R. *When Children Die: Improving Palliative and End-of-Life Care for Children and Their Families*; Institute of Medicine, Committee on Palliative and End-of-Life Care for Children and Their Families: Washington, DC, USA, 2004.
35. Jones, B.L.; Contro, N.; Koch, K.D. The duty of physicians to care for the family in pediatric palliative care: Context, communication, and caring. *Pediatrics* **2014**, *133* (Suppl. 1), S8–S15. [CrossRef] [PubMed]
36. Kazak, A.E.; Abrams, A.N.; Banks, J.; Christofferson, J.; DiDonato, S.; Grootenhuis, M.A.; Kabour, M.; Madan-Swain, A.; Patel, S.K.; Zadeh, S.; et al. Psychosocial Assessment as a Standard of Care in Pediatric Cancer: Psychosocial Assessment Standard. *Pediatr. Blood Cancer* **2015**, *62* (Suppl. 5), S426–S459. [CrossRef] [PubMed]
37. Kearney, J.A.; Byrne, M.W. Understanding parental behavior in pediatric palliative care: Attachment theory as a paradigm. *Palliat. Support. Care* **2015**, *13*, 1559–1568. [CrossRef] [PubMed]
38. Simons, L.E.; Goubert, L.; Vervoort, T.; Borsook, D. Circles of engagement: Childhood pain and parent brain. *Neurosci. Biobehav. Rev.* **2016**, *68* (Suppl. C), 537–546. [CrossRef] [PubMed]
39. Harper, F.W.K.; Penner, L.A.; Peterson, A.; Albrecht, T.L.; Taub, J. Children's Positive Dispositional Attributes, Parents' Empathic Responses, and Children's Responses to Painful Pediatric Oncology Treatment Procedures. *J. Psychosoc. Oncol.* **2012**, *30*, 593–613. [CrossRef] [PubMed]
40. Lynch, S.H.; Lobo, M.L. Compassion fatigue in family caregivers: A Wilsonian concept analysis. *J. Adv. Nurs.* **2012**, *68*, 2125–2134. [CrossRef] [PubMed]
41. Vogel, S.; Klumpers, F.; Krugers, H.J.; Fang, Z.; Oplaat, K.T.; Oitzl, M.S.; Joëls, M.; Fernández, G. Blocking the mineralocorticoid receptor in humans prevents the stress-induced enhancement of centromedial amygdala connectivity with the dorsal striatum. *Neuropsychopharmacology* **2015**, *40*, 947–956. [CrossRef] [PubMed]
42. Fagnano, M.; Berkman, E.; Wiesenthal, E.; Butz, A.; Halterman, J.S. Depression among caregivers of children with asthma and its impact on communication with health care providers. *Public Health* **2012**, *126*, 1051–1057. [CrossRef] [PubMed]
43. Gonzalez, A.V.; Siegel, J.T.; Alvaro, E.M.; O'Brien, E.K. The Effect of Depression on Physician–Patient Communication among Hispanic End-Stage Renal Disease Patients. *J. Health Commun.* **2013**, *18*, 485–497. [CrossRef] [PubMed]
44. Stephenson, E.; DeLongis, A.; Steele, R.; Cadell, S.; Andrews, G.S.; Siden, H. Siblings of Children with a Complex Chronic Health Condition: Maternal Posttraumatic Growth as a Predictor of Changes in Child Behavior Problems. *J. Pediatr. Psychol.* **2017**, *42*, 104–113. [CrossRef] [PubMed]
45. Tanco, K.; Park, J.C.; Cerana, A.; Sisson, A.; Sobti, N.; Bruera, E. A systematic review of instruments assessing dimensions of distress among caregivers of adult and pediatric cancer patients. *Palliat. Support. Care* **2017**, *15*, 110–124. [CrossRef] [PubMed]
46. Adler, N.E.; Page, A. *Cancer Care for the Whole Patient: Meeting Psychosocial Health Needs*; National Academies Press: Washington, DC, USA, 2008.
47. APOSW. Standards of Practice. Professional Resources. 2009. Available online: http://www.aposw.org/html/standards.php (accessed on 10 March 2018).

48. Arceci, R.; Ettinger, A.; Forman, E.; Haase, G.M.; Hammond, G.D.; Hoffman, R.; Kupst, M.J.; Link, M.P.; Lustig, C.P.; Traynor, D.S. National Action Plan for Childhood Cancer: Report of the National Summit Meetings on Childhood Cancer. *CA Cancer J. Clin.* **2002**, *52*, 377–379. [CrossRef] [PubMed]
49. National Comprehensive Cancer Network (NCCN). Distress management clinical practice guidelines. *J. Natl. Compr. Cancer Netw.* **2003**, *1*, 344–374.
50. Selove, R.; Kroll, T.; Coppes, M.; Cheng, Y. Psychosocial services in the first 30 days after diagnosis: Results of a web-based survey of Children's Oncology Group (COG) member institutions. *Pediatr. Blood Cancer* **2012**, *58*, 435–440. [CrossRef] [PubMed]
51. Feudtner, C.; Carroll, K.W.; Hexem, K.R.; Silberman, J.; Kang, T.I.; Kazak, A.E. Parental hopeful patterns of thinking, emotions, and pediatric palliative care decision making: A prospective cohort study. *Arch. Pediatr. Adolesc. Med.* **2010**, *164*, 831–839. [CrossRef] [PubMed]
52. Muscara, F.; McCarthy, M.C.; Thompson, E.J.; Heaney, C.M.; Hearps, S.J.C.; Rayner, M.; Burke, K.; Nicholson, J.M.; Anderson, V.A. Psychosocial, Demographic, and Illness-Related Factors Associated with Acute Traumatic Stress Responses in Parents of Children with a Serious Illness or Injury. *J. Trauma. Stress* **2017**, *30*, 237–244. [CrossRef] [PubMed]
53. Pritchard, M.; Burghen, E.; Srivastava, D.K.; Okuma, J.; Anderson, L.; Powell, B.; Furman, W.L.; Hinds, P.S. Cancer-Related Symptoms Most Concerning to Parents During the Last Week and Last Day of Their Child's Life. *Pediatrics* **2008**, *121*, e1301–e1309. [CrossRef] [PubMed]
54. Vollenbroich, R.; Borasio, G.D.; Duroux, A.; Grasser, M.; Brandstätter, M.; Führer, M. Listening to parents: The role of symptom perception in pediatric palliative home care. *Palliat. Support. Care* **2016**, *14*, 13–17. [CrossRef] [PubMed]
55. Hauer, J.M.; Wolfe, J. Supportive and palliative care of children with metabolic and neurological diseases. *Curr. Opin. Support. Palliat. Care* **2014**, *8*, 296–302. [CrossRef] [PubMed]
56. Wolfe, J.; Klar, N.; Grier, H.E.; Duncan, J.; Salem-Schatz, S.; Emanuel, E.J.; Weeks, J.C. Understanding of prognosis among parents of children who died of cancer: Impact on treatment goals and integration of palliative care. *JAMA* **2000**, *284*, 2469–2475. [CrossRef] [PubMed]
57. Contro, N.; Larson, J.; Scofield, S.; Sourkes, B.; Cohen, H. Family perspectives on the quality of pediatric palliative care. *Arch. Pediatr. Adolesc. Med.* **2002**, *156*, 14–19. [CrossRef] [PubMed]
58. Davies, B.; Conaughty, S. Pediatric end-of-life care: Lessons learned from parents. *J. Nurs. Adm.* **2002**, *32*, 5–7. [CrossRef] [PubMed]
59. Hinds, P.S.; Oakes, L.L.; Hicks, J.; Powell, B.; Srivastava, D.K.; Spunt, S.L.; Harper, J.; Baker, J.N.; West, N.K.; Furman, W.L. "Trying to be a good parent" as defined by interviews of parents who made phase I, terminal care, and resuscitation decisions for their child. *J. Clin. Oncol.* **2009**, *27*, 5979–5985. [CrossRef] [PubMed]
60. Epstein, R.M.; Street, R.L., Jr.; National Cancer Institute. *Patient-Centered Communication in Cancer Care: Promoting Healing and Reducing Suffering*; National Cancer Institute, U.S. Department of Health and Human Services, National Institutes of Health: Bethesda, MD, USA, 2007.
61. Jones, B.L.; Koch, K.D. Neonatal and pediatrics. In *Oxford Textbook of Palliative Care Communication*; Wittenberg, E., Ferrell, B.R., Goldsmith, J., Smith, T., Glajchen, M., Handzo, T.R.G.F., Eds.; Oxford University Press: New York, NY, USA, 2016; pp. 220–228.
62. Lam, H.S.; Wong, S.P.S.; Liu, F.Y.B.; Wong, H.L.; Fok, T.F.; Ng, P.C. Attitudes toward Neonatal Intensive Care Treatment of Preterm Infants with a High Risk of Developing Long-term Disabilities. *Pediatrics* **2009**, *123*, 1501–1508. [CrossRef] [PubMed]
63. October, T.W.; Fisher, K.R.; Feudtner, C.; Hinds, P.S. The parent perspective: "Being a good parent" when making critical decisions in the PICU. *Pediatr. Crit. Care Med.* **2014**, *15*, 291–298. [CrossRef] [PubMed]
64. Xafis, V.; Wilkinson, D.; Sullivan, J. What information do parents need when facing end-of-life decisions for their child? A meta-synthesis of parental feedback. *BMC Palliat. Care* **2015**, *14*, 19. [CrossRef] [PubMed]
65. Feudtner, C. Collaborative communication in pediatric palliative care: A foundation for problem-solving and decision making. *Pediatr. Clin. N. Am.* **2007**, *54*, 583–607. [CrossRef] [PubMed]
66. Goldman, A.; Hain, R.; Liben, S. *Oxford Textbook of Palliative Care for Children*, 2nd ed.; Oxford University Press, Inc.: New York, NY, USA, 2012.
67. Klick, J.C. Pediatric palliative care. *Curr. Probl. Pediatr. Adolesc. Health Care* **2010**, *40*, 120–151. [CrossRef] [PubMed]

68. Davies, B.; Steele, R.; Krueger, G.; Baird, J.; Bifirie, M.; Cadell, S.; Doane, G.; Garga, D.; Siden, H.; Strahlendorf, C.; et al. Best Practice in Provider/Parent Interaction. *Qual. Health Res.* **2017**, *27*, 406–420. [CrossRef] [PubMed]
69. Bluebond-Langner, M.; Hargrave, D.; Henderson, E.M.; Langner, R. 'I have to live with the decisions I make': Laying a foundation for decision making for children with life-limiting conditions and life-threatening illnesses. *Arch. Dis. Child.* **2017**, *102*, 468–471. [CrossRef] [PubMed]
70. Boss, R.D.; Hutton, N.; Sulpar, L.J.; West, A.M.; Donohue, P.K. Values Parents Apply to Decision-Making Regarding Delivery Room Resuscitation for High-Risk Newborns. *Pediatrics* **2008**, *122*, 583–589. [CrossRef] [PubMed]
71. Brooten, D.; Youngblut, J.M.; Seagrave, L.; Caicedo, C.; Hawthorne, D.; Hidalgo, I.; Roche, R. Parent's perceptions of health care providers actions around child ICU death: What helped, what did not. *Am. J. Hosp. Palliat. Care* **2013**, *30*, 40–49. [CrossRef] [PubMed]
72. Einarsdóttir, J. Emotional experts: Parents' views on end-of-life decisions for preterm infants in Iceland. *Med. Anthropol. Q.* **2009**, *23*, 34–50. [CrossRef] [PubMed]
73. Higgins, S.S. Parental role in decision making about pediatric cardiac transplantation: Familial and ethical considerations. *J. Pediatr. Nurs.* **2001**, *16*, 332–337. [CrossRef] [PubMed]
74. McHaffie, H.E.; Lyon, A.J.; Hume, R. Deciding on treatment limitation for neonates: The parents' perspective. *Eur. J. Pediatr.* **2001**, *160*, 339–344. [CrossRef] [PubMed]
75. Michelson, L.N.; Emanuel, L.; Carter, A.; Brinkman, P.; Clayman, M.L.; Frader, J. Pediatric intensive care unit family conferences: One mode of communication for discussing end-of-life care decisions. *Pediatr. Crit. Care Med.* **2011**, *12*, e336–e343. [CrossRef] [PubMed]
76. Slatter, A.; Francis, S.A.; Smith, F.; Bush, A. Supporting parents in managing drugs for children with cystic fibrosis. *Br. J. Nurs.* **2004**, *13*, 1135–1139. [CrossRef] [PubMed]
77. Sullivan, J.; Monagle, P.; Gillam, L. What parents want from doctors in end-of-life decision-making for children. *Arch. Dis. Child.* **2014**, *99*, 216–220. [CrossRef] [PubMed]
78. Carnevale, F.A.; Canoui, P.; Cremer, R.; Farrell, C.; Doussau, A.; Seguin, M.J.; Hubert, P.; Leclerc, F.; Lacroix, J. Parental involvement in treatment decisions regarding their critically ill child: A comparative study of France and Quebec. *Pediatr. Crit. Care Med.* **2007**, *8*, 337–342. [CrossRef] [PubMed]
79. Carnevale, F.A.; Benedetti, M.; Bonaldi, A.; Bravi, E.; Trabucco, G.; Biban, P. Understanding the private worlds of physicians, nurses, and parents: A study of life-sustaining treatment decisions in Italian paediatric critical care. *J. Child Health Care* **2011**, *15*, 334–349. [CrossRef] [PubMed]
80. Carnevale, F.A.; Canoui, P.; Hubert, P.; Farrell, C.; Leclerc, F.; Doussau, A.; Seguin, Ma.; Lacroix, J. The moral experience of parents regarding life-support decisions for their critically-ill children: A preliminary study in France. *J. Child Health Care* **2006**, *10*, 69–82. [CrossRef] [PubMed]
81. Gibson, B.E.; Teachman, G.; Wright, V.; Fehlings, D.; Young, N.L.; McKeever, P. Children's and parents' beliefs regarding the value of walking: Rehabilitation implications for children with cerebral palsy. *Child Care Health Dev.* **2012**, *38*, 61–69. [CrossRef] [PubMed]
82. Young, B.; Moffett, J.K.; Jackson, D.; McNulty, A. Decision-making in community-based paediatric physiotherapy: A qualitative study of children, parents and practitioners. *Health Soc. Care Commun.* **2006**, *14*, 116–124. [CrossRef] [PubMed]
83. Michelson, K.N.; Koogler, T.; Sullivan, C.; Ortega, M.; Hall, E.; Frader, J. Parental views on withdrawing life-sustaining therapies in critically ill children. *Arch. Pediatr. Adolesc. Med.* **2009**, *163*, 986–992. [CrossRef] [PubMed]
84. Young, B.; Dixon-Woods, M.; Windridge, K.; Heney, D. Managing communication with young people who have a potentially life threatening chronic illness: Qualitative study of patients and parents. *Br. Med. J.* **2003**, *326*, 305. [CrossRef]
85. Guerriere, D.N.; McKeever, P.; Llweellyn-Thomas, H.; Berrall, G. Mothers' decisions about gastrostomy tube insertion in children: Factors contributing to uncertainty. *Dev. Med. Child Neurol.* **2003**, *45*, 470–476. [CrossRef] [PubMed]
86. Kavanaugh, K.; Nantais-Smith, L.M.; Savage, T.; Schim, S.M.; Natarajan, G. Extended family support for parents faced with life-support decisions for extremely premature infants. *Neonatal Netw.* **2014**, *33*, 255–262. [CrossRef] [PubMed]

87. Pepper, D.; Rempel, G.; Austin, W.; Ceci, C.; Hendson, L. More than Information: A Qualitative Study of Parents' Perspectives on Neonatal Intensive Care at the Extremes of Prematurity. *Adv. Neonatal Care* **2012**, *12*, 303–309. [CrossRef] [PubMed]
88. Støre-Brinchmann, B.S.; Førde, R.; Nortvedt, P. What Matters to the Parents? A qualitative study of parents' experiences with life-and-death decisions concerning their premature infants. *Nurs. Ethics* **2002**, *9*, 388–404. [CrossRef] [PubMed]
89. Markward, M.J.; Benner, K.; Freese, R. Perspectives of parents on making decisions about the care and treatment of a child with cancer: A review of literature. *Fam. Syst. Health J. Collab. Fam. Healthc.* **2013**, *31*, 406–413. [CrossRef] [PubMed]
90. Roscigno, C.I.; Savage, T.A.; Kavanaugh, K.; Moro, T.T.; Kilpatrick, S.J.; Strassner, H.T.; Grobman, W.A.; Kimura, R.E. Divergent views of hope influencing communications between parents and hospital providers. *Qual. Health Res.* **2012**, *22*, 1232–1246. [CrossRef] [PubMed]
91. Ottawa Family Decision Guide. Available online: http://www.cheo.on.ca/uploads/Decision%20Services/OFDG.pdf (accessed on 15 March 2018).
92. Child Tracheostomy Decision Guide. Available online: http://www.wrha.mb.ca/extranet/eipt/files/EIPT-023-001.pdf (accessed on 12 February 2018).
93. American Academy of Pediatrics (AAP). Patient- and family-centered care coordination: A framework for integrating care for children and youth across multiple systems. *Pediatrics* **2014**, *133*, e1451–e1460.
94. Carosella, A.; Snyder, A.; Ward, E. What parents of children with complex medical conditions want their child's physicians to understand. *JAMA Pediatr.* **2018**, *172*, 315–316. [CrossRef] [PubMed]
95. Lutenbacher, M.; Karp, S.; Ajero, G.; Howe, D.; Williams, M. Crossing community sectors: Challenges faced by families of children with special health care needs. *J. Fam. Nurs.* **2005**, *11*, 162–182. [CrossRef] [PubMed]
96. Hamilton, L.J.; Lerner, C.F.; Presson, A.P.; Klitzner, T.S. Effects of a Medical Home Program for Children with Special Health Care Needs on Parental Perceptions of Care in an Ethnically Diverse Patient Population. *Matern. Child Health J.* **2013**, *17*, 463–469. [CrossRef] [PubMed]
97. Kuo, D.Z.; Cohen, E.; Agrawal, R.; Berry, J.; Casey, P. A National Profile of Caregiver Challenges Among More Medically Complex Children with Special Health Care Needs. *Arch. Pediatr. Adolesc. Med.* **2011**, *165*, 1020–1026. [CrossRef] [PubMed]
98. Lawson, K.A.; Bloom, S.R.; Sadof, M.; Stille, C.; Perrin, J.M. Care Coordination for Children with Special Health Care Needs: Evaluation of a State Experiment. *Matern. Child Health J.* **2011**, *15*, 993–1000. [CrossRef] [PubMed]
99. Jagt-van Kampen, C.T.; Colenbrander, D.A.; Bosman, D.K.; Grootenhuis, M.A.; Kars, M.C.; Schouten-van Meeteren, A.Y. Aspects and Intensity of Pediatric Palliative Case Management Provided by a Hospital-Based Case Management Team: A Comparative Study between Children with Malignant and Nonmalignant Disease. *Am. J. Hosp. Palliat. Care* **2018**, *35*, 123–131. [CrossRef] [PubMed]
100. Adams, S.; Cohen, E.; Mahant, S.; Friedman, J.N.; Macculloch, R.; Nicholas, D.B. Exploring the usefulness of comprehensive care plans for children with medical complexity (CMC): A qualitative study. *BMC Pediatr.* **2013**, *13*, 10. [CrossRef] [PubMed]
101. Kuo, D.Z.; Robbins, J.M.; Lyle, R.E.; Barrett, K.W.; Burns, K.H.; Casey, P.H. Parent-Reported Outcomes of Comprehensive Care for Children with Medical Complexity. *Fam. Syst. Health* **2013**, *31*, 132–141. [CrossRef] [PubMed]
102. Remedios, C.; Willenberg, L.; Zordan, R.; Murphy, A.; Hessel, G.; Philip, J. A pre-test and post-test study of the physical and psychological effects of out-of-home respite care on caregivers of children with life-threatening conditions. *Palliat. Med.* **2015**, *29*, 223–230. [CrossRef] [PubMed]
103. Smith, C.H.; Graham, C.A.; Herbert, A.R. Respite needs of families receiving palliative care. *J. Paediatr. Child Health* **2017**, *53*, 173–179. [CrossRef] [PubMed]
104. Meltzer, L.J.; Boroughs, D.S.; Downes, J.J. The Relationship between Home Nursing Coverage, Sleep, and Daytime Functioning in Parents of Ventilator-Assisted Children. *J. Pediatr. Nurs.* **2010**, *25*, 250–257. [CrossRef] [PubMed]
105. Pelentsov, L.J.; Laws, T.A.; Esterman, A.J. The supportive care needs of parents caring for a child with a rare disease: A scoping review. *Disabil. Health J.* **2015**, *8*, 475–491. [CrossRef] [PubMed]

106. Tsitsi, T.; Charalambous, A.; Papastavrou, E.; Raftopoulos, V. Effectiveness of a relaxation intervention (progressive muscle relaxation and guided imagery techniques) to reduce anxiety and improve mood of parents of hospitalized children with malignancies: A randomized controlled trial in Republic of Cyprus and Greece. *Eur. J. Oncol. Nurs.* **2016**, *26*, 9–18. [PubMed]
107. Kristjanson, L.; Hudson, P.; Oldham, L. Working with families. In *Palliative Care Nursing: A Guide to Practice*; O'Connor, M., Aranda, S., Eds.; Ausmed Publications: Melbourne, Austrilia, 2003; pp. 271–283.
108. Gupta, V.; Prescott, H. "That must be so hard"—Examining the impact of children's palliative care services on the psychological well-being of parents. *Clin. Child Psychol. Psychiatry* **2013**, *18*, 91–99. [CrossRef] [PubMed]
109. Wing, D.G.; Burge-Callaway, K.; Rose Clance, P.; Armistead, L. Understanding gender differences in bereavement following the death of an infant: Implications of or treatment. *Psychother. Theory Res. Pract. Train.* **2001**, *38*, 60–73. [CrossRef]
110. Cadell, S.; Hemsworth, D.; Quosai, T.S.; Steele, R.; Davies, E.; Liben, S.; Straatman, L.; Siden, H. Posttraumatic growth in parents caring for a child with a life-limiting illness: A structural equation model. *Am. J. Orthopsychiatry* **2014**, *84*, 123–133. [CrossRef] [PubMed]
111. Helgeson, V.S.; Jakubiak, B.; Van Vleet, M.; Zajdel, M. Communal Coping and Adjustment to Chronic Illness: Theory Update and Evidence. *Personal. Soc. Psychol. Rev.* **2018**, *22*, 170–195. [CrossRef] [PubMed]
112. Kramer, B.J. Expanding the Conceptualization of Caregiver Coping: The Importance of Relationship-Focused Coping Strategies. *Fam. Relat.* **1993**, *42*, 383–391. [CrossRef]
113. Jones, B.L.; Remke, S.S. Self care and sustainability for pediatric oncology providers. In *Pediatric Psychosocial Oncology: Textbook for Multi-Disciplinary Care*; Abrams, A., Muriel, A., Wiener, L., Eds.; Springer: Berlin/Heidelberg, Germany, 2016.
114. Whitehead, P.B.; Herbertson, R.K.; Hamric, A.B.; Epstein, E.G.; Fisher, J.M. Moral Distress among Healthcare Professionals: Report of an Institution-Wide Survey. *J. Nurs. Scholarsh.* **2015**, *47*, 117–125. [CrossRef] [PubMed]
115. Aycock, N.; Boyle, D. Interventions to manage compassion fatigue in oncology nursing. *Clin. J. Oncol. Nurs.* **2009**, *13*, 183–191. [CrossRef] [PubMed]
116. Jonas, D.F.; Bogetz, J.F. Identifying the Deliberate Prevention and Intervention Strategies of Pediatric Palliative Care Teams Supporting Providers during Times of Staff Distress. *J. Palliat. Med.* **2016**, *19*, 679–683. [CrossRef] [PubMed]
117. Stroebe, M.; Schut, H.; Stroebe, W. Health outcomes of bereavement. *Lancet* **2007**, *370*, 1960–1973. [CrossRef]
118. Li, J.; Stroebe, M.; Chan, C.; Chow, A. Guilt in bereavement: A review and conceptual framework. *Death Stud.* **2014**, *38*, 165–171. [CrossRef] [PubMed]
119. Kreicbergs, U.; Valdimarsdottir, U.; Onelov, E.; Henter, J.I.; Steineck, G. Anxiety and depression in parents 4–9 years after the loss of a child owing to a malignancy: A population-based follow-up. *Psychol. Med.* **2004**, *34*, 1431–1441. [CrossRef] [PubMed]
120. Lannen, P.K.; Wolfe, J.; Prigerson, H.G.; Onelov, E.; Kreicbergs, U.C. Unresolved Grief in a National Sample of Bereaved Parents: Impaired Mental and Physical Health 4 to 9 Years Later. *J. Clin. Oncol.* **2008**, *26*, 5870–5876. [CrossRef] [PubMed]
121. Alam, R.; Barrera, M.; D'Agostino, N.; Nicholas, D.B.; Schneiderman, G. Bereavement experiences of mothers and fathers over time after the death of a child due to cancer. *Death Stud.* **2012**, *36*, 1–22. [CrossRef] [PubMed]
122. Buckle, J.; Fleming, S. *Parenting after the Death of a Child: A practitioner's Guide*; CRC Press: New York, NY, USA, 2011.
123. Corden, A.; Sloper, P.; Sainsbury, R. Financial effects for families after the death of a disabled or chronically ill child: A neglected dimension of bereavement. *Child Care Health Dev.* **2002**, *28*, 199–204. [CrossRef] [PubMed]
124. Dutton, Y.C.; Zisook, S. Adaptation to Bereavement. *Death Stud.* **2005**, *29*, 877–903. [CrossRef] [PubMed]
125. O'Connor, M.F. Bereavement and the brain: Invitation to a conversation between bereavement researchers and neuroscientists. *Death Stud.* **2005**, *29*, 905–922. [CrossRef] [PubMed]
126. Stebbins, J.; Batrouney, T. *Beyond the Death of a Child: Social Impacts and Economic Costs of the Death of a Child*; The Compassionate Friends Victoria Inc.: Victoria, Australia, 2007.
127. Blackburn, P.; Dwyer, K. A Bereavement Common Assessment Framework in Palliative Care: Informing Practice, Transforming Care. *Am. J. Hosp. Palliat. Med.* **2017**, *34*, 677–684. [CrossRef] [PubMed]
128. Wynn, G.H.; Benedek, D.M.; Johnson, L.; Ursano, R. Chapter 22—Posttraumatic Stress Disorder A2. In *Conn's Translational Neuroscience*; Conn, P.M., Ed.; Academic Press: San Diego, CA, USA, 2017; pp. 499–515.

129. Djelantik, A.A.A.M.J.; Smid, G.E.; Kleber, R.J.; Boelen, P.A. Do prolonged grief disorder symptoms predict post-traumatic stress disorder symptoms following bereavement? A cross-lagged analysis. *Compr. Psychiatry* **2018**, *80*, 65–71. [CrossRef] [PubMed]
130. Ljungman, L.; Hoven, E.; Ljungman, G.; Cernvall, M.; von Essen, L. Does time heal all wounds? A longitudinal study of the development of posttraumatic stress symptoms in parents of survivors of childhood cancer and bereaved parents. *Psycho-Oncology* **2015**, *24*, 1792–1798. [CrossRef] [PubMed]
131. Lichtenthal, W.G.; Breitbart, W. The Central Role of Meaning in Adjustment to the Loss of a Child to Cancer: Implications for the Development of Meaning-Centered Grief Therapy. *Curr. Opin. Support. Palliat. Care* **2015**, *9*, 46–51. [CrossRef] [PubMed]
132. Endo, K.; Yonemoto, N.; Yamada, M. Interventions for bereaved parents following a child's death: A systematic review. *Palliat. Med.* **2015**, *29*, 590–604. [CrossRef] [PubMed]

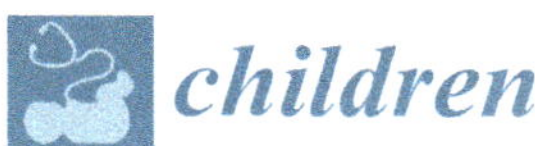

MDPI

Review

Children's Experience of Symptoms: Narratives through Words and Images †

Barbara M. Sourkes [1,2]

1 Division of Pediatric Critical Care Medicine, Stanford University School of Medicine, Palo Alto, CA 94304-5876, USA; bsourkes@stanford.edu

2 Pediatric Palliative Care Program, Lucile Packard Children's Hospital Stanford, Palo Alto, CA 94304-5731, USA

† This article is an abridged version of a paper presented as part of a pre-congress symposium: "Treating Distressing Symptoms in Children with Serious Illnesses" at the 3rd Congress on Paediatric Palliative Care: A Global Gathering in Rome, November 2016.

Received: 14 March 2018; Accepted: 29 March 2018; Published: 19 April 2018

Abstract: Children who live with a complex chronic or life-threatening illness face extraordinary challenges. Whether they are receiving disease-oriented treatment (aimed at potential cure or prolongation of life) or palliative treatment—or both concurrently—our challenge is to enhance their comfort and minimize their distress. Symptom management is thus a critical component of pediatric palliative care. Symptoms may be either physical or psychological in nature (or a confluence of both) and their effective management has a direct impact on the child's quality of life. This article provides an integrative overview of children's experience of selected physical and psychological symptoms, as expressed through their words and images. Understanding their perspectives is an essential component in the design and provision of optimal symptom management. Included, as well, are examples from siblings—a reminder of the profound impact of illness on these children who also "live" the experience, albeit in a different way. The symptoms that are described are pain, nausea and vomiting, fatigue, weakness, seizures, hair loss, depression, and anxiety. Although psychological symptoms are often inextricable from the physical, they may also present independently as part of the overall illness experience.

Keywords: pediatric palliative care; life-threatening illness; complex chronic illness; symptoms; experience; psychological; trauma

---

1. Introduction

Children who live with a complex chronic or life-threatening illness face extraordinary physical and psychological challenges. Many contend with hardship and terror as the illness wends its course into an uncertain future. Pediatric palliative care strives to optimize the quality of life of children living with serious illness, as well as to support the family. Whether children are receiving disease-oriented treatment (aimed at potential cure or prolongation of life) or palliative treatment—or both concurrently—our challenge is to enhance their comfort and minimize their distress.

The concept of psychic trauma lends itself to understanding children's experience of illness. Terr, a child psychiatrist, offers the following definition in her book *Too Scared to Cry*: "'Psychic trauma' occurs when a sudden, unexpected, overwhelmingly intense emotional blow or a series of blows assaults the person from outside. Traumatic events are external, but they quickly become incorporated into the mind. A person probably will not become fully traumatized unless he or she feels utterly helpless during the event or events." [1] (p. 8). This description certainly relates to the overwhelming sense of loss of control experienced by seriously-ill children: the shock of diagnosis, the indelible imprint of the sustained assault on the body and psyche, and the uncertainty of the outcome. Whereas "external" malevolence of intent characterizes many forms of trauma (e.g., abuse), the culprit in illness resides within the body itself and often in the inexplicable randomness of fate [2] (p. 4).

While many physical symptoms are a predictable manifestation of an underlying disease or disorder, the intensity and frequency of their occurrence can be highly variable. Psychological symptoms are often not as predictable and, as a result, may take longer to identify and address. Illness unfolds within the broader context of the "whole" child and family: thus social, cultural, and religious factors may all have an impact on how a child experiences and interprets a given symptom [3].

This article provides an integrative overview of children's experience of a range of physical and psychological symptoms, as expressed through their words and images. Understanding their perspectives is an essential component in the design and provision of optimal symptom management. Included, as well, are examples from siblings—a reminder of the profound impact of illness on these children who also "live" the experience, albeit in a different way. Although only the patient experiences the physical aspects of illness, the reverberations on the siblings may become a source of great distress, especially because they often go unacknowledged.

Many children in pediatric palliative care have diagnoses with cognitive, as well as physical, manifestations. The spectrum includes children with mild/moderate limitations to those with severe global developmental deficits and minimal awareness of the world around them. In addition are children who are cognitively normal, but may not be able to communicate effectively during certain phases of the illness. Thus, the children who "speak" in this article may be seen as the expressive voice for many others who suffer similar symptoms but are unable to report their experience.

The selected symptoms to be described are pain, nausea and vomiting, fatigue, weakness, seizures, hair loss, depression, and anxiety. Although psychological symptoms are often inextricable from the physical, they may also present independently as part of the overall illness experience.

2. Pain

The term "pain" [4–7] has many meanings, ranging from the physical to the psychological and, most often, a confluence of the two. In this section are examples of stark depictions of physical pain, bearing pain for the sake of living, and pain associated with death.

2.1. Depictions of Physical Pain

> Psychologist: If you could choose one word to describe the time since your diagnosis, what would it be?
>
> Child (without hesitation): PAIN. Once I felt as if an I.V. was exploding in my arm! [8] (p. 23)

The child then described the excruciating pain he had felt when someone tripped over his IV pole that then came crashing down (Figure 1). The boldly colored, nightmarish image with foreboding slashes of black conveys the extreme pain and the associated anxiety and vulnerability. At the bottom of the picture—totally overwhelmed by the chaos—is his arm, the site of the pain.

In response to the question: "What is the scariest feeling, thought or experience you have had since you sister became ill?" a healthy sibling drew her response: "Dreaming of my sister in pain . . . ." (Figure 2) [8] (p. 23). She depicted herself as a diminutive brown figure in a small bed, overwhelmed by the dream image of her sister in bright orange—screaming "OW." Her image testifies to the powerful impact on siblings of witnessing the patient's suffering. Even as they are spared the physical pain of illness, they are unshielded from a sense of fear and overwhelming helplessness. Therein lies the source of the siblings' trauma, in counterpoint to the patients'.

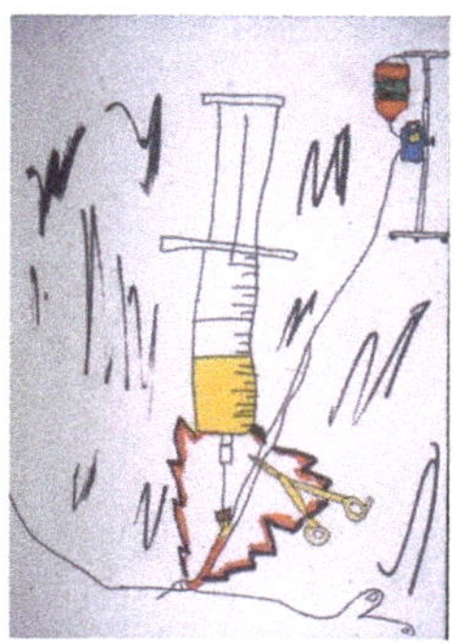

Figure 1. Intravenous (IV) exploding in my arm.

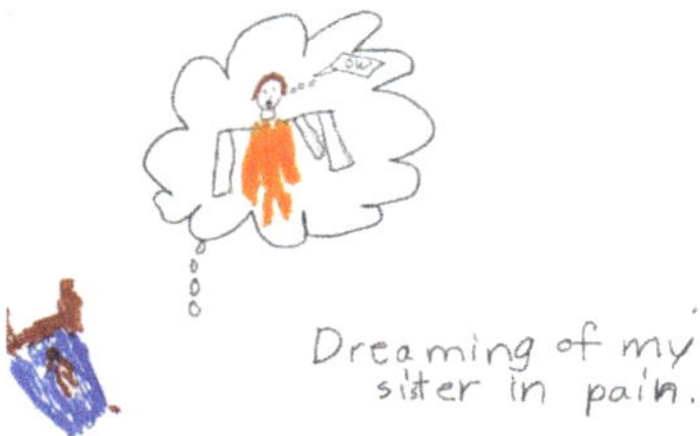

Figure 2. Dreaming of my sister in pain.

2.2. *Bearing Pain for the Sake of Living*

Children are well aware that, despite everyone's best efforts, certain life-prolonging or curative treatments may cause them distress or pain. They can perceive the cost/benefit exchange: what they are willing to withstand on an ongoing basis in order to achieve the goal of living.

A teenager with end-stage renal disease depicted his absolute dependence on hemodialysis to live. He complained about many levels of discomfort: from the disruption to his life caused by the dialysis schedule to increasing pain associated with the treatment itself. He entitled his drawing (in French) "MA machine" ("MY machine"). (Figure 3) [8] (p. 23), with the emphasis on "MA/MY". The possessiveness is an indication of its critical importance to him in sustaining his life. One hand is literally plugged into the machine, while the other is in a "thumbs up" gesture. His facial expression is ambiguous—triumph, horror, or a combination of the two.

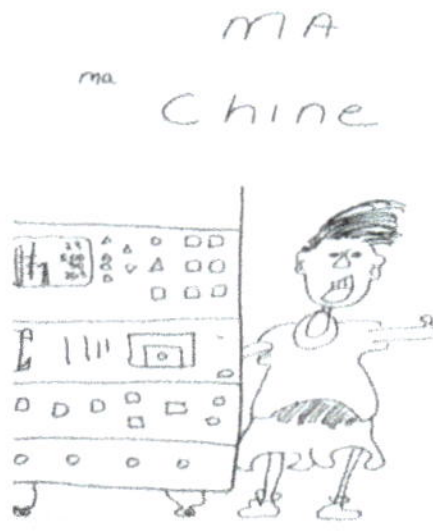

Figure 3. MA machine.

2.3. Pain Associated with Death

For some children, the experience of pain is directly associated with the fear of death. This occurs even in children whose prognosis is good, and although death is a threat, it is by no means a certain outcome. The child who drew the image of the skull and crossbones leering above a bone marrow aspiration needle (Figure 4) [2] (pp. 114–115) had an excellent prognosis. In an image that *explicitly* links pain with the thought of death (Figure 5) [2] (pp. 114–115) a child stated: "When I'm just lying in bed in the hospital and in pain, this (pointing to his drawing) is what I think about." (R.I.P. stands for "Rest in Peace").

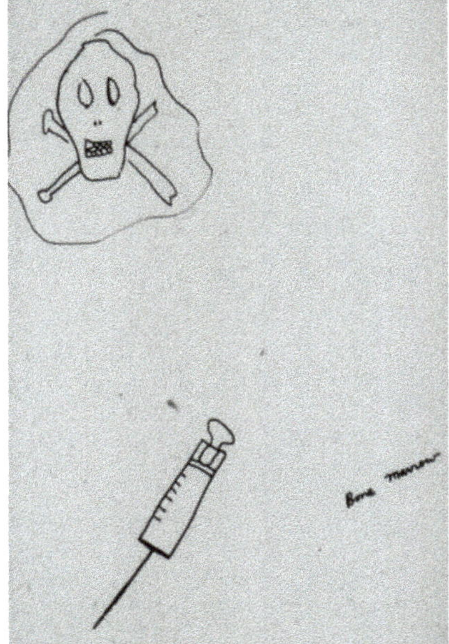

Figure 4. Bone marrow aspiration needle.

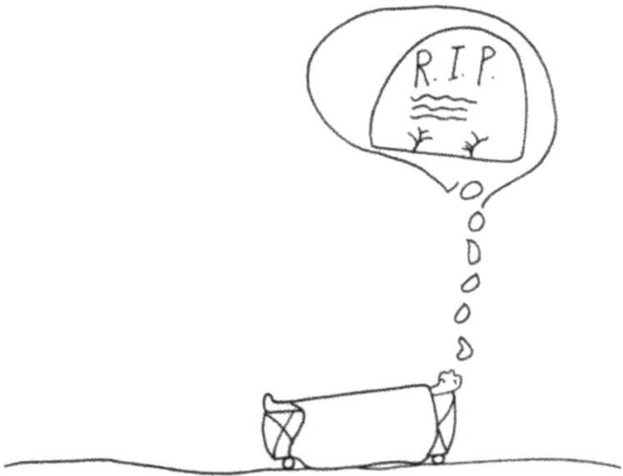

Figure 5. Tombstone.

3. Nausea and Vomiting

Nausea and vomiting [9,10] can be highly stressful for children on many levels. Very young children may be frightened by the unpredictability of vomiting and retching. Older children respond to the pervasive (and intrusive) nature of nausea: "I can't even think straight when I feel like throwing up. It blocks out everything." Or, as a sibling stated matter-of-factly: "I hate when he pukes all the time. It sounds bad and it stinks." The fact that nausea is antithetical to having an appetite for food can be distressing for both children and parents. On a "medical" level, there is the worry about the child not getting adequate nutrition. On an emotional level, nausea precludes food as a source of pleasure and comfort for a child, as well as taking away an important avenue for parents to provide that comfort.

In preparation for learning relaxation/hypnosis techniques as an antidote to nausea, a child composed the following image involving her favorite stuffed animal, Nutty the Squirrel. Like many children, she yearned for the nausea to end so that she could eat her favorite foods (Figure 6): "This is me lying in a field of flowers on a warm, sunny day with Nutty the Squirrel. I am barefoot, wearing overalls. We would have a picnic basket filled with both our favorite foods: nut soup, chicken rice soup, sandwiches, lasagna, cookies, candy, ice cream, apples and milk." [2] (p. 63).

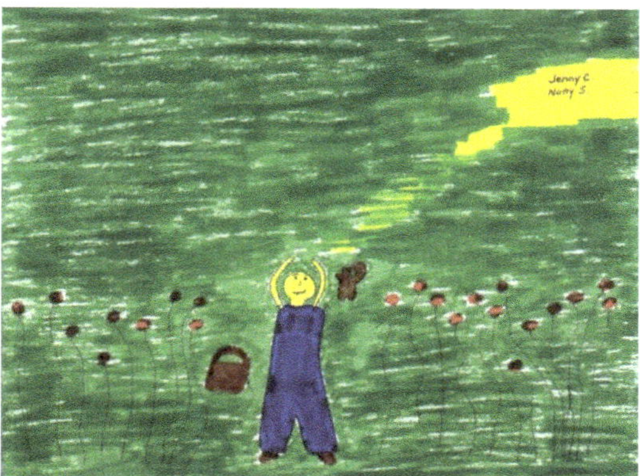

Figure 6. Relaxation scene.

4. Fatigue

Fatigue [11]—a child's complaint of "always feeling tired"—is now recognized as an independent symptom in and of itself, rather than simply being taken for granted as a "given" of the effects of illness or activity. For adolescents who want to be out in the world with their peers, fatigue is a huge impediment to their quality of life. In the words of a teenager: "When I am feeling sick, I am sick—that's it. But when I am feeling okay, I hate being too tired to do anything. It makes me feel like an old person".

Fatigue can also be an intrinsic part of the dying process, and in that context, it may actually bring a measure of peace.

A child did her last drawing, a color-feeing mandala, four days before her death (Figure 7) [12] (p. 31). She was calm and deliberate, although very weak, as she described "How I am feeling today: tired (medium blue), happy (medium—deep blue "wave" to right of tired), angry (dark green inset), cruddy (pale blue)." Her one comment on the deepening shades of blue in her mandala was: "I wanted to put in more "happy" but I am too tired to draw anymore ... I am happy with my family." She spoke quietly and smiled. Her image and words provided the opening for a conversation with her parents, who told her that they recognized her tiredness, and that it was all right for her to "let go".

Terd
HAPPY
ANGRy
Grubby
ACTUAL SIZE

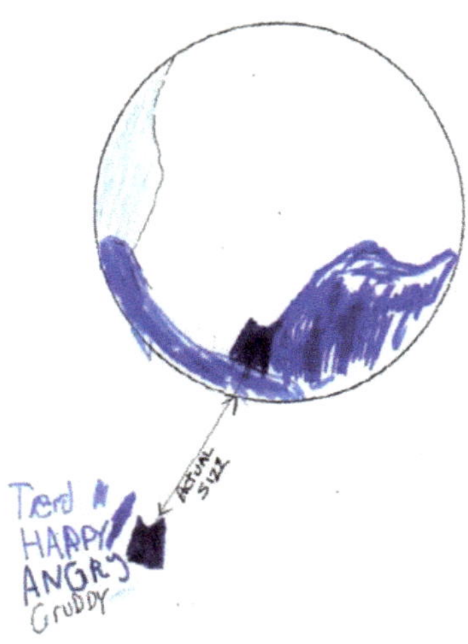

Figure 7. Tired.

5. Weakness

While generalized weakness may be a symptom of many diseases, it is a very specific symptom (and omen) in degenerative disorders.

"A child with muscular dystrophy was tripping and falling constantly, but adamantly refused to use a wheelchair, protesting that he did not need it. His older brother with the same disease was already severely compromised. In a family drawing, (Figure 8) the child portrayed himself jumping and smiling; he drew his brother as an incomplete almost ghost-like figure at the computer. The extremities of all four family members are distorted or missing. This child's awareness—and attempted denial—of his own progressive deterioration as well as his brother's status (and thus his own in the future) are embedded in the drawing" [8] (p. 25).

In a thematically-related drawing (Figure 9), a child from a different family drew her mother, her sister, and herself working in their hillside yard; she described her brother as "*playing* [author's italics] falling down the hill." Although she had been told that his weakness was actually a symptom of disease, she was still hopeful that it was not of any serious import.

BROther
at the computer
mother
she cooks
father
he draws with me
ME
I am jumping

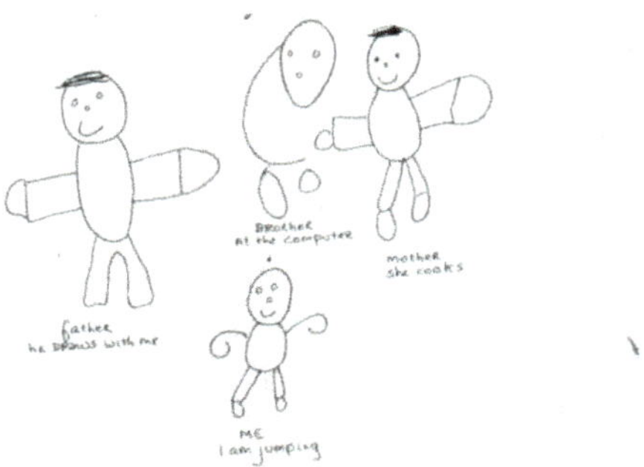

Figure 8. I am jumping.

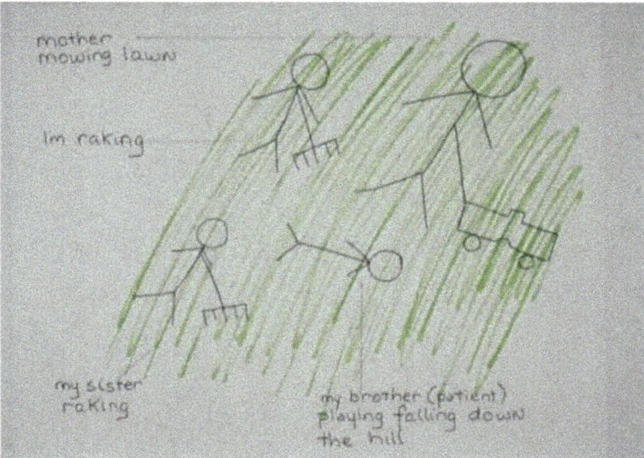

Figure 9. My brother playing falling down the hill.

6. Seizures

Seizures [13,14] are a symptom that—over and above their physical properties—carry a great deal of emotional, social, and cultural impact. For children with severe neurological deficits and minimal awareness, the primary focus is on medical management of their seizures. However, for children who are more functional, the unpredictability of seizures can undermine their confidence in venturing out in the world. They are aware that the dramatic presentation of some types of seizures is frightening and mysterious to others, and they fear social stigmatization. As a sibling of a child with absence seizures (petit mal) reflected (Figure 10): "I hate when my sister suddenly stares in the middle of us playing or talking. It makes her weird".

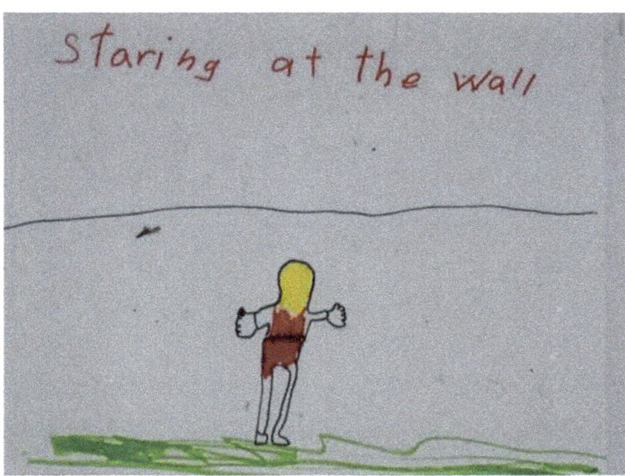

Figure 10. Staring at the wall.

7. Hair Loss

Acceptance of the temporary hair loss secondary to chemotherapy is initially difficult for most children, regardless of age. Reactions of fear and sadness are common. Even young children recognize its significance, from the cosmetic surface through to the evidence of the gravity of the illness. A child stated that losing her hair been the hardest part of the illness for her (Figure 11) [2] (p. 45). She portrays herself in her drawing as stripped and vulnerable.

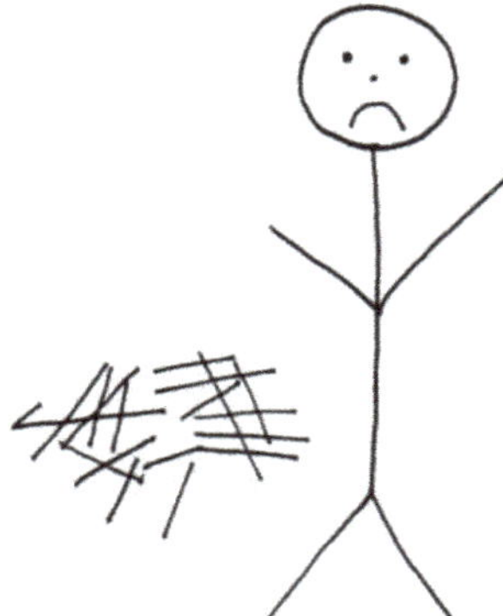

Figure 11. Losing my hair.

Over time, matter-of-fact comments about the baldness—even humor—surface.

A child who had been bald most of her life because of continuous treatment stated: "I don't have hair because I take very strong medicine. Sometimes people laugh at me. It's not very fair. It makes me mad." She proceeded to draw a picture with the following explanation: "This is Mr. Snail, the groom. He is going to his wedding. He had to brush his hair, so he's late." (Figure 12) [2] (p. 46). Her identification with the snail was clear, since her own head was smooth and shiny and often covered with an interesting hat.

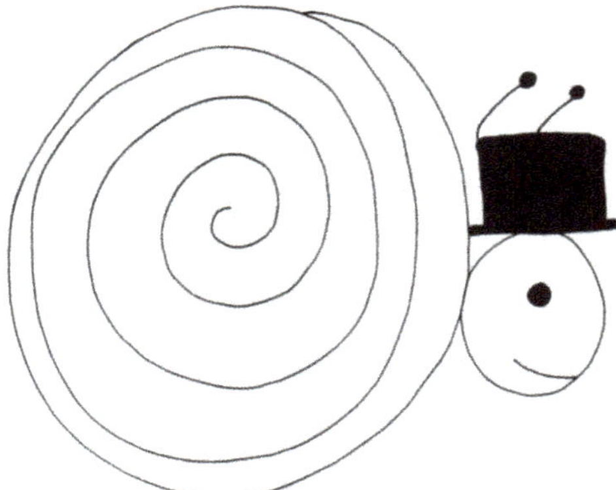

Figure 12. Mr. Snail.

8. Depression and Anxiety

Depression and anxiety [15,16] were once considered as an inevitable part of children's reaction to serious illness and were accorded little attention. Fortunately, these psychological symptoms are now recognized as symptoms in and of themselves that are as important to address as physical distress. Psychotherapy and psychotropic medication may become part of an integrated treatment plan.

"Although many psychological problems may be categorized as adjustment reactions, more severe psychopathology can emerge. This is especially true in children with preexistent vulnerabilities, or when there is a prior psychiatric history in a family member. While it is important not to overemphasize psychopathology, there is also a risk in minimizing or not recognizing it. Any psychological response, however benign initially, can develop into a more complex symptom under the sustained stress of illness. Thus, the severity of symptoms, particularly in terms of intensity and duration, must be continually assessed relative to the child's current reality" [2] (p. 9). Furthermore, psychological symptoms often present in ways that, at least initially, appear indistinguishable from physical distress (e.g., fatigue may in fact be indicative of depression). It often takes highly skilled medical and psychological evaluation to differentiate the source of the distress.

Children's drawings can be clues to identifying psychological symptoms.

The following two images drawn by hospitalized children (Figure 13 [2] (p. 64) and Figure 14 [2] (p. 65) are striking for their emptiness and isolation. In Figure 14, the stark isolation is 'relieved" only by an ominous-looking television. Contrast these two images with Figure 15. Although this artist was older (an adolescent), it is not only age that accounts for the difference in what his drawing communicates. Despite being alone in the hospital room, there is a sense of involvement in life. The door has a window, there are two beds suggesting the possibility of a roommate, and the boy is engrossed in (ironically) a popular hospital series. His favorite stuffed animal sits at the foot of his bed. While a diagnosis cannot be based on drawings alone, the first two images certainly raise the question of depression in these children and can furnish an opening in a psychological evaluation or psychotherapy.

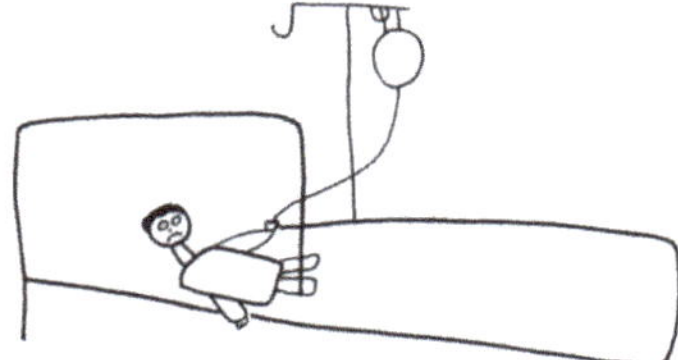

Figure 13. Sad boy in the hospital.

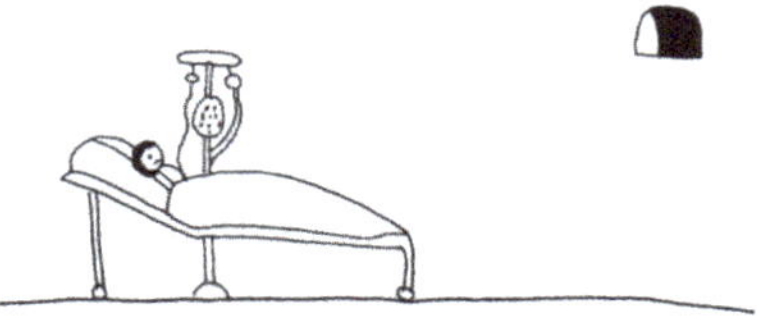

Figure 14. Alone in the hospital.

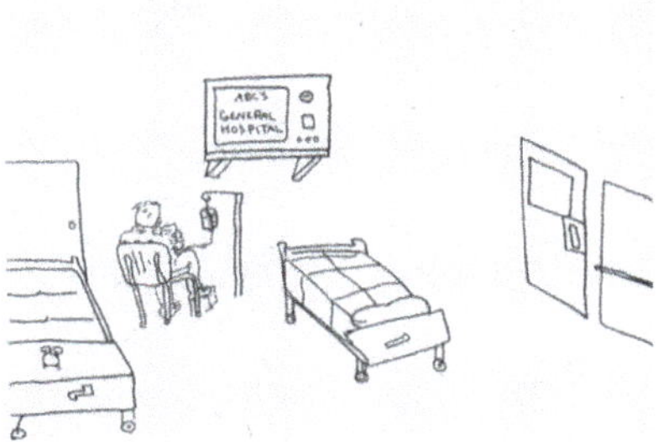

Figure 15. Being in the hospital.

Occasionally children will name the symptom explicitly; in Figure 16 [8] (p. 27), a sibling describes the intensity of her feelings regarding the illness of her younger sister and includes depression in the triad of emotions.

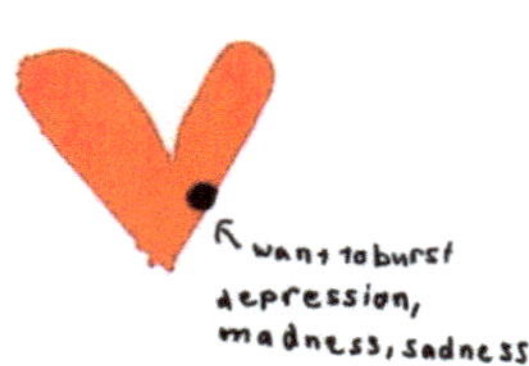

Figure 16. A heart that wants to burst.

Distinguishing the clinical disorder of depression from sadness or anticipatory grief in seriously-ill children can be a poignant challenge. Thus, in Figure 17 [2] (p. 49), a child who had a large tumor in her cheek (thus the bands across the little figure's face) entitled her implicit self-portrait: "From me to everybody." The image reflected not depression, but rather her sadness and grief—her separateness from everyone—as she faced death.

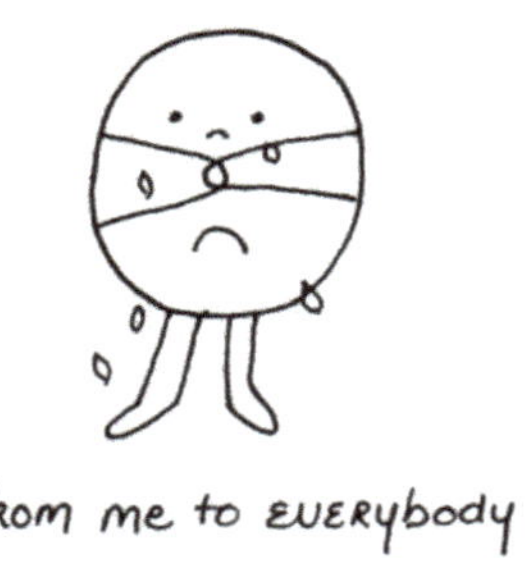

Figure 17. From me to everybody.

Anxiety can emerge in many contexts, from specific triggers (e.g., procedure related) to a generalized sense of foreboding. It is the latter that can be difficult to identify and address in children. A four-year-old child being cared for in home-hospice would not verbally acknowledge that he had any symptoms of any kind. However, he described a dark and threatening drawing as "a batman tunnel. It's completely dark, but I wasn't scared" (Figure 18) [17] (p. 85). This image certainly connotes anxiety or distress—especially in contrast with his earlier bright pictures (Figure 19) [17] (p. 85).

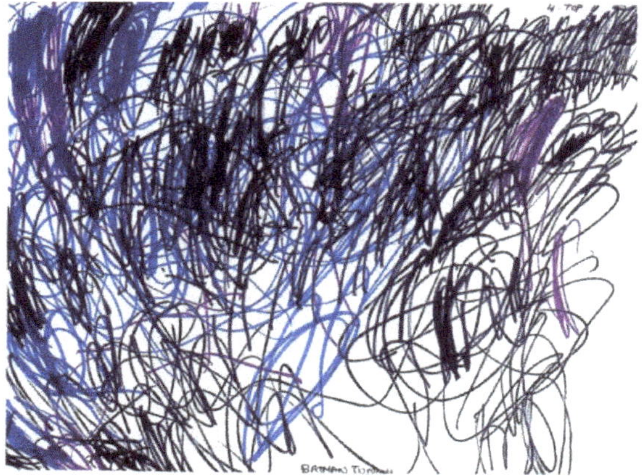

Figure 18. Batman tunnel.

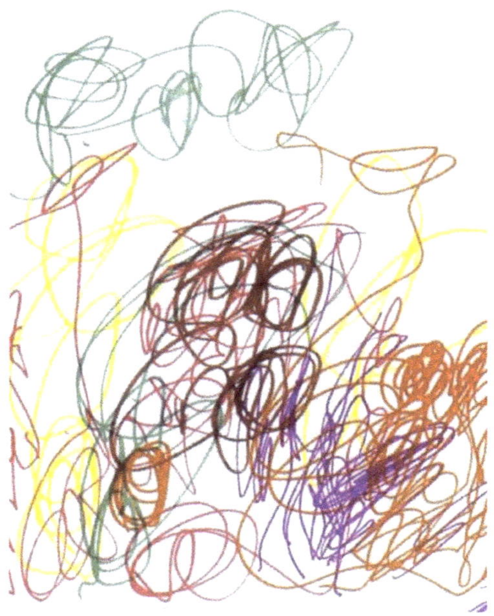

Figure 19. Untitled.

Nightmares are not uncommon manifestations of anxiety. Thus, this interchange:

> Psychologist: What are your bad dreams about?
>
> Child: Monsters, a snake biting....
>
> Psychologist: When you have those bad dreams, what do you think you are worried about?
>
> Child: You dying. Everyone dying in the world and leaving me alone.... [2] (p. 122–123)

In a drawing by another child (Figure 20) [2] (p. 123), he portrayed himself in bed, overwhelmed by a grotesque monster who seems to be "breathing terror" toward him. The boldly printed word "EEEK" was the only verbal accompaniment that the child could offer.

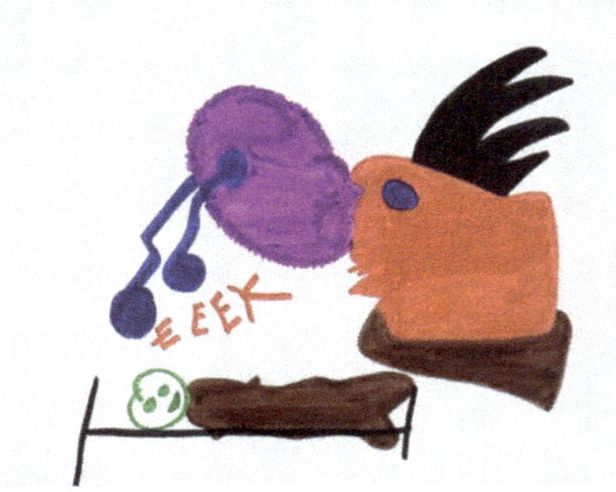

Figure 20. Nightmare.

9. Conclusions

Many children are capable of describing symptoms vividly, whether in words or images, even at times offering an explanation or interpretation as to their significance. These selected narratives underscore the inextricable nature of the physical and psychological in the expression of many symptoms. Their complexity is testimony to the crucial need for an interdisciplinary treatment team and the paramount importance of ongoing communication among the children, families, and professionals who care for them.

Conflicts of Interest: The author declares no conflict of interest.

References

1. Terr, L. *Too Scared to Cry*; Basic Books: New York, NY, USA, 1990.
2. Sourkes, B. *Armfuls of Time: The Psychological Experience of the Child with a Life-Threatening Illness*; University of Pittsburgh Press: Pittsburgh, PA, USA, 1995.
3. Rajapakse, D.; Cormac, M. Symptoms in Life-Threatening Illness: Overview and Assessment. In *Oxford Textbook of Palliative Care for Children*, 2nd ed.; Goldman, A., Hain, R., Liben, S., Eds.; Oxford University Press: Oxford, UK, 2012; pp. 167–177.
4. Collins, J.; Berde, C.; Frost, J. Pain assessment and management. In *Textbook of Interdisciplinary Pediatric Palliative Care*; Wolfe, J., Hinds, P., Sourkes, B., Eds.; Elsevier: Philadelphia, PA, USA, 2011; pp. 18–29, ISBN 978-1-4377-0262-0.
5. Bioy, A.; Wood, C. Introduction to Pain. In *Oxford Textbook of Palliative Care for Children*, 2nd ed.; Goldman, A., Hain, R., Liben, S., Eds.; Oxford University Press: Oxford, UK, 2012; pp. 192–203.
6. Hunt, A. Pain Assessment. In *Textbook of Palliative Care for Children*, 2nd ed.; Goldman, A., Hain, R., Liben, S., Eds.; Oxford University Press: Oxford, UK, 2012; pp. 204–217.
7. Kuttner, L. *A Child in Pain: What Health Professionals Can Do to Help*; Crown House: Wales, UK, 2010.
8. Muriel, A.; Case, C.; Sourkes, B. Children's Voices: Experiences of Patients and Their Siblings. In *Textbook of Interdisciplinary Pediatric Palliative Care*; Wolfe, J., Hinds, P., Sourkes, B., Eds.; Elsevier Saunders: Philadelphia, PA, USA, 2011.
9. Friedrichsdorf, S.; Drake, R.; Webster, L. Gastrointestinal symptoms. In *Textbook of Interdisciplinary Pediatric Palliative Care*; Wolfe, J., Hinds, P., Sourkes, B., Eds.; Elsevier Saunders: Philadelphia, PA, USA, 2011; pp. 311–334.

10. Miller, M.; Karwacki, M. Management of the Gastrointestinal Tract in Paediatric Palliative Medicine. In *Oxford Textbook of Palliative Care for Children*, 2nd ed.; Goldman, A., Hain, R., Liben, S., Eds.; Oxford University Press: Oxford, UK, 2012; pp. 271–283.
11. Hesselgrave, J.; Hockenberry, M. Fatigue. In *Textbook of Interdisciplinary Pediatric Palliative Care*; Wolfe, J., Hinds, P., Sourkes, B., Eds.; Elsevier Saunders: Philadelphia, PA, USA, 2011; pp. 266–271.
12. Sourkes, B. Pediatric Palliative Care: An Overview. In *Insights: A Publication of the National Hospice and Palliative Care Association*; National Hospice and Palliative Care Association: Alexandria, VA, USA, 2011; pp. 28–33.
13. Hain, R.; Douglas, H. Neurological Symptoms. In *Textbook of Interdisciplinary Pediatric Palliative Care*; Wolfe, J., Hinds, P., Sourkes, B., Eds.; Elsevier Saunders: Philadelphia, PA, USA, 2011; pp. 239–250.
14. Hauer, J.; Faulkner, K. Neurological and Neuromuscular Conditions and Symptoms. In *Oxford Textbook of Palliative Care for Children*, 2nd ed.; Goldman, A., Hain, R., Liben, S., Eds.; Oxford University Press: Oxford, UK, 2012; pp. 295–308.
15. Pao, M.; Wiener, L. Psychological symptoms. In *Oxford Textbook of Interdisciplinary Pediatric Palliative Care*; Wolfe, J., Hinds, P., Sourkes, B., Eds.; Elsevier Saunders: Philadelphia, PA, USA, 2011; pp. 229–238.
16. Muriel, A.; McCulloch, R.; Hammel, J. Depression, Anxiety and Delirium. In *Oxford Textbook of Palliative Care for Children*, 2nd ed.; Goldman, A., Hain, R., Liben, S., Eds.; Oxford University Press: Oxford, UK, 2012; pp. 309–318.
17. Aldridge, J.; Sourkes, B. The Psychological Impact of Life-Limiting Conditions on the Child. In *Oxford Textbook of Palliative Care for Children*, 2nd ed.; Goldman, A., Hain, R., Liben, S., Eds.; Oxford University Press: Oxford, UK, 2012; pp. 78–89.

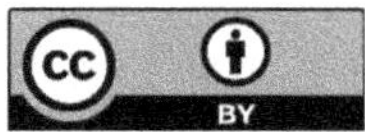

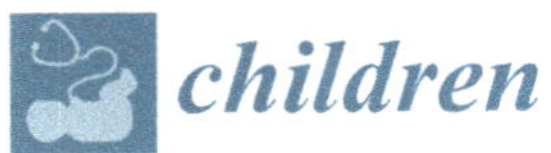 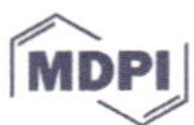

Review

Emerging Methodologies in Pediatric Palliative Care Research: Six Case Studies

Katherine E. Nelson [1,2], James A. Feinstein [3,4], Cynthia A. Gerhardt [5,6], Abby R. Rosenberg [7,8], Kimberley Widger [1,9], Jennifer A. Faerber [10] and Chris Feudtner [11,12,*]

1 Pediatric Advanced Care Team, Department of Paediatrics, Hospital for Sick Children, Toronto, ON M5G 1X8, Canada; katherine.nelson@sickkids.ca (K.E.N.); kim.widger@utoronto.ca (K.W.)
2 Institute of Health Policy, Management, and Evaluation, University of Toronto, Toronto, ON M5T 3M6, Canada
3 Adult and Child Consortium for Health Outcomes Research and Delivery Science, Children's Hospital Colorado, Aurora, CO 80045, USA; james.feinstein@ucdenver.edu
4 Division of General Pediatrics, University of Colorado Anschutz Medical Campus, Aurora, CO 80045, USA
5 Center for Biobehavioral Health, The Research Institute at Nationwide Children's Hospital, Columbus, OH 43205, USA; cynthia.gerhardt@nationwidechildrens.org
6 Departments of Pediatrics and Psychology, The Ohio State University, Columbus, OH 43210, USA
7 Department of Pediatrics, University of Washington School of Medicine; Cancer and Blood Disorders Center, Seattle Children's Hospital, Seattle, WA 98105, USA; abby.rosenberg@seattlechildrens.org
8 Treuman Katz Center for Pediatric Bioethics, Seattle Children's Research Institute, Seattle, WA 98101, USA
9 Lawrence S. Bloomberg Faculty of Nursing, University of Toronto, Toronto, ON M5T 1P8, Canada
10 Department of Pediatrics, The Children's Hospital of Philadelphia, Philadelphia, PA 19104, USA; faerberj@email.chop.edu
11 Pediatric Advanced Care Team, The Children's Hospital of Philadelphia, Philadelphia, PA 19104, USA
12 Department of Pediatrics, The Perelman School of Medicine at the University of Pennsylvania, Philadelphia, PA 19104, USA
* Correspondence: feudtner@email.chop.edu; Tel.: +1-267-426-5032

Received: 9 January 2018; Accepted: 16 February 2018; Published: 26 February 2018

Abstract: Given the broad focus of pediatric palliative care (PPC) on the physical, emotional, and spiritual needs of children with potentially life-limiting illnesses and their families, PPC research requires creative methodological approaches. This manuscript, written by experienced PPC researchers, describes issues encountered in our own areas of research and the novel methods we have identified to target them. Specifically, we discuss potential approaches to: assessing symptoms among nonverbal children, evaluating medical interventions, identifying and treating problems related to polypharmacy, addressing missing data in longitudinal studies, evaluating longer-term efficacy of PPC interventions, and monitoring for inequities in PPC service delivery.

Keywords: pediatric palliative care; research methods; outcomes

---

1. Introduction

Pediatric palliative care (PPC) has an expansive mission. In our care of children with potentially life-limiting illnesses, we take into consideration the physical, emotional, spiritual, and relational needs of children and their families [1]. From a clinical perspective, the task of identifying and addressing needs in so many domains is difficult; developing a research agenda that includes all relevant areas of study is equally challenging. There are many important questions that we need to answer as a field. While identifying the question is usually straightforward, designing a high-quality study to answer that question is often tricky. Fortunately, the science of research design is evolving, and novel methodologic approaches can make the barriers to PPC research less daunting. As experienced PPC researchers, we have each faced the gap between defining the question of interest and identifying how best to study it. For this manuscript, we have selected challenges that we have encountered in our own work and identified potential methodologic approaches to address each of them. Our objective is to describe approaches to a broad range of issues encountered in PPC research, but the list is based on our own areas of expertise, and as such, is not comprehensive. We have highlighted other palliative care studies (adult or pediatric) that utilize the proposed methods whenever possible. Specifically, this manuscript describes approaches to: assessing symptoms among nonverbal children, evaluating medical interventions, identifying and treating problems related to polypharmacy, addressing missing data in longitudinal studies, evaluating longer-term efficacy of PPC interventions, and monitoring for inequities in PPC service delivery. The goal of this paper is to motivate novice and experienced researchers by highlighting specific examples of state of the art methods to address some of the current challenges in PPC research.

2. How Can We Assess Pain and Other Symptoms in Nonverbal Children?

2.1. Significance of the Issue

Symptom burden is a persistent problem among children receiving PPC, necessitating better assessment, communication, and management. Children near end of life experience both physical (such as fatigue, pain, dyspnea, cachexia, and nausea [2–4]) and emotional symptoms (for example, sadness, anxiety, and irritability [4,5]). Progressive metabolic conditions may have organic behavioral symptoms that can become increasingly difficult to treat [6]. Further, symptoms often overlap [2,3,5], with fatigue and pain occurring in nearly all children at end of life [2,7,8]. Accurate symptom assessment is the first step toward better management. However, some children are unable to communicate verbally, which complicates this assessment. Inaccurate evaluation of symptoms may result in inadequate treatment and/or unnecessary interventions and polypharmacy. Furthermore, poorly managed symptoms can affect quality of life, satisfaction with care, and parent well-being years later [9–13].

2.2. Methodologic Challenges

Methodologic issues have impeded progress in symptom assessment among children receiving PPC. A major barrier is the lack of standardized tools with established psychometric properties. Historically, symptom measures have been created for a specific study or extrapolated from work with adults. Often the format and content are not tailored to the child's condition or developmental level. Nor have studies consistently reported on other aspects of the symptom (such as type, frequency, severity, or degree of distress [4]). Most studies focus on cancer and rely heavily on symptom tallies from chart reviews or retrospective mother and nurse report. The views of fathers are usually absent, and only one study has included child self-report [14]. While nurses often assume the primary role for symptom assessment and management, nursing and parental reports of children's symptoms are rarely compared. Additionally, we need to better understand symptom trajectories and identify predictive associations with other quality indicators (such as quality of life/death, satisfaction with care, and parent outcomes).

2.3. State of Art or Novel Approaches to Surmount Challenges

Methodologically rigorous research is essential to lessen symptom burden among children receiving PPC. Measures should: (a) be standardized; (b) include multiple informants, particularly children, mothers, and fathers; (c) encompass diverse health conditions; and (d) be collected prospectively. Obtaining patient-reported outcomes may be difficult for children who are nonverbal due to developmental level, disease progression, or treatment (for example, tracheotomy, pain medication). However, training research staff to assist children using accommodative strategies (such as reading questions aloud, utilizing communication boards/electronic touch pads/adaptive devices) can minimize problems due to fatigue, cognitive deficits, or physical ability. Direct observation and brief ecological momentary assessment through phone call, texting, or short online surveys can also help. If children cannot reliably report, proxy-reports of parents or nurses may be required. A mixed method and multi-informant approach is typically recommended.

Pediatric palliative care research to characterize symptomatology, identify associations with other outcomes, and evaluate interventions is now underway. The study Charting the Territory includes longitudinal symptom assessment among children with progressive, metabolic, neurological, or chromosomal conditions [15]. The Pediatric Quality of Life and Evaluation of Symptoms Technology (PediQUEST) study has examined the efficacy of providing real-time feedback to providers about electronic patient-reported outcomes on symptom burden and quality of life in children with advanced cancer [14,16]. With continued efforts and attention to methodological rigor, we can achieve meaningful progress in symptom management for children with life-limiting conditions.

3. How Can We Assess the Impact of Medical Interventions on Children with Serious Illness?

3.1. Significance of the Issue

One challenge in providing PPC is the limited evidence base for treatments [17]. We often rely on the adult literature about effective interventions and therapies, despite the potential risks associated with "off-label" medication use [18] and challenges in translating adult data for pediatric use [19]. Similarly, the adoption of procedures may outpace the evidence base. For example, a 2013 Cochrane review of gastrostomy tube feeding in children with cerebral palsy did not identify any studies meeting inclusion criteria, concluding that "considerable uncertainty about the effects of gastrostomy tube feeding for children with cerebral palsy remains" [20]. Despite this uncertainty, gastrostomy tubes are common: in two population-based studies of children with neurologic impairment, approximately 10% had gastrostomy tubes [21,22].

3.2. Methodologic Challenges

While ideally every intervention would be subjected to a large, high quality pediatric randomized controlled trial, ethical challenges, identification of adequately sized samples, and funding issues often interfere [23,24]. Also, children with complex medical conditions may not meet inclusion criteria for many trials [25]. A study of clinical trials in adolescent depression found that nearly 70% excluded children with "any current significant physical condition" [26]. Recruiting families for PPC-specific trials can also be difficult [27]. For these reasons, health administrative data has emerged as an appealing alternative for bolstering the evidence base for treatments in pediatrics [28]. However, this alternative is not without its challenges. While these data sources are population-based—with real-world outcomes and large samples, even for relatively rare diseases—they also pose challenges. For children with complex disease or multiple comorbidities, the granular clinical details necessary to identify comparable intervention and control groups are often lacking. Therefore, in PPC studies using health administrative data, population heterogeneity is often a significant issue.

3.3. State of Art or Novel Approaches to Surmount Challenges

Among several options for managing heterogeneous populations in health administrative data are two fairly new methodologies that may be helpful in PPC research design. First, since identifying an appropriate control group is often impossible, one option is to use each individual as his or her own control. In an exposure-crossover design, the rate of a recurrent outcome is compared before and after an exposure [29]. Because every individual has the same profile of fixed characteristics before and after the exposure, the design itself controls all patient-level factors that are stable over time. Self-matching is useful for estimating population-wide effects but has limited ability to evaluate the influence of clinical characteristics, which can vary over time. For these situations, longitudinal models that allow the values of clinical covariates to change over time are required. Second, in a heterogeneous population the question is often about differential effects across subgroups. In latent class analysis and other mixture models, the statistical model can group individuals into classes based on clusters of traits that predict outcomes [30]. In traditional regression models, the independent effect of each trait on the outcome is estimated, whereas latent class analysis identifies patterns in the combined effects of multiple traits on the outcome, allowing a richer description of subgroups within a heterogeneous population [31], as exemplified in two recent PPC studies [32,33]. Latent class analysis can identify potential subgroups of patients, sharing similar observed characteristics, who might experience different effects from a given treatment. This approach is similar to traditional subgroup analysis but surmounts some of the methodological challenges of sub-group analyses, including low statistical power, falling prey to type I errors, and failing to identify higher-order treatment effect interactions [31]. Thus, methodologies like the exposure-crossover design and latent class analysis can be helpful to manage population heterogeneity in studies evaluating the effectiveness of interventions among children receiving PPC.

4. How Do We Monitor and Manage the Problems Arising from Polypharmacy?

4.1. Significance of the Issue

The goal of pharmacotherapy in children receiving PPC is to alleviate existing symptoms while minimizing side effects. Children receiving PPC may have increasing polypharmacy as their physical symptoms progress [34]. Children with polypharmacy may take five or more medications simultaneously, and in PPC these regimens frequently include multiple high-risk medications (such as opioids, psychotherapeutics, and anticonvulsants) [34–37]. Problems from polypharmacy may include increased risk for side effects, adverse drug events, drug-drug interactions, and drug-disease interactions [36–40]. Evidence to guide pharmacotherapy for children receiving PPC is limited for single medications and almost non-existent for complicated regimens.

4.2. Methodologic Challenges

Methodologic challenges complicate detection and management of problems from polypharmacy. First, few population-level data sources contain information about exposures (medications) and outcomes (adverse drug events). Infrequent adverse drug events represent "needles in the haystack," and large comprehensive data sources are required to complete pharmacoepidemiologic studies in populations with rare conditions. Second, identifying outcomes is challenging in both population and clinical studies. Few outcome measures—either case definitions of adverse drug events or patient-reported outcome measures—are available in pediatrics, let alone for children receiving PPC. Third, children receiving PPC may experience multiple treatment- and condition-related symptoms, and this overlap complicates the detection of adverse drug events. Finally, even when evidence exists to support management strategies, translating generalized recommendations to unique and complex PPC patients is difficult [41,42].

4.3. State of Art or Novel Approaches to Surmount Challenges

Fortunately, recognition of the risks of polypharmacy has driven the development of new approaches to meet these challenges. Enhanced data sources now permit population-level pharmacoepidemiologic studies, including in ambulatory settings [35–37]. National data sources provide large enough sample sizes to analyze patterns of medication exposure in patients with rare diseases [43], and the increasing availability of integrated clinical data may allow for better detection of adverse drug events. Furthermore, big data algorithms allow for the assessment of exposures—including exposures to multiple drug combinations—at increasingly smaller intervals (such as on a daily or even hourly basis) [35]. Improved temporal resolution will increase our ability to understand the sequence of events leading to problematic polypharmacy, allowing us to target interventions toward periods of increased risk.

Limited availability of objective patient data complicates the identification of adverse drug events in clinical studies. The Food and Drug Administration's Best Pharmaceuticals for Children Act has prioritized the development of outcome measures of drug safety and efficacy in children with intellectual and developmental disabilities [38,44]. Patient- and proxy-reported symptom assessments developed for PPC patients [14,16] are now being studied for their specific utility in assessing symptom variation before and after medication changes. Patient-Reported Outcomes Measurement Information System (PROMIS) is also expanding the availability of pediatric-specific patient-reported outcome measures, even for those children with neurologic impairment [45,46]. Utilization of these measures may identify changing symptomatology, which can guide therapeutic decisions and enhance medication safety [14,47]. Ultimately, evolving multi-center PPC research networks will enable more rigorous evaluations of medication management strategies specific to PPC patients [41,48].

5. How Can We Address Problems Arising from Missing Data in Longitudinal Studies?

5.1. Significance of the Issue

Longitudinal studies of PPC patients are particularly prone to missing data because PPC patients have a high level of morbidity and mortality, and are thus often unable to complete assessments, especially as their illness advances or their symptoms worsen. The subsequent presence of missing data in these studies erodes precision and threatens the validity of results. Said differently, the loss of precision results in decreased statistical power to detect meaningful differences in effects, and reasons why the data are missing can introduce potential biases in the estimation of effects [49]. If we ignore the presence of missing data in a PPC study, and children who are sicker are more likely to have missing data, inferences made based on data from the remaining less-ill or less-symptomatic participants can be misleading, failing to reflect what happened to all the participants, and may over- or under-estimate associations or treatment effects.

5.2. Methodologic Challenges

Analytic approaches for handling missing data are all based on three different possible assumptions about the mechanisms that can result in missing data: missing completely at random (MCAR), missing at random (MAR), and missing not at random (MNAR). The analytic approach of last observation carried forward is easy to implement but should be avoided even when missing data are MCAR [50]. The analytic approaches of complete-case analysis and unweighted generalized estimating equations make a strong assumption that the data are MCAR (that is, missing data is independent of both observed and unobserved data [51]), an assumption that is unrealistic in a PPC study of patients with high-levels of symptom burden, psychosocial stress, and death. MCAR methods might be sufficiently valid with a small amount of missing data (<5%) but otherwise can lead to serious bias and loss of precision [52]. If the data is assumed to be MAR (that is, missingness depends only on observed data), there are several practical approaches for handling missing data [53], including multiple imputation (MI), weighted procedures that adjust for drop out, and maximum likelihood model-based approaches, such as mixed-effects models. Of note, for these approaches to be accurate, other assumptions (such as no model misspecification) need to be met, and MI requires large sample sizes and strong covariates [49]. Methods exist to test whether the data are MCAR or MAR using data from the study but, importantly, no test exists to rule out the possibility that the data are actually MNAR (that is, missingness is related to unobserved characteristics, such as an unexpected progression of disease or worsening of symptoms, even after accounting for observed data). Importantly, if the missing data is believed to be MNAR—which is most often likely—the missing data mechanism should not be ignored [49].

5.3. State of Art or Novel Approaches to Surmount Challenges

Ideally, the impact and potential bias of missing data is reduced by how the study is designed [52]. This can be done by enabling multiple ways to collect not only the primary data regarding participants, but also auxiliary data. By this phrase "auxiliary data," we mean data collected expressly to address problems that will arise from the expected degree of missingness of primary data elements. Auxiliary data need to be associated with the outcome and should be easier or more feasible to collect than the outcome data. Some approaches to gathering auxiliary data include administration of a short assessment containing only three to five items that are presumed to be highly correlated with the primary outcomes; obtaining assessments from other informants; and measuring variables that might be surrogate outcomes (which is to say, an outcome that is not the most valued main outcome, such as reduction in the level of a symptom, but instead a proxy outcome or a process measure that is strongly associated with the valued main outcome, such as a biomarker or the receipt of an effective symptom ameliorating medication) [49,52].

If the missing data might be MNAR, the methods described above under the MAR assumptions can be used for the primary analysis of incomplete longitudinal data, as these models are robust to departures from MAR [50], but additional analyses using MNAR models should be performed to examine the extent to which inferences from the primary outcome model vary across the different scenarios for missing data. There are three main approaches to performing these sensitivity analyses [54]: selection models [51], pattern-mixture models [55,56], and shared random effects models. These methods pose their own challenges [57], but we believe that the combination of MAR models and sensitivity analyses using MNAR models is the best way to advance our knowledge and understanding in the face of missing data in PPC studies.

6. How Can We Assess Longer-Term Outcomes of Interventions?

6.1. Significance of the Issue

Studies comparing children with and without PPC involvement suggest that PPC results in improved symptom management, fewer invasive procedures, and more comprehensive anticipatory end-of-life guidance [58–60]. The few published randomized controlled trials (RCTs) evaluating PPC interventions also demonstrate improved symptom burden and quality of life, clearer adolescent goals of care, and improved parental mood [16,61–63]. All studies included outcome measurements at specific time-points after the intervention. Among the RCTs, the longest follow-up was 9 months, and investigators observed substantial participant-attrition over time [16,48]. Although proximal efficacy is important, the lack of long-term observation represents a crucial gap in knowledge [64]. Trajectories of serious pediatric illness are long-lasting and characterized by fluctuating and/or chronic symptoms, varying acuity and needs, and diverse psychosocial sequelae [17,34,65–67]. Furthermore, parents and healthy siblings are also at risk for delayed consequences (such as poor mental health and risky health behaviors) [68–71]. Improving these outcomes demands that we also evaluate the durability of PPC interventions among patients and their families.

6.2. Methodologic Challenges

Demonstrating long-term benefit will not be easy. First, adult studies suggest palliative care interventions may have short-lived effects; a recent meta-analysis of RCTs showed improved quality of life and symptom burden at 3-months, but not at 6-months [72]. Second, measuring quality of life among children with serious illness is challenging, particularly since validated instruments are limited [73]. Third, outcomes beyond quality of life are important; we also wonder about patients' functional outcomes (for example, return to school), parent and sibling outcomes (such as caregiver burden), sibling outcomes (such as adjustment), and experience-specific sequelae (such as bereavement outcomes). Fourth, relevant follow-up times depend on patient trajectories, which vary across individuals and diagnoses. Additionally, the possibility of external factors modifying outcomes increases with longer follow-up times. Finally, if findings suggest minimal long-term efficacy, the appropriate response is unclear: are improved short-term outcomes sufficient to warrant implementation, or do we delay implementation until we develop boosters to extend efficacy?

6.3. State of Art or Novel Approaches to Surmount Challenges

Addressing these challenges requires a multi-faceted approach. We should determine what is important to stakeholders, when it is important, and how we can best measure it, which may require the development of new instruments. Due to variability in patient and family- experiences, studies must be longitudinal and include repeated measures. Rather than describing scores at isolated time-points, novel approaches might include "areas under the curve" or comparisons of trajectories between patients who do or do not receive interventions. Investigators should consider interdisciplinary and community partnerships to facilitate longer-term follow-up (for example, partnering with teachers to assess bereaved siblings [70]). Lastly, we must leverage cooperative research groups to enroll sufficient numbers of children and families. Serious illness in children endures. It is time to determine if and how the impact of PPC interventions endures too.

7. How Do We Monitor for Inequities in the Provision of PPC?

7.1. Significance of the Issue

The World Health Organization promotes a "vision of a future in which all people have access to health services that are provided in a way that are coordinated around their needs, respects their preferences, and are safe, effective, timely, affordable, and of acceptable quality" [74]. Unfortunately, in PPC we face many unanswered questions about inequities in PPC provision. International research indicates that not all children who might benefit from PPC receive it. Reported PPC referral rates for children who died after any life-threatening condition vary widely across countries and institutions, with reported rates ranging from 8% to 39% [75–80]. Among children with cancer, rates tend to be higher, with a 63% referral rate reported in one Canadian study [80]. The evaluation of characteristics between children who do and do not receive PPC identifies concerning inequities. Referral rates are lower among children living in rural areas or low-income neighborhoods [80] as well as for African-American children and those without private insurance [76]. Studies show that in child health overall [81], as well as in PPC [82], barriers to accessing appropriate services are multilevel, requiring intervention at the level of the child and family, healthcare provider, health system, and broader society [81,82].

7.2. Methodologic Challenges

Inequities in receipt of PPC have been identified primarily through the use of population-based health administrative data [76]. However, administrative data are not available everywhere, and they do not show the origin of the disparity (for example, healthcare providers may preferentially offer PPC or certain families may be more likely to decline PPC involvement). Misclassification is also possible: families might receive excellent PPC through community providers, and this care may not be identified in administrative data. Additionally, for families who decline PPC, we know little about individual-level (such as lack of knowledge) or societal-level (such as general distrust of the healthcare system) factors that may affect their decision-making [81].

7.3. State of Art or Novel Approaches to Surmount Challenges

Despite the limitations of currently available health administrative data, continued use of these data will help assess the effect of interventions to address disparities. Locally, or where administrative data are not available, comparing demographic characteristics (such as ethnicity, race, language spoken, income, geographic area) among referred children to those of the population served by the institution may highlight potential inequities [83]. Alternatively, as part of morbidity and mortality rounds for children who die within an institution, differences in demographic characteristics between children who did and did not receive PPC could be examined. Further evaluation of disparities in PPC provision may also be facilitated by development, implementation, and validation of "trigger" systems through electronic medical records to identify children who have been diagnosed with a life-threatening condition based on published International Classification of Diseases, Tenth Revision (ICD-10) codes [39,84–87], or other disease- or family-related factors [88]. Such systems may help overcome referral biases among health professionals. They also offer the opportunity to explore decision-making when the system is triggered but a referral does not happen. Qualitative research to explore the views of health providers and families when referrals do not happen would allow for the identification of contributing factors, which could further help with the monitoring and guiding of efforts to reduce inequities.

8. Conclusions

As PPC providers, we pride ourselves in finding creative solutions to seemingly intractable clinical challenges. To address the seemingly unanswerable research questions that are ubiquitous in PPC, we should apply the same "think outside the box" approach to our methodologies. Pushing the boundaries of research design will help us provide the best possible care to children with potentially life-limiting illnesses and their families.

Acknowledgments: K.N. and K.W. receive support from the Canadian Child Health Clinician Scientist Training Program. K.N. receives support from the Clinician Scientist Training Program at the Hospital for Sick Children, Toronto, Canada. J.F. receives support from the *Eunice Kennedy Shriver* National Institute for Child Health and Human Development (Grant K23HD091295).

Author Contributions: C.F. conceived the review and co-authored a section with J.F.; K.N. contributed a section and drafted the manuscript; J.F., C.G., A.R., and K.W. each contributed a section. All authors evaluated, revised, and have approved the final manuscript.

Conflicts of Interest: The authors declare no conflicts of interest. No funding sources played any role in the conception, drafting, or review of this article.

References

1. Himelstein, B.P.; Hilden, J.M.; Boldt, A.M.; Weissman, D. Pediatric palliative care. *N. Engl. J. Med.* **2004**, *350*, 1752–1762. [CrossRef] [PubMed]
2. Wolfe, J.; Grier, H.E.; Klar, N.; Levin, S.B.; Ellenbogen, J.M.; Salem-Schatz, S.; Emanuel, E.J.; Weeks, J.C. Symptoms and suffering at the end of life in children with cancer. *N. Engl. J. Med.* **2000**, *342*, 326–333. [CrossRef] [PubMed]
3. Jalmsell, L.; Kreicbergs, U.; Onelöv, E.; Steineck, G.; Henter, J.-I. Symptoms affecting children with malignancies during the last month of life: A nationwide follow-up. *Pediatrics* **2006**, *117*, 1314–1320. [CrossRef] [PubMed]
4. Hongo, T.; Watanabe, C.; Okada, S.; Inoue, N.; Yajima, S.; Fujii, Y.; Ohzeki, T. Analysis of the circumstances at the end of life in children with cancer: symptoms, suffering and acceptance. *Pediatr. Int.* **2003**, *45*, 60–64. [CrossRef] [PubMed]
5. Collins, J.J.; Byrnes, M.E.; Dunkel, I.J.; Lapin, J.; Nadel, T.; Thaler, H.T.; Polyak, T.; Rapkin, B.; Portenoy, R.K. The Measurement of Symptoms in Children with Cancer. *J. Pain Symptom Manag.* **2000**, *19*, 363–377. [CrossRef]
6. Drake, R.; Frost, J.; Collins, J.J. The symptoms of dying children. *J. Pain Symptom Manag.* **2003**, *26*, 594–603. [CrossRef]
7. Malcolm, C.; Forbat, L.; Anderson, G.; Gibson, F.; Hain, R. Challenging symptom profiles of life-limiting conditions in children: A survey of care professionals and families. *Palliat. Med.* **2011**, *25*, 357–364. [CrossRef] [PubMed]
8. Theunissen, J.M.J.; Hoogerbrugge, P.M.; van Achterberg, T.; Prins, J.B.; Vernooij-Dassen, M.J.F.J.; van den Ende, C.H.M. Symptoms in the palliative phase of children with cancer. *Pediatr. Blood Cancer* **2007**, *49*, 160–165. [CrossRef] [PubMed]

9. Van der Geest, I.M.M.; Darlington, A.-S.E.; Streng, I.C.; Michiels, E.M.C.; Pieters, R.; van den Heuvel-Eibrink, M.M. Parents' experiences of pediatric palliative care and the impact on long-term parental grief. *J. Pain Symptom Manag.* **2014**, *47*, 1043–1053. [CrossRef] [PubMed]
10. Vollenbroich, R.; Borasio, G.D.; Duroux, A.; Grasser, M.; Brandstätter, M.; Führer, M. Listening to parents: The role of symptom perception in pediatric palliative home care. *Palliat. Support. Care* **2016**, *14*, 13–19. [CrossRef] [PubMed]
11. Rosenberg, A.R.; Orellana, L.; Ullrich, C.; Kang, T.I.; Geyer, J.R.; Feudtner, C.; Dussel, V.; Wolfe, J. Quality of life in children with advanced cancer: A report from the PediQUEST Study. *J. Pain Symptom Manag.* **2016**, *52*, 243–253. [CrossRef] [PubMed]
12. Jalmsell, L.; Kreicbergs, U.; Onelöv, E.; Steineck, G.; Henter, J.-I. Anxiety is contagious—Symptoms of anxiety in the terminally ill child affect long-term psychological well-being in bereaved parents. *Pediatr. Blood Cancer* **2010**, *54*, 751–757. [CrossRef] [PubMed]
13. Kreicbergs, U.; Valdimarsdóttir, U.; Onelöv, E.; Björk, O.; Steineck, G.; Henter, J.-I. Care-related distress: A nationwide study of parents who lost their child to cancer. *J. Clin. Oncol.* **2005**, *23*, 9162–9171. [CrossRef] [PubMed]
14. Wolfe, J.; Orellana, L.; Ullrich, C.; Cook, E.F.; Kang, T.I.; Rosenberg, A.; Geyer, R.; Feudtner, C.; Dussel, V. Symptoms and distress in children with advanced cancer: Prospective patient-reported outcomes from the PediQUEST Study. *J. Clin. Oncol.* **2015**, *33*, 1928–1935. [CrossRef] [PubMed]
15. Siden, H.; Steele, R.; Brant, R.; Cadell, S.; Davies, B.; Straatman, L.; Widger, K.; Andrews, G.S. Designing and implementing a longitudinal study of children with neurological, genetic or metabolic conditions: Charting the territory. *BMC Pediatr.* **2010**, *10*, 67. [CrossRef] [PubMed]
16. Wolfe, J.; Orellana, L.; Cook, E.F.; Ullrich, C.; Kang, T.I.; Geyer, J.R.; Feudtner, C.; Weeks, J.C.; Dussel, V. Improving the care of children with advanced cancer by using an electronic patient-reported feedback intervention: Results from the PediQUEST randomized controlled trial. *J. Clin. Oncol.* **2014**, *32*, 1119–1126. [CrossRef] [PubMed]
17. Miller, E.G.; Levy, C.; Linebarger, J.S.; Klick, J.C.; Carter, B.S. Pediatric palliative care: Current evidence and evidence gaps. *J. Pediat.* **2015**, *166*, 1536–1540. [CrossRef] [PubMed]
18. Pandolfini, C.; Bonati, M. A literature review on off-label drug use in children. *Eur. J. Pediatr.* **2005**, *164*, 552–558. [CrossRef] [PubMed]
19. Dunne, J.; Rodriguez, W.J.; Murphy, M.D.; Beasley, B.N.; Burckart, G.J.; Filie, J.D.; Lewis, L.L.; Sachs, H.C.; Sheridan, P.H.; Starke, P.; et al. Extrapolation of Adult Data and Other Data in Pediatric Drug-Development Programs. *Pediatrics* **2011**, *128*, e1242–e1249. [CrossRef] [PubMed]
20. Gantasala, S.; Sullivan, P.B.; Thomas, A.G. Gastrostomy feeding versus oral feeding alone for children with cerebral palsy. *Cochrane Database Syst. Rev.* **2013**, *7*. [CrossRef] [PubMed]
21. Cohen, E.; Berry, J.G.; Camacho, X.; Anderson, G.; Wodchis, W.; Guttmann, A. Patterns and Costs of Health Care Use of Children with Medical Complexity. *Pediatrics* **2012**, *130*, e1463–e1470. [CrossRef] [PubMed]
22. Stone, B.; Hester, G.; Jackson, D.; Richardson, T.; Hall, M.; Gouripeddi, R.; Butcher, R.; Keren, R.; Srivastava, R. Effectiveness of Fundoplication or Gastrojejunal Feeding in Children with Neurologic Impairment. *Hosp. Pediatr.* **2017**, *7*, 140–148. [CrossRef] [PubMed]
23. Bourgeois, F.T.; Murthy, S.; Pinto, C.; Olson, K.L.; Ioannidis, J.P.A.; Mandl, K.D. Pediatric Versus Adult Drug Trials for Conditions with High Pediatric Disease Burden. *Pediatrics* **2012**, *130*, 285–292. [CrossRef] [PubMed]
24. Cohen, E.; Shaul, R.Z. Beyond the therapeutic orphan: Children and clinical trials. *Pediatric Health* **2008**, *2*, 151–159. [CrossRef]
25. Cohen, E.; Kuo, D.Z.; Agrawal, R.; Berry, J.G.; Bhagat, S.K.M.; Simon, T.D.; Srivastava, R. Children with medical complexity: An emerging population for clinical and research initiatives. *Pediatrics* **2011**, *127*, 529–538. [CrossRef] [PubMed]
26. Blanco, C.; Hoertel, N.; Franco, S.; Olfson, M.; He, J.-P.; López, S.; González-Pinto, A.; Limosin, F.; Merikangas, K.R. Generalizability of Clinical Trial Results for Adolescent Major Depressive Disorder. *Pediatrics* **2017**, *140*, e20161701. [CrossRef] [PubMed]
27. Bensink, M.E.; Armfield, N.R.; Pinkerton, R.; Irving, H.; Hallahan, A.R.; Theodoros, D.G.; Russell, T.; Barnett, A.G.; Scuffham, P.A.; Wootton, R. Using videotelephony to support paediatric oncology-related palliative care in the home: From abandoned RCT to acceptability study. *Palliat. Med.* **2009**, *23*, 228–237. [CrossRef] [PubMed]

28. McDonald, K.M.; Davies, S.M.; Haberland, C.A.; Geppert, J.J.; Ku, A.; Romano, P.S. Preliminary Assessment of Pediatric Health Care Quality and Patient Safety in the United States Using Readily Available Administrative Data. *Pediatrics* **2008**, *122*, e416–e425. [CrossRef] [PubMed]
29. Redelmeier, D.A. The exposure-crossover design is a new method for studying sustained changes in recurrent events. *J. Clin. Epidemiol* **2013**, *66*, 955–963. [CrossRef] [PubMed]
30. Muthén, B.; Muthén, L.K. Integrating person-centered and variable-centered analyses: Growth mixture modeling with latent trajectory classes. *Alcohol. Clin. Exp. Res.* **2000**, *24*, 882–891. [CrossRef] [PubMed]
31. Lanza, S.T.; Rhoades, B.L. Latent Class Analysis: An Alternative Perspective on Subgroup Analysis in Prevention and Treatment. *Prev. Sci.* **2011**, *14*, 157–168. [CrossRef] [PubMed]
32. Madrigal, V.N.; Carroll, K.W.; Faerber, J.A.; Walter, J.K.; Morrison, W.E.; Feudtner, C. Parental Sources of Support and Guidance When Making Difficult Decisions in the Pediatric Intensive Care Unit. *J. Pediat.* **2016**, *169*, 221–226. [CrossRef] [PubMed]
33. Lindley, L.C.; Mack, J.W.; Bruce, D.J. Clusters of Multiple Complex Chronic Conditions: A Latent Class Analysis of Children at End of Life. *J. Pain Symptom Manag.* **2016**, *51*, 868–874. [CrossRef] [PubMed]
34. Feudtner, C.; Kang, T.I.; Hexem, K.R.; Friedrichsdorf, S.J.; Osenga, K.; Siden, H.; Friebert, S.E.; Hays, R.M.; Dussel, V.; Wolfe, J. Pediatric Palliative Care Patients: A Prospective Multicenter Cohort Study. *Pediatrics* **2011**, *127*, 1094–1101. [CrossRef] [PubMed]
35. Feinstein, J.A.; Feudtner, C.; Valuck, R.J.; Kempe, A. The depth, duration, and degree of outpatient pediatric polypharmacy in Colorado fee-for-service Medicaid patients. *Pharmacoepidemiol. Drug Saf.* **2015**, *24*, 1049–1057. [CrossRef] [PubMed]
36. Feinstein, J.; Dai, D.; Zhong, W.; Freedman, J.; Feudtner, C. Potential drug-drug interactions in infant, child, and adolescent patients in children's hospitals. *Pediatrics* **2015**, *135*, e99–108. [CrossRef] [PubMed]
37. Dai, D.; Feinstein, J.A.; Morrison, W.E.; Zuppa, A.F.; Feudtner, C. Epidemiology of Polypharmacy and Potential Drug–Drug Interactions Among Pediatric Patients in ICUs of U.S. Children's Hospitals. *Pediatr. Crit. Care Med.* **2016**, *17*, e218–e228. [CrossRef] [PubMed]
38. Feinstein, J.A.; Morrato, E.H.; Feudtner, C. Prioritizing Pediatric Drug Research Using Population-Level Health Data. *JAMA Pediatr.* **2017**, *171*, 7–8. [CrossRef] [PubMed]
39. Feudtner, C.; Feinstein, J.A.; Zhong, W.; Hall, M.; Dai, D. Pediatric complex chronic conditions classification system version 2: Updated for ICD-10 and complex medical technology dependence and transplantation. *BMC Pediatr.* **2014**, *14*, 199. [CrossRef] [PubMed]
40. Feinstein, J.A.; Feudtner, C.; Kempe, A. Adverse Drug Event-Related Emergency Department Visits Associated with Complex Chronic Conditions. *Pediatrics* **2014**, *133*, e1575–e1585. [CrossRef] [PubMed]
41. Feudtner, C.; Freedman, J.; Kang, T.I.; Womer, J.W.; Dai, D.; Faerber, J. Comparative effectiveness of Senna to prevent problematic constipation in pediatric oncology patients receiving opioids: A multicenter study of clinically detailed administrative data. *J. Pain Symptom Manag.* **2014**, *48*, 272–280. [CrossRef] [PubMed]
42. Blackmer, A.B.; Feinstein, J.A. Management of Sleep Disorders in Children with Neurodevelopmental Disorders: A Review. *Pharmacotherapy* **2016**, *36*, 84–98. [CrossRef] [PubMed]
43. Institute of Medicine. *Dying in America: Improving Quality and Honoring Individual Preferences Near the End of Life*; The National Academies Press: Washington, DC, USA, 2015.
44. National Institutes of Health Best Pharmaceuticals for Children Act (BPCA) Priority List of Needs in Pediatric Therapeutics. Available online: https://urldefense.proofpoint.com/v2/url?u=http-3A__www.webcitation.org_6w6TBjpO7&d=DwIDAw&c=Sj806OTFwmuG2UO1EEDr-2uZRzm2EPz39TfVBG2Km-o&r=hCtRmhaXCNElmg7tzNohbAfk6UpCYSLjij0FFxe5rdc&m=Jyl39bOW_Ls_GdjfohyH9Tt9Mh6lg_vBx2B7YMXx3Ag&s=8HInzoXlPNwPDwNfnVGcCf5XlOgmelju31Qex0WZC-M&e= (accessed on 30 December 2017).
45. Available PROMIS® Measures for Pediatric Self-Report (Ages 8–17) and Parent Proxy Report (Ages 5–17). Available online: https://urldefense.proofpoint.com/v2/url?u=http-3A__www.webcitation.org_6w6TVGEkS&d=DwIDAw&c=Sj806OTFwmuG2UO1EEDr-2uZRzm2EPz39TfVBG2Km-o&r=hCtRmhaXCNElmg7tzNohbAfk6UpCYSLjij0FFxe5rdc&m=XYRSLI5eBKo30Q_e54g5A7dtDt9OxQ18AIvCfLweQF4&s=_qBm6X7yEcME_VrfUGFcTXsfwEe0_zt3E7R2gNnhzi0&e= (accessed on 30 December 2017).

46. Lai, J.-S.; Nowinski, C.; Victorson, D.; Bode, R.; Podrabsky, T.; McKinney, N.; Straube, D.; Holmes, G.L.; McDonald, C.M.; Henricson, E.; et al. Quality-of-life measures in children with neurological conditions: Pediatric Neuro-QOL. *Neurorehabil. Neural Repair* **2012**, *26*, 36–47. [CrossRef] [PubMed]
47. Joyce, B.T.; Lau, D.T. Hospice experiences and approaches to support and assess family caregivers in managing medications for home hospice patients: A providers survey. *Palliat. Med.* **2013**, *27*, 329–338. [CrossRef] [PubMed]
48. Dussel, V.; Orellana, L.; Soto, N.; Chen, K.; Ullrich, C.; Kang, T.I.; Geyer, J.R.; Feudtner, C.; Wolfe, J. Feasibility of Conducting a Palliative Care Randomized Controlled Trial in Children with Advanced Cancer: Assessment of the PediQUEST Study. *J. Pain Symptom Manag.* **2015**, *49*, 1059–1069. [CrossRef] [PubMed]
49. Bell, M.L.; Fairclough, D.L. Practical and statistical issues in missing data for longitudinal patient-reported outcomes. *Stat. Methods Med. Res.* **2014**, *23*, 440–459. [CrossRef] [PubMed]
50. Molenberghs, G.; Thijs, H.; Jansen, I.; Beunckens, C.; Kenward, M.G.; Mallinckrodt, C.; Carroll, R.J. Analyzing incomplete longitudinal clinical trial data. *Biostatistics* **2004**, *5*, 445–464. [CrossRef] [PubMed]
51. Little, R.J.A.; Rubin, D.B. *Statistical. Analysis with Missing Data*, 2nd ed.; John Wiley & Sons: New York, NY, USA, 1987; pp. 3–349.
52. Fairclough, D.L. *Design. and Analysis of Quality of Life Studies in Clinical Trials*, 2nd ed.; Chapman & Hall/CRC Press: Boca Raton, FL, USA, 2010; pp. 1–357.
53. Fitzmaurice, G.M.; Laird, N.M.; Ware, J.H. *Applied. Longitudinal Analysis*, 2nd ed.; John Wiley & Sons: Hoboken, NJ, USA, 2011; pp. 1–654.
54. Ibrahim, J.G.; Molenberghs, G. Missing data methods in longitudinal studies: A review. *Test (Madr.)* **2009**, *18*, 1–43. [PubMed]
55. Little, R.J.A. A class of pattern-mixture models for normal incomplete data. *Biometrika* **1994**, *81*, 471–483. [CrossRef]
56. Little, R.J.A. Pattern-Mixture Models for Multivariate Incomplete Data. *J. Am. Stat. Assoc.* **1993**, *88*, 125.
57. Little, R.J.A. Selection and Pattern-mixture models. (Chapter 18). In *Longitudinal Data Analysis*; Chapman & Hall/CRC Press: Boca Raton, FL, USA, 2009; pp. 409–429.
58. Osenga, K.; Postier, A.; Dreyfus, J.; Foster, L.; Teeple, W.; Friedrichsdorf, S.J. A Comparison of Circumstances at the End of Life in a Hospital Setting for Children with Palliative Care Involvement Versus Those Without. *J. Pain Symptom Manag.* **2016**, *52*, 673–680. [CrossRef] [PubMed]
59. Kassam, A.; Skiadaresis, J.; Alexander, S.; Wolfe, J. Differences in end-of-life communication for children with advanced cancer who were referred to a palliative care team. *Pediatr. Blood Cancer* **2015**, *62*, 1409–1413. [CrossRef] [PubMed]
60. Ullrich, C.K.; Lehmann, L.; London, W.B.; Guo, D.; Sridharan, M.; Koch, R.; Wolfe, J. End-of-Life Care Patterns Associated with Pediatric Palliative Care among Children Who Underwent Hematopoietic Stem Cell Transplant. *Biol. Blood Marrow Transplant.* **2016**, *22*, 1049–1055. [CrossRef] [PubMed]
61. Lyon, M.E.; Jacobs, S.; Briggs, L.; Cheng, Y.I.; Wang, J. Family-Centered Advance Care Planning for Teens with Cancer. *JAMA Pediatr.* **2013**, *167*, 460–467. [CrossRef] [PubMed]
62. Lyon, M.E.; D'Angelo, L.J.; Dallas, R.H.; Hinds, P.S.; Garvie, P.A.; Wilkins, M.L.; Garcia, A.; Briggs, L.; Flynn, P.M.; Rana, S.R.; et al. A randomized clinical trial of adolescents with HIV/AIDS: Pediatric advance care planning. *AIDS Care* **2017**, *29*, 1287–1296. [CrossRef] [PubMed]
63. Sahler, O.J.Z.; Dolgin, M.J.; Phipps, S.; Fairclough, D.L.; Askins, M.A.; Katz, E.R.; Noll, R.B.; Butler, R.W. Specificity of problem-solving skills training in mothers of children newly diagnosed with cancer: Results of a multisite randomized clinical trial. *J. Clin. Oncol.* **2013**, *31*, 1329–1335. [CrossRef] [PubMed]
64. Rosenberg, A.R.; Wolfe, J. Approaching the third decade of paediatric palliative oncology investigation: Historical progress and future directions. *Lancet Child Adolesc. Health.* **2017**, *1*, 56–67. [CrossRef]
65. Hain, R.; Devins, M.; Hastings, R.; Noyes, J. Paediatric palliative care: Development and pilot study of a "Directory" of life-limiting conditions. *BMC Palliative Care* **2013**, *12*, 43. [CrossRef] [PubMed]
66. Ananth, P.; Melvin, P.; Feudtner, C.; Wolfe, J.; Berry, J.G. Hospital Use in the Last Year of Life for Children with Life-Threatening Complex Chronic Conditions. *Pediatrics* **2015**, *136*, 938–946. [CrossRef] [PubMed]
67. Smith, A.G.; Andrews, S.; Bratton, S.L.; Sheetz, J.; Feudtner, C.; Zhong, W.; Maloney, C.G. Pediatric Palliative Care and Inpatient Hospital Costs: A Longitudinal Cohort Study. *Pediatrics* **2015**, *135*, 694–700. [CrossRef] [PubMed]
68. Janvier, A.; Farlow, B.; Baardsnes, J.; Pearce, R.; Barrington, K.J. Measuring and communicating meaningful outcomes in neonatology: A family perspective. *Semin. Perinatol.* **2016**, *40*, 571–577. [CrossRef] [PubMed]

69. Rosenberg, A.R.; Postier, A.; Osenga, K.; Kreicbergs, U.; Neville, B.; Dussel, V.; Wolfe, J. Long-Term Psychosocial Outcomes Among Bereaved Siblings of Children with Cancer. *J. Pain Symptom Manag.* **2015**, *49*, 55–65. [CrossRef] [PubMed]
70. Gerhardt, C.A.; Fairclough, D.L.; Grossenbacher, J.C.; Barrera, M.; Gilmer, M.J.; Foster, T.L.; Compas, B.E.; Davies, B.; Hogan, N.S.; Vannatta, K. Peer relationships of bereaved siblings and comparison classmates after a child's death from cancer. *J. Pediatr. Psychol.* **2012**, *37*, 209–219. [CrossRef] [PubMed]
71. Rosenberg, A.R.; Baker, K.S.; Syrjala, K.; Wolfe, J. Systematic review of psychosocial morbidities among bereaved parents of children with cancer. *Pediatr. Blood Cancer* **2012**, *58*, 503–512. [CrossRef] [PubMed]
72. Kavalieratos, D.; Corbelli, J.; Zhang, D.; Dionne-Odom, J.N.; Ernecoff, N.C.; Hanmer, J.; Hoydich, Z.P.; Ikejiani, D.Z.; Klein-Fedyshin, M.; Zimmermann, C.; et al. Association Between Palliative Care and Patient and Caregiver Outcomes: A Systematic Review and Meta-analysis. *JAMA* **2016**, *316*, 2104–2114. [CrossRef] [PubMed]
73. Coombes, L.H.; Wiseman, T.; Lucas, G.; Sangha, A.; Murtagh, F.E. Health-related quality-of-life outcome measures in paediatric palliative care: A systematic review of psychometric properties and feasibility of use. *Palliat. Med.* **2016**, *30*, 935–949. [CrossRef] [PubMed]
74. WHO Framework on Integrated People-Centred Health Services. Available online: https://urldefense.proofpoint.com/v2/url?u=http-3A__www.webcitation.org_6w6Vhur8c&d=DwIDAw&c=Sj806OTFwmuG2UO1EEDr-2uZRzm2EPz39TfVBG2Km-o&r=hCtRmhaXCNElmg7tzNohbAfk6UpCYSLjij0FFxe5rdc&m=x8_mpOyGJseAl4wojph16pQ-O6XtwZ_S1RUQToospNM&s=Zd_0V18RBXrx39jLIDxSe_wx72-unLMTCYYPC6qoOrM&e= (accessed on 30 December 2017).
75. Fraser, L.K.; Miller, M.; McKinney, P.A.; Parslow, R.C.; Feltbower, R.G. Referral to a specialist paediatric palliative care service in oncology patients. *Pediatr. Blood Cancer* **2011**, *56*, 677–680. [CrossRef] [PubMed]
76. Keele, L.; Keenan, H.T.; Sheetz, J.; Bratton, S.L. Differences in characteristics of dying children who receive and do not receive palliative care. *Pediatrics* **2013**, *132*, 72–78. [CrossRef] [PubMed]
77. Chang, E.; MacLeod, R.; Drake, R. Characteristics influencing location of death for children with life-limiting illness. *Arch. Dis. Child.* **2013**, *98*, 419–424. [CrossRef] [PubMed]
78. Widger, K.; Davies, D.; Rapoport, A.; Vadeboncoeur, C.; Liben, S.; Sarpal, A.; Stenekes, S.; Cyr, C.; Daoust, L.; Gregoire, M.C.; et al. Pediatric palliative care in Canada in 2012: A cross-sectional descriptive study. *CMAJ Open* **2016**, *4*, E562–E568. [CrossRef] [PubMed]
79. Keele, L.; Keenan, H.T.; Bratton, S.L. The Effect of Palliative Care Team Design on Referrals to Pediatric Palliative Care. *J. Pall Med.* **2016**, *19*, 286–291. [CrossRef] [PubMed]
80. Widger, K.; Sutradhar, R.; Rapoport, A.; Vadeboncoeur, C.; Zelcer, S.; Kassam, A.; Nelson, K.E.; Liu, Y.; Wolfe, J.; Earle, C.C.; et al. Predictors of Specialized Pediatric Palliative Care Involvement and Impact on Patterns of End-of-Life Care in Children With Cancer. *J. Clin. Oncol.* **2018**, JCO2017756312. [CrossRef] [PubMed]
81. Ridgeway, J.L.; Wang, Z.; Finney Rutten, L.J.; van Ryn, M.; Griffin, J.M.; Murad, M.H.; Asiedu, G.B.; Egginton, J.S.; Beebe, T.J. Conceptualising paediatric health disparities: A metanarrative systematic review and unified conceptual framework. *BMJ Open* **2017**, *7*, e015456. [PubMed]
82. Linton, J.M.; Feudtner, C. What accounts for differences or disparities in pediatric palliative and end-of-life care? A systematic review focusing on possible multilevel mechanisms. *Pediatrics* **2008**, *122*, 574–582. [CrossRef] [PubMed]
83. Chin, M.H.; Alexander-Young, M.; Burnet, D.L. Health care quality-improvement approaches to reducing child health disparities. *Pediatrics* **2009**, *124* (Suppl. 3), S224–S236. [CrossRef] [PubMed]
84. Fraser, L.K.; Jarvis, S.; Moran, N.; Aldridge, J.; Parslow, R.; Beresford, B. *Children in Scotland Requiring Palliative Care*; University of York: York, UK, 2015; p. 46.
85. Simon, T.D.; Cawthon, M.L.; Stanford, S.; Popalisky, J.; Lyons, D.; Woodcox, P.; Hood, M.; Chen, A.Y.; Rita Mangione-Smith for the Center of Excellence on Quality of Care Measures for Children with Complex Needs (COE4CCN) Medical Complexity Working Group. Pediatric Medical Complexity Algorithm: A New Method to Stratify Children by Medical Complexity. *Pediatrics* **2014**, *133*, e1647–e1654. [CrossRef] [PubMed]
86. Berry, J.G.; Hall, M.; Cohen, E.; O'Neill, M.; Feudtner, C. Ways to Identify Children with Medical Complexity and the Importance of Why. *J. Pediat.* **2015**, *167*, 229–237. [CrossRef] [PubMed]

87. Friebert, S.; Osenga, K. Pediatric Palliative Care Referral Criteria. Available online: https://urldefense.proofpoint.com/v2/url?u=http-3A__www.webcitation.org_6xCh24iqm&d=DwIDAw&c=Sj806OTFwmuG2UO1EEDr-2uZRzm2EPz39TfVBG2Km-o&r=hCtRmhaXCNElmg7tzNohbAfk6UpCYSLjij0FFxe5rdc&m=ro98t5YdoLzY-mFoUWhMZ8_3k4j0RBcCZEMk0idOD-o&s=nPGEm3cYtA4-KHCRep61S53wPv7tpyPHjsgW9KQIqDc&e= (accessed on 13 February 2018).
88. Kaye, E.C.; Rubenstein, J.; Levine, D.; Baker, J.N.; Dabbs, D.; Friebert, S.E. Pediatric palliative care in the community. *CA Cancer J. Clin.* **2015**, *65*, 316–333. [CrossRef] [PubMed]

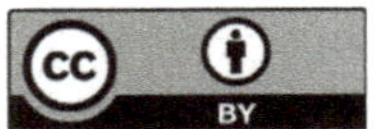

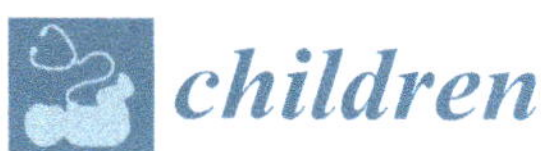

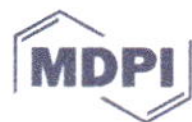

Article

From the Child's Word to Clinical Intervention: Novel, New, and Innovative Approaches to Symptoms in Pediatric Palliative Care

Katharine E. Brock [1,2,3], Joanne Wolfe [4,5] and Christina Ullrich [4,5,*]

1 Aflac Cancer and Blood Disorders Center of Children's Healthcare of Atlanta, Atlanta, GA 30322, USA; Katharine.brock@choa.org
2 Pediatric Palliative Care, Children's Healthcare of Atlanta, Atlanta, GA 30322, USA
3 Department of Pediatrics, Division of Pediatric Hematology/Oncology, Emory University, Atlanta, GA 30322, USA
4 Department of Psychosocial Oncology and Palliative Care, Dana-Farber Cancer Institute, Boston, MA 02215, USA; Joanne_Wolfe@dfci.harvard.edu
5 Department of Pediatric Hematology/Oncology, Dana-Farber Cancer Institute, Boston Children's Hospital Cancer and Blood Disorders Center, Boston, MA 02215, USA
* Correspondence: Christina_Ullrich@dfci.harvard.edu; Tel.: +1-617-632-4997

Received: 19 December 2017 Accepted: 21 March 2018; Published: 28 March 2018

Abstract: Despite vast improvements in disease-based treatments, many children live with life-threatening disorders that cause distressing symptoms. These symptoms can be difficult to comprehensively assess and manage. Yet, frequent and accurate symptom reporting and expert treatment is critical to preserving a patient's physical, psychological, emotional, social, and existential heath. We describe emerging methods of symptom and health-related quality-of-life (HRQOL) assessment through patient-reported outcomes (PROs) tools now used in clinical practice and novel research studies. Computer-based and mobile apps can facilitate assessment of symptoms and HRQOL. These technologies can be used alone or combined with therapeutic strategies to improve symptoms and coping skills. We review technological advancements, including mobile apps and toys, that allow improved symptom reporting and management. Lastly, we explore the value of a pediatric palliative care interdisciplinary team and their role in assessing and managing distressing symptoms and minimizing suffering in both the child and family. These methods and tools highlight the way that novel, new, and innovative approaches to symptom assessment and management are changing the way that pediatrics and pediatric palliative care will be practiced in the future.

Keywords: pediatric palliative care; quality of life; symptom management; hospice; patient-reported outcomes; mobile apps

1. Introduction

Over 400,000 US children live with life-threatening or chronic, complex conditions [1,2]. Over 12,400 children are diagnosed with cancer annually in the United States [3]. Despite vast improvement in overall survival, less attention has been focused on comprehensively assessing and treating symptoms. Even with a bevy of new cancer-directed therapies, children continue to suffer from distressing symptoms such as pain, fatigue, nausea/vomiting, decreased appetite, anxiety, and depression [4–6]. Symptoms may arise from the disease itself, or commonly from the treatments prescribed. Many of the symptoms children suffer through are experienced in the home setting, away from the hospital, contributing to the perception of few treatment options [7]. Numerous factors lead to poor symptom control at the patient, parent, healthcare team, and system levels [8]. These include a lack of provider time and skill in addressing symptoms, infrequent use of systematic assessment tools, and provider uncertainty around the accuracy of pediatric patient-reported symptoms [8,9]. Patient forgetfulness, the desire to be a "good patient", and the belief that one needs to experience symptoms for better chance of cure also impact symptom reporting [10,11]. System challenges include lack of sufficient integrative medicine, chronic pain, psychiatry, psychology, and palliative care resources to meet patients' needs [12–14]. Multiple interventions have been attempted to improve the reporting of symptoms by patients and families, such as improved outpatient screening [15], frequent monitoring [8,16,17], increased use of patient-reported outcomes (PROs) [5,18], technological advances [8,16,17], and embedding palliative care experts within oncology centers [19]. In this article, we describe the current state of symptom assessment and management within pediatric palliative care, with a focus on pediatric oncology. We also describe emerging and novel approaches to symptom assessment for patients with serious and complex illness.

2. Technological Advances for Symptom Assessment, Reporting, and Management

Technology use in America is ubiquitous. Ninety-five percent of Americans own a cellphone [20]; 70% own a smartphone, up from 35% in 2011 [20]. Of US adults aged 18–29 years, 100% own a cellphone, with 92% owning a smartphone [20]; among 12–17 year-olds, nearly three-quarters own a smartphone [21]. Along with mobile phones, Americans own a range of other devices; nearly 80% of US adults own a computer, and 51% own tablet devices [20]. Roughly three-quarters have internet access in the home [22]. Of teens and adults ages 18–29 years, nearly 100% use the internet regularly [21,22], and 71–86% are social media users, often accessing sites daily [21,23]. Notably, the use of these devices has extended into the healthcare setting. Technology has changed how patients and clinicians communicate with each other outside of the hospital and how patients or parents connect with other families online. Patients utilize technology to remember appointments, instructions, and enhance their medication adherence [24,25].

As technology plays a larger role in children, patients, and families lives, hospitals, clinicians, and researchers have attempted to utilize technology for symptom assessment and integrate reports into the medical record. In technology's most simple form, patients can be called or emailed symptom questionnaires to complete. This can be done while patients are in the hospital or waiting room, yet an important application is for longitudinal symptom tracking while patients are at home. Systems must be reliable, accurate, and permit efficient collection of symptom and health-related quality of life (HRQOL) data.

Electronic systems, usually employing a handheld computer and touch screen, are quite acceptable to patients [26–29]. While relatively little comparison of technology-based versus paper-based modes of administration has been conducted, one study found data equivalence between app-based and other delivery methods [30]. Another (n = 19) study of children with or without a speech or voice disorder also found that the scores did not differ between paper and pencil and electronic handheld device groups. However, the percentage of children who made answering errors or omissions was significantly smaller in the group who used an electronic handheld device. The device also permitted more efficient collection and manipulation of data [31].

Increasing in complexity, survey results can be fed back to the research team and physician in real time. Electronic methods of collecting data from patients have also allowed the presentation of real-time symptom and HRQOL measurements to clinicians, at the time of the clinical encounter with the patient. Feedback to clinicians is viewed favorably by patients [32,33] and clinicians alike [33]. Moreover, this strategy is feasible in busy oncology practices [34], does not increase consultation time, facilitates patient-clinician communication about symptoms or HRQOL, and increases the likelihood that symptom issues are addressed [33,35–38]. Many technology-based PRO collection systems permit assessment of symptoms and HRQOL in between clinic visits, at times that the clinician would not otherwise understand the patient's condition. This is especially important since patients may be unwilling to call the office, and routine PRO assessment may provide opportunities to attend to symptoms before they escalate.

3. Assessment of Child Symptoms and Health-Related Quality of Life

The Science of Self and Proxy Reporting

Accurate symptom reporting, timely assessment, and expert treatment are critical to preventing additional decrements to the patient's physical, psychological, emotional, social, and existential domains of heath. Child self-report is considered the gold standard for assessing symptom burden and HRQOL, as parents and clinicians tend to under-report the severity and number of symptoms children are experiencing [39,40]. Discrepancies among reporters have been demonstrated in several disease groups, including children with cancer, congenital cardiac disease, and those who are status-post bone marrow transplantation [41–43]; however, the direction of this association can vary. For example, parents of children with sickle cell disease have been shown to give worse ratings of their child's HRQOL compared with the child's ratings [44].

In general, concordance is better (informant discrepancy is less) with physical symptoms compared with psychological symptoms [45,46]. This difference was recently demonstrated to be true in a population of children who received a pediatric palliative care consult and may be explained by the fact that physical symptoms are more readily assessed based on biomedical or behavioral changes [47]. Parent ratings can also be affected by their own life experiences, mental state, and distress levels [43,45,48–50]. Considerations around use of child self-report versus parent or clinician proxy-report are summarized in Table 1. In the end, the best approach to differing perspectives is to take advantage of their diversity, incorporating all viewpoints to provide a more global picture of the child's experience [43].

Table 1. Considerations around use of self, parent and clinician report when assessing child symptoms and health-related quality-of-life (HRQOL).

Self-Report	Parent Report	Clinician Report
• For subjective outcomes (e.g., symptoms, HRQOL), the person experiencing the outcomes is the expert. Thus, self-report is considered the gold standard	• Parent often has a longstanding and nuanced knowledge of child; besides the child, is often considered "the expert" regarding the child's experience	• May or may not be familiar with child, which can impact ratings
• Various factors (e.g., medical, developmental, cognitive) may influence self-report	• When child unable to self-report, parent report is often considered the next best alternative	• Valuable when the child cannot self-report due to developmental considerations or illness
• Young and seriously ill children may be limited in their ability to self-report at all	• In general, greater agreement with child ratings for observable functioning (e.g., physical symptoms and HRQOL) and less for functioning that cannot be observed (e.g., emotional symptoms and HRQOL)	• Like all raters, reports may be colored by the rater's own experiences, beliefs, skill level, academic interests, expectations and points of reference
	• May be influenced by parent factors, such as parent anxiety or distress (generally associated with worse ratings) as well as parent expectations and points of reference	• Clinicians may have the experience of caring for many children under similar circumstances, which can shape their views about a particular child's experience
	• Parent proxies can also provide input regarding the parent and family experience	

Since child self-report is taken to be the gold standard when it comes to assessing their symptoms, novel methods are needed to obtain symptom assessments from children of all ages and developmental stages, validate additional pediatric measures across a wider variety of patient populations, understand patient-reported outcomes, translate results to the treating teams, and change supportive care therapies when warranted.

4. Patient-Reported Outcomes Assessment

A patient-reported outcome (PRO) is "any report of the status of a patient's health condition that comes directly from the patient, without interpretation of the patient's response by a clinician or anyone else" [51]. Medical outcomes have historically focused on biomedical or physiologic endpoints (e.g., progression free survival in oncology, overall survival). However, these outcomes do not capture a person's experience of living with a medical condition or illness, such as side effects of the illness and its treatment, and treatment burden. To gain a better understanding of a patient's lived experience, assessment of PRO that capture outcomes such as functional status, as well as aspects of HRQOL, including physical symptoms and functioning, emotional symptoms and social functioning are imperative. Adult oncologists endorse the utility of PRO collection, with clinical measures such as performance status being most important. PRO becomes even more important when multiple treatments options are under consideration, in the setting of advanced or incurable disease, or for patients receiving palliative care [52].

In recent years, systematic collection of PRO has also become an integral part of the assessment of new therapies and interventions [51,53]. Basch and colleagues demonstrated that patient self-reports of symptomatic adverse events (toxicities) were highly feasible (overall adherence of 93%) in a large, multicenter trial of 361 adults with cancer. Moreover, participants reported more toxicities than did investigators, indicating that this collection strategy utilizing PRO may enhance the precision of symptomatic toxicity collection in trials [54]. In both the clinical and research settings, PRO assessment is advantageous to patients, practitioners, and investigators alike, and therefore, integration of PRO assessment into clinical workflows and investigations will likely accelerate.

Patient-Reported Outcomes Assessment with Feedback

With regard to clinical outcomes, feedback of PRO to clinicians in the aforementioned study conducted by Basch and colleagues resulted in fewer emergency room visits and hospitalizations [55]. Feedback also resulted in improved survival [56]. Whether this was due to improved symptom control and mitigation/prevention of worsening toxicity or enhanced tolerance of continued treatment warrants additional study. PRO data can improve care delivered by informing patient and clinician expectations, catalyzing communication about important issues, and promoting shared decision-making such that interventions meeting a patient's specific needs and goals are chosen. Recent experience with PRO reporting to clinicians in a large health care system also suggests that it enhances physician satisfaction and prevents burnout by enhancing physician-patient relationships, increasing workflow efficiency and enabling crucial conversations that otherwise may not occur [57]. Suggestions for PRO assessment and feedback to clinicians are presented in Table 3.

Table 2. Suggestions for use of patient-reported outcomes (PRO) and feedback reports in the clinical setting.

Aspects of Patient-Reported Outcomes and Feedback Reports	Considerations
Choice of measures and outcomes	Outcomes should be meaningful and important to the patient. When possible, select standardized measures. Utilize instruments that have been evaluated by members of the target audience. If available and pending context (research vs clinical), consider use of condition-specific measures which may be more sensitive to intervention effects. Carefully select frequency and timing of assessments to avoid survey fatigue, ensure that assessment points are clinically meaningful and provide results that can be acted upon in future clinical visits.

Table 2. *Cont.*

Aspects of Patient-Reported Outcomes and Feedback Reports	Considerations
Data presentation	Make displays intuitive using pie graphs and line charts showing trends in function and symptoms. Make reports easily accessible to viewers [58]. Present a defined, carefully selected set of data (avoid presenting too much). Present current scores and recent trends. Correlation of trends with recent clinical events (e.g., chemotherapy, hospitalization) is also helpful. Make scores easy to interpret for patients and clinicians. Provide context for clinicians who may not be familiar with symptom or HRQOL scores and meaningful changes in scores. Other strategies to effectively present results to patients and clinicians have recently been described [59,60].
Clinician Use	Make reports available at the point of care in electronic format via website, emailed to clinicians, and incorporated within the electronic medical record. The optimal mode will depend upon the clinical practice. Link reports to supportive care guidelines/recommendations for intervention Minimize disruption to the clinical workflow.
Implementation	Ensure buy-in from patients/families and clinicians alike when embarking on the study. Ensure patient interface is easy to use. Minimize time burden for all users. Ensure processes for responding to reports in a timely manner. Ensure adequate networks, software and properly configured devices for data collection.

5. Patient-Reported Outcomes in Pediatrics

Collection of PRO in pediatrics lags-behind the adult realm in both the clinical and research realm. For example, within the research realm, a review of clinical trials listed in ClinicalTrials.gov [61] and involving children with chronic conditions revealed that only 36 of 495 trials included patient and family-important outcomes, with these outcomes being particularly rare in drug trial and early phase trials [62]. The National Cancer Institute's Common Terminology Criteria for Adverse Events (CTCAE) is a well-established system by which adverse events are gleaned from the medical record, potentially missing subjective symptoms that are reported by the patient and not reliably contained in the medical record. The Pediatric Patient-Reported Outcomes version of the CTCAE, or PRO-CTCAE, builds on the established CTCAE, allowing the child's (or proxy's) voice to be a routine trial endpoint. While not yet publicly available, the hope is that through the Pediatric- and Proxy PRO-CTCAE measures, the impact of an investigational treatment on a child can be more fully understood and addressed [63,64]. This continues to be a research- and clinical trial–focused tool rather than for use in routine clinical care settings.

Regarding clinical use, pediatric oncologists report that routine assessment of PRO would be useful in their practice, particularly those focused on pain, feeling sad or depressed, overall physical symptoms, problems with therapy adherence, and emotional issues [65]. When PROs are collected frequently and routinely, the process is normalized. It conveys a message to patients and families that their perspectives and experiences are valued. This, of course, means that clinicians must respond to PRO collected data in the clinical setting so that child reports are not ignored.

Pediatric Patient-Reported Outcome Instrumentation

Pediatric PRO collection has historically been challenged by the number of instruments developed for collection of PRO from children as well as their inconsistent use. Many of these instruments are not based on a similar conceptual foundation (i.e., instrument content and domains are founded on different conceptual frameworks). Pediatric PRO instruments have also been developed with the use of different psychometric methods and properties (e.g., cross-sectional versus longitudinal). As a result, a wide range of instruments exist, with varying degrees of reliability, validity, and comparability [66]. Recent systematic reviews assessing PROs for children with cancer confirmed that substantial heterogeneity exists in content and distribution of items (e.g., which aspects of health are assessed and whether individual questions focus on function versus well-being) [67,68].

To address these issues, the National Institutes of Health (NIH)-sponsored PROMIS (Patient-Reported Outcomes Measurement Information System) measures, including pediatrics-specific measures, were developed in recent years as part of the NIH Roadmap for Medical Research Initiative [69–72]. Publicly available, PROMIS measures assess domains such as physical, emotional, and social health as well as symptoms (e.g., pain). PROMIS measures are designed to assess symptoms and function in the general population and in individuals living with chronic conditions with a brief completion time. Pediatric self-report PROMIS measures are available for ages 8–17 years and parent-proxy versions are available for children aged 5–17 years, in English, Spanish, and other languages. They are psychometrically sound, having undergone extensive testing using modern test theory, in both cross-sectional and longitudinal analyses (e.g., responsiveness, test-retest reliability) [73,74]. In addition, short forms and compatibility with computer adaptive testing make them highly usable. An additional strength of the PROMIS measures is that child and adult emotional distress measures are linked, allowing both populations to be evaluated within studies or for children to be followed into adulthood in longitudinal studies [75].

An innovative technological approach to instrumentation and collection of PRO is that of computer adaptive technology (CAT). In CAT, each question presented is selected based on a respondent's previous response. This permits generation of an accurate score based on fewer numbers of questions than standard item administration would require. Developed in Europe, the Kids-CAT system has been validated as a system for measuring physical and psychological well-being, parent relations, social support and peers, and school well-being in children with asthma, diabetes, or rheumatoid arthritis. In addition to providing greater measurement precision and lower test burden compared to conventional tests, it provides immediate feedback reports to clinicians [76–78].

6. Novel Tools, Apps, and Toys for Symptom Assessment and Management

6.1. Online or Computer-Based Tools

Online tools are being developed both in a research context, and also in a patient-focused manner. One example of a research-focused tool is PediQUEST [5]. Evaluated in the first randomized controlled trial of a supportive care intervention for children with advanced cancer, PediQUEST is a web-based PRO data collection system that prospectively and longitudinally collected child self-reported and parent proxy-reported symptoms and HRQOL at three large cancer centers [79]. The PediQUEST study demonstrated that collection of PRO from children with advanced cancer was highly feasible. For example, among 708 potential child administrations (i.e., assessments of children old enough to self-report), 98% were provided a report [80]. This is of particular importance given that child participants had advanced illness. When reports were sent to clinicians, both parents and clinicians valued the reports. Reports facilitated communication about symptoms and HRQOL and resulted in improved emotional symptoms and well-being [5].

KLIK (Kwaliteit van Leven In Kaart (Quality of Life in Clinical Practice) is another online tool for pediatric PRO reporting that was developed in the Netherlands, and evaluated in large studies with thousands of patients [81,82]. The KLIK website generates an e-mail several days before an appointment that allows children (8–18 years old) or parents (for children age 0–7 years old) to complete PRO measures [81]. KLIK transforms child responses into an ePROfile which is shared with the child's health care provider via a central website [83]. In a randomized multicenter study of children with juvenile idiopathic arthritis, reports were reviewed during a routine appointment (intervention group). In this group, psychosocial topics were discussed more often, and clinicians were more satisfied with the care provided [82]. Similar studies in the pediatric oncology population also revealed that psychosocial issues were more frequently raised among those who received the reports, without increasing the duration of the clinical encounter [84,85]. Of note, participants were prompted by email to complete assessments, suggesting that, at least in these pediatric populations, remote (i.e., not clinic-based) assessments are feasible.

Other online tools have been marketed in a direct to consumer fashion. My Quality (My Quality, Ltd., United Kingdom) is an online tool that allows families with children with life-limiting illness to designate and monitor parameters that they identify as impacting their quality of life [86]. Initial testing of the site revealed that it was highly usable and feasible, and the site's graphic representation of change over time facilitated collaboration in the child's care. Moreover, families who used the site had greater empowerment over time [87].

6.2. Mobile Apps

An increasing number of mobile apps designed for smart phones have also been developed for symptom tracking, symptom reporting, and symptom management, with some combining multiple focuses. Apps can be used by parents to report their young or non-verbal child's symptoms. Apps are particularly attractive for adolescent and young adults, who may not reliably report their symptoms in clinic, notably around sensitive topics such as sexual dysfunction or body image. Some apps are focused on one symptom, such as PainSquad+ for pain [16] or SyMon-SAYS for fatigue [8], while others such as Symple (Symple Health, Andover, United Kingdom) may assess a broader range of symptoms, including fatigue, nausea, and mental health issues [88]. Another smartphone app allows tracking of child pain and interference caused by pain while simultaneously tracking parent response to their pain. Such a strategy allows analysis of the inter-relationships between the child's pain experience and caregiver responses, such as how a child's pain and pain interference changes after a given type of caregiver responses (protective versus minimizing responses) and whether caregiver responses to pain is predicted by child factors, pain, or caregiver mood [89]. The validated measures utilized within these apps are varied, making it difficult to compare one to another. However, instituting app-based symptom tracking within a clinic or small group of providers is an area ripe for quality improvement research.

More advanced apps, such as Pain Buddy [17], are starting to couple assessment with analysis and targeted intervention. Instead of solely tracking symptoms and distress over time, apps now have the capability to generate reports, send alerts to physicians, and deliver a focused intervention to the user. This allows a physician to plan for pharmacologic therapies and the user to receive immediate non-pharmacologic treatment, including mindfulness or breathing techniques. Other publicly available apps designed for children and adolescents manage symptoms using non-pharmacologic therapies and by teaching coping skills for managing pain, symptoms ,and stress [90]. Some examples are Healing Buddies Comfort Kit (Children's Hospitals and Clinics of Minnesota, Ridgeview Medical Center, and DesignWise Medical, Version 1.1, Minneapolis, MN, USA) [91], Mindfulness for Children (Mindfulness for Children, Version 1.2, Niva, Denmark) [92], and Positive Penguins [93] (HR INSIDE PTY LTD, Version 2.0, Melbourne, Australia).

6.3. Therapeutic Toys

One emerging area in pain management for children is the use of therapeutic toys. Toys are a fun incentive and can promote social, emotional, and intellectual development [94]. In medicine, toys and play have often been employed as a method of distraction during procedures, such as suturing or IV sticks, or to promote education, such as dolls to prepare children for port-a-cath or gastrostomy tube placement.

As toy technology advances, they can also be utilized as a therapeutic alternative, helping to reduce pain, stress, fear, and anxiety. Some hospitals are already utilizing advanced sensory rooms or machines which engage a patient's senses—smell, touch, sight, and sound. This can assist in having a calming effect and provide symptom relief without utilizing medication. Mixed-media toys may have both a physical toy and a mobile app that pairs with the toy to vibrate, feel emotions, and transport children to a soothing soundscape. One example is Jerry the Bear, a comforting companion for children with type 1 diabetes (Sproutel, Inc, Version 1.2.0, Providence, RI, USA) [95]. Similar comforting companions and apps can be designed to entertain, comfort, educate, connect, and mimic a child's experience.

While there are many limitations and practical challenges in using web-based mobile apps and toys to assess symptoms and improve a child's quality of life, this is also an opportunity to involve patients and families in developing technology that is user-friendly. Children are incredibly creative and technology-savvy. Engaging children around the development of these programs, apps, and toys may empower them to take control over their symptoms by providing valuable perspectives on living through illness, hospitalizations, and procedures.

7. Meeting Patients Where They Are: Integration of Palliative Care in the Clinic Setting to Address Symptoms

Integration of palliative care principles and services into routine outpatient care for children with high-risk cancer disease is associated with improved symptom management for patients and quality of life (QOL) for both children and families [19,96–103]. Adult cancer centers have already demonstrated that integrating palliative care into the care of patients with cancer improved patient's pain, fatigue, depression, anxiety, and sleep [104,105]. Currently, this model is becoming recognized in pediatrics [19,99,106]. Several oncology or palliative care clinics have integrated web-based, computerized symptom assessments and PROs with validated tools [107]. For example, the Memorial Symptoms Assessment Scale, Pediatric Quality of Life inventory, and PROMIS forms have been utilized in both a clinical context and in research studies [5,17].

Perhaps most importantly, an interdisciplinary team-based assessment of a patient and family often yields additional information that cannot be gleaned from a survey. While integration or embedding within specialty clinics, such as oncology or cardiology, can be difficult and logistically challenging, there is value to a specialty palliative care team assessing, treating, and following the patient and family over time [19,98]. While a physician, nurse practitioner or nurse is extremely valuable in symptom assessment and treatment, the perspective of other team members should not be discounted. In fact, it is the experience of many palliative care teams that the social worker, chaplain, psychologist, child life specialist, or clinical pharmacist can be incredibly beneficial in assessing and managing physical symptoms, psychological symptoms, spiritual distress, and psychosocial pain [108–111]. The rationale for this is that many discussions are not about the symptom itself, but the meaning behind the symptom. This can include uncertainty about the cause or the future and whether this means diminished function [112]. When a patient's concern about a symptom is routed to a medical provider, a physician tends to give scientific medical responses, while the patient may desire a listening ear, reassurance and empathy. See Table 3 for an overview of the symptom assessment methods.

Table 3. Methods of pediatric symptom assessment.

Assessment	Strengths	Weaknesses	Application to PPC
Patient-reported outcomes (PROs)	• Can be adapted to a number of electronic interfaces, including EMR and direct-to- clinician reports • Variety of choices for different symptoms, HRQOL measures • Valid and reliable measures for pediatric research studies • Can be fed back to clinical team for improved symptom management	• Long forms can be time-consuming • Need to consider child self-report vs. proxy report • PROs lacking for non-malignant conditions and within pediatric research • Limitation of PROs in patients at end-of life, or who are non-verbal	• Can be incorporated prior to and within symptom management visits • PROs can be completed at home, with hospice providers and sent to hospital-based team • Allows for multi-site research studies

Table 3. *Cont.*

Assessment	Strengths	Weaknesses	Application to PPC
Online tools (e.g., KLIK, PediQUEST, MyQuality) [5,80,81,83,86]	• Utilize a variety of PROs • Applicable in research and clinical settings • Surveys prior to physician appointments increased psychosocial discussions • Improves parent and clinician satisfaction	• Initial investment into development and technology • Need for interface between electronic assessments and EMR	• Allows families to choose the measures of importance • Easier communication with busy clinicians • Feasible for children with advanced disease
Mobile apps	• Can be used by parent, child or both allowing inter-relationship analysis across a variety of symptoms • Direct reporting to clinicians • Ability to provide targeted interventions focusing on non-pharmacologic therapies	• Measures within apps vary, making it hard for clinicians to understand results or compare across apps • Availability only on some operating systems (e.g., Apple (Apple Inc., Cupertino, CA, USA) vs Android (Google, Mountain View, CA, USA))	• Teaches and enhances patient coping skills • Ability to teach mindfulness, guided imagery, and breathing techniques • Applicable for research on pain, fatigue, etc.
Therapeutic toys	• Promote social, emotional development • Can reduce pain, stress, fear • Mixed-media capability with toy and mobile app • Engaged children who can assist in design ideas	• Can be expensive to acquire for hospitals or patients/parents • Toys must meet many hospital safety and compliance regulations • Few options available	• Utilized as distraction for procedures • Engages a patient's senses of smell, touch • Children can use toys to communicate emotions and feelings
Interdisciplinary Pediatric Palliative Care team	• Ease of assessment in inpatient and outpatient settings • Benefit of multiple member assessment (physician, nursing, social work, chaplain, child life) • Data supporting improved patient/family outcomes	• Less feasible when patients are home • Increased personnel and time needed • Not available at all pediatric centers	• Provides human connection for families • Have ability to combine with any other strategy • Provides medical opinion and puts treatment plan in place

EMR: electronic medical record, HRQOL: health-related quality of life.

8. Discussion

Recent innovations in addressing symptoms hold great promise in improving the care of children with serious illness. PROs, computer-based mobile apps, and toys are innovative solutions to the challenge of accurate pediatric symptom assessment and management. At the same time, they highlight areas in which future efforts are needed to advance care. One such area is that of symptom and HRQOL assessment methodology. Appreciation for the way in which a global view of a child's experience is best obtained by self-report in conjunction with proxy-report is mounting. However, this must be accompanied by better understanding of what drives differences between these reporters, and how each perspective can best be understood in the context of the child's total experience. As described in this paper, further instrument development is also imperative to improve psychometrics and standardization. With regard to the latter, this will require some consensus pertaining to the most important outcomes to capture. Within palliative care, PRO research that captures a child's end-of-life experience is a particular need. Challenges to such work do exist; the child may be too sick to self-report during times of very advanced illness and highly emotionally charged circumstances. That being said, sensitivity, combined with a rigorous approach to this research, can overcome these challenges.

While still relatively early in development, systems for eliciting symptom and HRQOL data exist to facilitate efficient collection of longitudinal data and optimal medical care. Through technology-based collection of PRO, care is enhanced, including shared decision-making, effective communication and patient-centered care. At the same time we must guard against the possibility of moving from "high touch" to "high tech" care. Electronic medical records are gradually becoming more compatible with routine PRO assessment, allowing integration of reports. If PRO assessments are not tied to clinical encounters, systems and resources to address patient reports outside of clinical appointments in a timely manner will also be necessary.

We are just now scratching the surface of other PRO applications that extend beyond the point of care, such as evaluation of care quality, effectiveness, and value. These aspects of care have historically been measured in terms of care processes or downstream outcomes (e.g., readmission rates). In this age of value-based medicine, reimbursement is increasingly tied to patient outcomes as opposed to procedure or visit-based reimbursement. With value-based care placing greater emphasis on patient experience, such as patient well-being, now is the time for the incorporation of standardized measurement of PRO. PRO can thus become important indicators (performance measures) of provider and organizational performance, complementing other performance measures based in clinical outcomes and health care processes. Use of PRO in this regard further highlights the need to integrate PRO collection into electronic medical records.

Availing ourselves of the potential opportunities afforded by PRO assessment will necessitate overcoming barriers. First, optimal practices with regard to electronic administration of assessments (e.g., online versus app-based) must be delineated. The chosen methods must possess protections for patient privacy and confidentiality. Ideally these methods will also remain viable and compatible in the face of rapidly changing technology. Clinician buy-in to use these technologies can be achieved through involvement of clinicians in the development of PRO assessment practices as well as clinician education and staff training for maximum efficiency. A greater challenge may be organizational in nature. For example, a recent survey of pediatricians from 52 countries revealed largely organizational barriers to their assessment and use in clinical practice, including time, insufficient staff, logistical challenges, and financial resources [65].

Similar barriers will exist to more widespread use of computer-based or mobile apps. As patients, families, and clinicians have an increasing variety and number of choices to track and manage symptoms, it will become difficult to understand the measures, science, and methods behind each app. It would also become impractical for a physician to link with patients across multiple different sites. In starting to use a technology, collaboration with industry partners and information technology services may be needed to assist with installation and patient/clinician efficiency. Once mobile utilization has started, continual effort will be required to limit practice variation through quality improvement research and initiatives.

While all of the former methods are highly reliant upon technology incorporation into standard clinical practice, routinely integrating pediatric palliative care into the care of children will shift the culture of care to one emphasizing comfort and quality of life, regardless of treatment plan or outcome. Despite an increasing body of literature supporting pediatric palliative care integration as a standard of care for many children with complex, chronic, and life-threatening illness, utilization in practice has been slow. Several limitations remain to better integration including the size of the pediatric palliative care workforce, the comfort and knowledge of the pediatric clinicians, the system-level support, a billing infrastructure that values quality, and the ability to collaborate with local and state community organizations. When palliative care is better integrated, the lives of patients and families can be improved by focusing on symptom control, enhancing quality of life, and communicating well to enrich care coordination. Pediatric palliative care consultation combined with patient PRO may be an even more powerful approach to improving child HRQOL and should be investigated.

To the degree that disease-based screening, assessments, and treatments have improved over the years, the same attention needs to be paid to the patient experience. Novel approaches to improve the reporting of symptoms by patients and families, and the interpretation and management skills of clinicians are on the horizon. Yet, continued development and study of technological and team-based methods to improve symptom assessment and control are needed to drive palliative care forward.

Author Contributions: J.W. and C.U. conceived of the manuscript, K.E.B. and C.U. developed the manuscript outline, obtained references, and wrote the paper. The final manuscript was edited, reviewed, and agreed upon by all authors.

Conflicts of Interest: The authors declare no conflict of interest.

References

1. Feudtner, C.; Christakis, D.A.; Connell, F.A. Pediatric deaths attributable to complex chronic conditions: A population-based study of Washington State, 1980–1997. *Pediatrics* **2000**, *106*, 205–209. [PubMed]
2. Behrman, R.E.; Field, M.J. *When Children Die: Improving Palliative and End-of-Life Care for Children and Their Families—Summary*; The National Academies Press: Washington, DC, USA, 2003; p. 712.
3. Ries, L.A.G.; Smith, M.A.; Gurney, J.G.; Linet, M.; Tamra, T.; Young, J.L.; Bunin, G.R. *Cancer Incidence and Survival among Children and Adolescents: United States SEER Program 1975–1995*; NIH Pub. No.99-4649; National Cancer Institute: Rockville, MD, USA, 1999.
4. Kestler, S.A.; LoBiondo-Wood, G. Review of symptom experiences in children and adolescents with cancer. *Cancer Nurs.* **2012**, *35*, E31–E49. [CrossRef] [PubMed]
5. Wolfe, J.; Orellana, L.; Ullrich, C.; Cook, E.F.; Kang, T.I.; Rosenberg, A.; Geyer, R.; Feudtner, C.; Dussel, V. Symptoms and distress in children with advanced cancer: Prospective Patient-reported outcomes from the PediQUEST Study. *J. Clin. Oncol. Off. J. Am. Soc. Clin. Oncol.* **2015**, *33*, 1928–1935. [CrossRef] [PubMed]
6. Ruland, C.M.; Hamilton, G.A.; Schjodt-Osmo, B. The complexity of symptoms and problems experienced in children with cancer: A review of the literature. *J. Pain Symptom Manag.* **2009**, *37*, 403–418. [CrossRef] [PubMed]
7. Fortier, M.A.; Sender, L.S.; Kain, Z.N. Management of pediatric oncology pain in the home setting: The next frontier. *J. Pediatr. Hematol. Oncol.* **2011**, *33*, 249–250. [CrossRef] [PubMed]
8. Lai, J.S.; Yount, S.; Beaumont, J.L.; Cella, D.; Toia, J.; Goldman, S. A patient-centered symptom monitoring and reporting system for children and young adults with cancer (SyMon-SAYS). *Pediatr. Blood Cancer* **2015**, *62*, 1813–1818. [CrossRef] [PubMed]
9. Cleeland, C.S. Cancer-related symptoms. *Semin. Radiat. Oncol.* **2000**, *10*, 175–190. [CrossRef] [PubMed]
10. Aronson, L. "Good" patients and "difficult" patients-rethinking our definitions. *N. Engl. J. Med.* **2013**, *369*, 796–797. [CrossRef] [PubMed]
11. Woodgate, R.L.; Degner, L.F. Expectations and beliefs about children's cancer symptoms: Perspectives of children with cancer and their families. *Oncol. Nurs. Forum* **2003**, *30*, 479–491. [CrossRef] [PubMed]
12. Adams, D.; Schiffgen, M.; Kundu, A.; Dagenais, S.; Clifford, T.; Baydala, L.; King, W.J.; Vohra, S. Patterns of utilization of complementary and alternative medicine in 2 pediatric gastroenterology clinics. *J. Pediatr. Gastroenterol. Nutr.* **2014**, *59*, 334–339. [CrossRef] [PubMed]
13. Muriel, A.C.; Hwang, V.S.; Kornblith, A.; Greer, J.; Greenberg, D.B.; Temel, J.; Schapira, L.; Pirl, W. Management of psychosocial distress by oncologists. *Psychiatr. Serv.* **2009**, *60*, 1132–1134. [CrossRef] [PubMed]
14. Johnston, D.L.; Nagel, K.; Friedman, D.L.; Meza, J.L.; Hurwitz, C.A.; Friebert, S. Availability and use of palliative care and end-of-life services for pediatric oncology patients. *J. Clin. Oncol. Off. J. Am. Soc. Clin. Oncol.* **2008**, *26*, 4646–4650. [CrossRef] [PubMed]
15. Williams, P.D.; Williams, A.R.; Kelly, K.P.; Dobos, C.; Gieseking, A.; Connor, R.; Ridder, L.; Potter, N.; Del Favero, D. A symptom checklist for children with cancer: The Therapy-Related Symptom Checklist-Children. *Cancer Nurs.* **2012**, *35*, 89–98. [CrossRef] [PubMed]
16. Jibb, L.A.; Stevens, B.J.; Nathan, P.C.; Seto, E.; Cafazzo, J.A.; Johnston, D.L.; Hum, V.; Stinson, J.N. Implementation and preliminary effectiveness of a real-time pain management smartphone app for adolescents with cancer: A multicenter pilot clinical study. *Pediatr. Blood Cancer* **2017**, *64*, e26554. [CrossRef] [PubMed]
17. Fortier, M.A.; Chung, W.W.; Martinez, A.; Gago-Masague, S.; Sender, L. Pain buddy: A novel use of m-health in the management of children's cancer pain. *Comput. Biol. Med.* **2016**, *76*, 202–214. [CrossRef] [PubMed]
18. Pinheiro, L.C.; McFatrich, M.; Lucas, N.; Walker, J.S.; Withycombe, J.S.; Hinds, P.S.; Sung, L.; Tomlinson, D.; Freyer, D.R.; Mack, J.W.; et al. Child and adolescent self-report symptom measurement in pediatric oncology research: A systematic literature review. *Qual. Life Res.* **2017**, *27*, 291–319. [CrossRef] [PubMed]
19. Kaye, E.C.; Friebert, S.; Baker, J.N. Early Integration of palliative care for children with high-risk cancer and their families. *Pediatr. Blood Cancer* **2016**, *63*, 593–597. [CrossRef] [PubMed]
20. Pew Research Center, Washington, D.C. Mobile Fact Sheet. Available online: http://www.pewinternet.org/fact-sheet/mobile/ (accessed on 15 November 2017).

21. Lenhart, A. Teens, Social Media & Technology Overview. 2015. Available online: http://www.pewinternet.org/2015/04/09/teens-social-media-technology-2015/#fn-13190-1 (accessed on 21 January 2018).
22. Pew Research Center, Washington, D.C. Internet/Broadband Fact Sheet. Available online: http://www.pewinternet.org/fact-sheet/internet-broadband/ (accessed on 15 November 2017).
23. Pew Research Center, Washington, D.C. Social Media Fact Sheet. Available online: http://www.pewinternet.org/fact-sheet/social-media/ (accessed on 15 November 2017).
24. Gurol-Urganci, I.; de Jongh, T.; Vodopivec-Jamsek, V.; Atun, R.; Car, J. Mobile phone messaging reminders for attendance at healthcare appointments. *Cochrane Database Syst. Rev.* **2013**, *12*, CD007458. [CrossRef] [PubMed]
25. De Jongh, T.; Gurol-Urganci, I.; Vodopivec-Jamsek, V.; Car, J.; Atun, R. Mobile phone messaging for facilitating self-management of long-term illnesses. *Cochrane Database Syst. Rev.* **2012**, *12*, CD007459. [CrossRef] [PubMed]
26. Velikova, G.; Wright, E.P.; Smith, A.B.; Cull, A.; Gould, A.; Forman, D.; Perren, T.; Stead, M.; Brown, J.; Selby, P.J. Automated collection of quality-of-life data: A comparison of paper and computer touch-screen questionnaires. *J. Clin. Oncol. Off. J. Am. Soc. Clin. Oncol.* **1999**, *17*, 998–1007. [CrossRef] [PubMed]
27. Wolpin, S.; Berry, D.; Austin-Seymour, M.; Bush, N.; Fann, J.R.; Halpenny, B.; Lober, W.B.; McCorkle, R. Acceptability of an Electronic Self-Report Assessment Program for patients with cancer. *Comput. Inform. Nurs.* **2008**, *26*, 332–338. [CrossRef] [PubMed]
28. Erharter, A.; Giesinger, J.; Kemmler, G.; Schauer-Maurer, G.; Stockhammer, G.; Muigg, A.; Hutterer, M.; Rumpold, G.; Sperner-Unterweger, B.; Holzner, B. Implementation of computer-based quality-of-life monitoring in brain tumor outpatients in routine clinical practice. *J. Pain Symptom Manag.* **2010**, *39*, 219–229. [CrossRef] [PubMed]
29. Abernethy, A.P.; Herndon, J.E., II; Wheeler, J.L.; Day, J.M.; Hood, L.; Patwardhan, M.; Shaw, M.; Lyerly, H.K. Feasibility and acceptability to patients of a longitudinal system for evaluating cancer-related symptoms and quality of life: Pilot study of an e/Tablet data-collection system in academic oncology. *J. Pain Symptom Manag.* **2009**, *37*, 1027–1038.
30. Belisario, J.S.M.; Jamsek, J.; Huckvale, K.; O'Donoghue, J.; Morrison, C.P.; Car, J. Comparison of self-administered survey questionnaire responses collected using mobile apps versus other methods. *Cochrane Database Syst. Rev.* **2015**, *7*, MR000042. [CrossRef] [PubMed]
31. Vinney, L.A.; Grade, J.D.; Connor, N.P. Feasibility of using a handheld electronic device for the collection of patient reported outcomes data from children. *J. Commun. Disord.* **2012**, *45*, 12–19. [CrossRef] [PubMed]
32. Velikova, G.; Keding, A.; Harley, C.; Cocks, K.; Booth, L.; Smith, A.B.; Wright, P.; Selby, P.J.; Brown, J.M. Patients report improvements in continuity of care when quality of life assessments are used routinely in oncology practice: Secondary outcomes of a randomised controlled trial. *Eur. J. Cancer* **2010**, *46*, 2381–2388. [CrossRef] [PubMed]
33. Detmar, S.B.; Muller, M.J.; Schornagel, J.H.; Wever, L.D.; Aaronson, N.K. Health-related quality-of-life assessments and patient-physician communication: A randomized controlled trial. *J. Am. Med. Assoc.* **2002**, *288*, 3027–3034. [CrossRef]
34. Carlson, L.E.; Speca, M.; Hagen, N.; Taenzer, P. Computerized quality-of-life screening in a cancer pain clinic. *J. Palliat. Care* **2001**, *17*, 46–52. [PubMed]
35. Velikova, G.; Booth, L.; Smith, A.B.; Brown, P.M.; Lynch, P.; Brown, J.M.; Selby, P.J. Measuring quality of life in routine oncology practice improves communication and patient well-being: A randomized controlled trial. *J. Clin. Oncol. Off. J. Am. Soc. Clin. Oncol.* **2004**, *22*, 714–724. [CrossRef] [PubMed]
36. Taenzer, P.; Bultz, B.D.; Carlson, L.E.; Speca, M.; DeGagne, T.; Olson, K.; Doll, R.; Rosberger, Z. Impact of computerized quality of life screening on physician behaviour and patient satisfaction in lung cancer outpatients. *Psycho-Oncology* **2000**, *9*, 203–213. [CrossRef]
37. Mark, T.L.; Fortner, B.; Johnson, G. Evaluation of a tablet PC technology to screen and educate oncology patients. *Support. Care Cancer Off. J. Multinatl. Assoc. Support. Care Cancer* **2008**, *16*, 371–378. [CrossRef] [PubMed]
38. Ruland, C.M.; White, T.; Stevens, M.; Fanciullo, G.; Khilani, S.M. Effects of a computerized system to support shared decision making in symptom management of cancer patients: Preliminary results. *J. Am. Med. Inform. Assoc.* **2003**, *10*, 573–579. [CrossRef] [PubMed]

39. Hockenberry, M.J.; Hinds, P.S.; Barrera, P.; Bryant, R.; Adams-McNeill, J.; Hooke, C.; Rasco-Baggott, C.; Patterson-Kelly, K.; Gattuso, J.S.; Manteuffel, B. Three instruments to assess fatigue in children with cancer: The child, parent and staff perspectives. *J. Pain Symptom Manag.* **2003**, *25*, 319–328. [CrossRef]
40. Glaser, A.W.; Davies, K.; Walker, D.; Brazier, D. Influence of proxy respondents and mode of administration on health status assessment following central nervous system tumours in childhood. *Qual. Life Res.* **1997**, *6*, 43–53. [CrossRef] [PubMed]
41. Drakouli, M.; Petsios, K.; Giannakopoulou, M.; Patiraki, E.; Voutoufianaki, I.; Matziou, V. Determinants of quality of life in children and adolescents with CHD: A systematic review. *Cardiol. Young* **2015**, *25*, 1027–1036. [CrossRef] [PubMed]
42. Amedro, P.; Dorka, R.; Moniotte, S.; Guillaumont, S.; Fraisse, A.; Kreitmann, B.; Borm, B.; Bertet, H.; Barrea, C.; Ovaert, C.; et al. Quality of Life of Children with Congenital Heart Diseases: A Multicenter Controlled Cross-Sectional Study. *Pediatr. Cardiol.* **2015**, *36*, 1588–1601. [CrossRef] [PubMed]
43. Ullrich, C.K.; Rodday, A.M.; Bingen, K.M.; Kupst, M.J.; Patel, S.K.; Syrjala, K.L.; Harris, L.L.; Recklitis, C.J.; Chang, G.; Guinan, E.C.; et al. Three sides to a story: Child, parent, and nurse perspectives on the child's experience during hematopoietic stem cell transplantation. *Cancer* **2017**, *123*, 3159–3166. [CrossRef] [PubMed]
44. Panepinto, J.A.; O'Mahar, K.M.; DeBaun, M.R.; Loberiza, F.R.; Scott, J.P. Health-related quality of life in children with sickle cell disease: Child and parent perception. *Br. J. Haematol.* **2005**, *130*, 437–444. [CrossRef] [PubMed]
45. Rajmil, L.; Lopez, A.R.; Lopez-Aguila, S.; Alonso, J. Parent-child agreement on health-related quality of life (HRQOL): A longitudinal study. *Health Qual. Life Outcomes* **2013**, *11*, 101. [CrossRef] [PubMed]
46. Eiser, C.; Morse, R. Can parents rate their child's health-related quality of life? Results of a systematic review. *Qual. Life Res.* **2001**, *10*, 347–357. [CrossRef] [PubMed]
47. Weaver, M.S.; Darnall, C.; Bace, S.; Vail, C.; MacFadyen, A.; Wichman, C. Trending Longitudinal Agreement between Parent and Child Perceptions of Quality of Life for Pediatric Palliative Care Patients. *Children* **2017**, *4*, 65. [CrossRef] [PubMed]
48. Rapp, M.; Eisemann, N.; Arnaud, C.; Ehlinger, V.; Fauconnier, J.; Marcelli, M.; Michelsen, S.I.; Nystrand, M.; Colver, A.; Thyen, U. Predictors of parent-reported quality of life of adolescents with cerebral palsy: A longitudinal study. *Res. Dev. Disabil.* **2017**, *62*, 259–270. [CrossRef] [PubMed]
49. Aspesberro, F.; Mangione-Smith, R.; Zimmerman, J.J. Health-related quality of life following pediatric critical illness. *Intensive Care Med.* **2015**, *41*, 1235–1246. [CrossRef] [PubMed]
50. Rodday, A.M.; Terrin, N.; Leslie, L.K.; Graham, R.J.; Parsons, S.K. Understanding the Relationship Between Child Health-Related Quality of Life and Parent Emotional Functioning in Pediatric Hematopoietic Stem Cell Transplant. *J. Pediatr. Psychol.* **2017**, *42*, 804–814. [CrossRef] [PubMed]
51. U.S. Food and Drug Administration. Guidance for Industry: Patient-reported outcome measures-Use in medical product development to support labeling claims. *Fed. Regist.* **2009**, *74*, 65132–65133.
52. Meldahl, M.L.; Acaster, S.; Hayes, R.P. Exploration of oncologists' attitudes toward and perceived value of patient-reported outcomes. *Qual. Life Res.* **2013**, *22*, 725–731. [CrossRef] [PubMed]
53. Patient-Reported Outcomes Version of the Common Terminology Criteria for Adverse Events (PRO-CTCAE). Available online: https://healthcaredelivery.cancer.gov/pro-ctcae/ (accessed on 21 November 2017).
54. Basch, E.; Dueck, A.C.; Rogak, L.J.; Minasian, L.M.; Kelly, W.K.; O'Mara, A.M.; Denicoff, A.M.; Seisler, D.; Atherton, P.J.; Paskett, E.; et al. Feasibility Assessment of patient reporting of symptomatic adverse events in multicenter cancer clinical trials. *JAMA Oncol.* **2017**, *3*, 1043–1050. [CrossRef] [PubMed]
55. Basch, E.; Deal, A.M.; Kris, M.G.; Scher, H.I.; Hudis, C.A.; Sabbatini, P.; Rogak, L.; Bennett, A.V.; Dueck, A.C.; Atkinson, T.M.; et al. Symptom Monitoring with patient-reported outcomes during routine cancer treatment: A randomized controlled trial. *J. Clin. Oncol. Off. J. Am. Soc. Clin. Oncol.* **2016**, *34*, 557–565. [CrossRef] [PubMed]
56. Basch, E.; Deal, A.M.; Dueck, A.C.; Scher, H.I.; Kris, M.G.; Hudis, C.; Schrag, D. Overall Survival results of a trial assessing patient-reported outcomes for symptom monitoring during routine cancer treatment. *J. Am. Med. Assoc.* **2017**, *318*, 197–198. [CrossRef] [PubMed]
57. Rotenstein, L.S.; Huckman, R.S.; Wagle, N.W. Making Patients and doctors happier—The Potential of patient-reported outcomes. *N. Engl. J. Med.* **2017**, *377*, 1309–1312. [CrossRef] [PubMed]

58. Brundage, M.; Blackford, A.; Tolbert, E.; Smith, K.; Bantug, E.; Snyder, C.; Board, P.D. Presenting comparative study PRO results to clinicians and researchers: Beyond the eye of the beholder. *Qual. Life Res.* **2018**, *27*, 75–90. [CrossRef] [PubMed]
59. Bantug, E.T.; Coles, T.; Smith, K.C.; Snyder, C.F.; Rouette, J.; Brundage, M.D.; Board, P.D. Graphical displays of patient-reported outcomes (PRO) for use in clinical practice: What makes a pro picture worth a thousand words? *Patient Educ. Couns.* **2016**, *99*, 483–490. [CrossRef] [PubMed]
60. Dobrozsi, S.; Panepinto, J. Child and parent preferences for graphical display of patient-reported outcome data. *Pediatr. Blood Cancer* **2017**, *64*. [CrossRef] [PubMed]
61. U.S. National Library of Medicine. Available online: https://clinicaltrials.gov/ (accessed on 26 March 2018).
62. Fayed, N.; de Camargo, O.K.; Elahi, I.; Dubey, A.; Fernandes, R.M.; Houtrow, A.; Cohen, E. Patient-important activity and participation outcomes in clinical trials involving children with chronic conditions. *Qual. Life Res.* **2014**, *23*, 751–757. [CrossRef] [PubMed]
63. Reeve, B.B.; Edwards, L.J.; Jaeger, B.C.; Hinds, P.S.; Dampier, C.; Gipson, D.S.; Selewski, D.T.; Troost, J.P.; Thissen, D.; Barry, V.; et al. Assessing responsiveness over time of the PROMIS pediatric symptom and function measures in cancer, nephrotic syndrome, and sickle cell disease. *Qual. Life Res.* **2017**, *27*, 249–257. [CrossRef] [PubMed]
64. Reeve, B.B.; McFatrich, M.; Pinheiro, L.C.; Weaver, M.S.; Sung, L.; Withycombe, J.S.; Baker, J.N.; Mack, J.W.; Waldron, M.K.; Gibson, D.; et al. Eliciting the child's voice in adverse event reporting in oncology trials: Cognitive interview findings from the Pediatric Patient-Reported Outcomes version of the Common Terminology Criteria for Adverse Events initiative. *Pediatr. Blood Cancer* **2017**, *64*, e26261. [CrossRef] [PubMed]
65. Schepers, S.A.; Haverman, L.; Zadeh, S.; Grootenhuis, M.A.; Wiener, L. Healthcare Professionals' Preferences and Perceived Barriers for Routine Assessment of Patient-Reported Outcomes in Pediatric Oncology Practice: Moving Toward International Processes of Change. *Pediatr. Blood Cancer* **2016**, *63*, 2181–2188. [CrossRef] [PubMed]
66. Huang, I.C.; Revicki, D.A.; Schwartz, C.E. Measuring pediatric patient-reported outcomes: Good progress but a long way to go. *Qual. Life Res.* **2014**, *23*, 747–750. [CrossRef] [PubMed]
67. Anthony, S.J.; Selkirk, E.; Sung, L.; Klaassen, R.J.; Dix, D.; Scheinemann, K.; Klassen, A.F. Considering quality of life for children with cancer: A systematic review of patient-reported outcome measures and the development of a conceptual model. *Qual. Life Res.* **2014**, *23*, 771–789. [CrossRef] [PubMed]
68. Janssens, A.; Thompson Coon, J.; Rogers, M.; Allen, K.; Green, C.; Jenkinson, C.; Tennant, A.; Logan, S.; Morris, C. A systematic review of generic multidimensional patient-reported outcome measures for children, part I: Descriptive characteristics. *Value Health* **2015**, *18*, 315–333. [CrossRef] [PubMed]
69. PROMIS. Available online: http://www.healthmeasures.net/explore-measurement-systems/promis (accessed on 29 November 2017).
70. DeWitt, E.M.; Stucky, B.D.; Thissen, D.; Irwin, D.E.; Langer, M.; Varni, J.W.; Lai, J.S.; Yeatts, K.B.; Dewalt, D.A. Construction of the eight-item patient-reported outcomes measurement information system pediatric physical function scales: Built using item response theory. *J. Clin. Epidemiol.* **2011**, *64*, 794–804. [CrossRef] [PubMed]
71. Irwin, D.E.; Stucky, B.D.; Thissen, D.; Dewitt, E.M.; Lai, J.S.; Yeatts, K.; Varni, J.W.; DeWalt, D.A. Sampling plan and patient characteristics of the PROMIS pediatrics large-scale survey. *Qual. Life Res.* **2010**, *19*, 585–594. [CrossRef] [PubMed]
72. Varni, J.W.; Stucky, B.D.; Thissen, D.; Dewitt, E.M.; Irwin, D.E.; Lai, J.S.; Yeatts, K.; Dewalt, D.A. PROMIS Pediatric Pain Interference Scale: An item response theory analysis of the pediatric pain item bank. *J. Pain* **2010**, *11*, 1109–1119. [CrossRef] [PubMed]
73. Quinn, H.; Thissen, D.; Liu, Y.; Magnus, B.; Lai, J.S.; Amtmann, D.; Varni, J.W.; Gross, H.E.; DeWalt, D.A. Using item response theory to enrich and expand the PROMIS(R) pediatric self report banks. *Health Qual. Life Outcomes* **2014**, *12*, 160. [CrossRef] [PubMed]
74. Irwin, D.E.; Gross, H.E.; Stucky, B.D.; Thissen, D.; DeWitt, E.M.; Lai, J.S.; Amtmann, D.; Khastou, L.; Varni, J.W.; DeWalt, D.A. Development of six PROMIS pediatrics proxy-report item banks. *Health Qual. Life Outcomes* **2012**, *10*, 22. [CrossRef] [PubMed]

75. Reeve, B.B.; Thissen, D.; DeWalt, D.A.; Huang, I.C.; Liu, Y.; Magnus, B.; Quinn, H.; Gross, H.E.; Kisala, P.A.; Ni, P.; et al. Linkage between the PROMIS(R) pediatric and adult emotional distress measures. *Qual. Life Res.* **2016**, *25*, 823–833. [CrossRef] [PubMed]
76. Barthel, D.; Fischer, K.I.; Nolte, S.; Otto, C.; Meyrose, A.K.; Reisinger, S.; Dabs, M.; Thyen, U.; Klein, M.; Muehlan, H.; et al. Implementation of the Kids-CAT in clinical settings: A newly developed computer-adaptive test to facilitate the assessment of patient-reported outcomes of children and adolescents in clinical practice in Germany. *Qual. Life Res.* **2016**, *25*, 585–594. [CrossRef] [PubMed]
77. Devine, J.; Otto, C.; Rose, M.; Barthel, D.; Fischer, F.; Muhlan, H.; Nolte, S.; Schmidt, S.; Ottova-Jordan, V.; Ravens-Sieberer, U. A new computerized adaptive test advancing the measurement of health-related quality of life (HRQoL) in children: The Kids-CAT. *Qual. Life Res.* **2015**, *24*, 871–884. [CrossRef] [PubMed]
78. Barthel, D.; Otto, C.; Nolte, S.; Meyrose, A.K.; Fischer, F.; Devine, J.; Walter, O.; Mierke, A.; Fischer, K.I.; Thyen, U.; et al. The validation of a computer-adaptive test (CAT) for assessing health-related quality of life in children and adolescents in a clinical sample: Study design, methods and first results of the Kids-CAT study. *Qual. Life Res.* **2017**, *26*, 1105–1117. [CrossRef] [PubMed]
79. Wolfe, J.; Orellana, L.; Cook, E.F.; Ullrich, C.; Kang, T.; Geyer, J.R.; Feudtner, C.; Weeks, J.C.; Dussel, V. Improving the care of children with advanced cancer by using an electronic patient-reported feedback intervention: Results from the PediQUEST randomized controlled trial. *J. Clin. Oncol. Off. J. Am. Soc. Clin. Oncol.* **2014**, *32*, 1119–1126. [CrossRef] [PubMed]
80. Dussel, V.; Orellana, L.; Soto, N.; Chen, K.; Ullrich, C.; Kang, T.I.; Geyer, J.R.; Feudtner, C.; Wolfe, J. Feasibility of Conducting a Palliative Care Randomized Controlled Trial in Children With Advanced Cancer: Assessment of the PediQUEST Study. *J. Pain Symptom Manag.* **2015**, *49*, 1059–1069. [CrossRef] [PubMed]
81. Haverman, L.; van Oers, H.; Limperg, P.F.L.; Hijmans, C.T.; Schepers, S.A.; Sint Nicolas, S.M.; Verhaak, C.M.; Bouts, A.H.M.; Fijnvandraat, K.; Peters, M.; et al. Implementation of Electronic Patient Reported Outcomes in Pediatric Daily Clinical Practice: The KLIK Experience. *Clin. Pract. Pediatr. Psychol.* **2014**, *2*, 50–67. [CrossRef]
82. Haverman, L.; van Rossum, M.A.; van Veenendaal, M.; van den Berg, J.M.; Dolman, K.M.; Swart, J.; Kuijpers, T.W.; Grootenhuis, M.A. Effectiveness of a web-based application to monitor health-related quality of life. *Pediatrics* **2013**, *131*, e533–e543. [CrossRef] [PubMed]
83. Haverman, L.; Engelen, V.; van Rossum, M.A.; Heymans, H.S.; Grootenhuis, M.A. Monitoring health-related quality of life in paediatric practice: Development of an innovative web-based application. *BMC Pediatr.* **2011**, *11*, 3. [CrossRef] [PubMed]
84. Engelen, V.; van Zwieten, M.; Koopman, H.; Detmar, S.; Caron, H.; Brons, P.; Egeler, M.; Kaspers, G.J.; Grootenhuis, M. The influence of patient reported outcomes on the discussion of psychosocial issues in children with cancer. *Pediatr. Blood Cancer* **2012**, *59*, 161–166. [CrossRef] [PubMed]
85. Engelen, V.; Detmar, S.; Koopman, H.; Maurice-Stam, H.; Caron, H.; Hoogerbrugge, P.; Egeler, R.M.; Kaspers, G.; Grootenhuis, M. Reporting health-related quality of life scores to physicians during routine follow-up visits of pediatric oncology patients: Is it effective? *Pediatr. Blood Cancer* **2012**, *58*, 766–774. [CrossRef] [PubMed]
86. My Quality Ltd. My Quality. Available online: https://my-quality.Net/ (accessed on 26 March 2018).
87. Harris, N.; Beringer, A.; Fletcher, M. Families' priorities in life-limiting illness: Improving quality with online empowerment. *Arch. Dis. Child.* **2016**, *101*, 247–252. [CrossRef] [PubMed]
88. Symple health, Inc. Symple. https://www.Sympleapp.com/ (accessed on 26 March 2018).
89. Connelly, M.; Bromberg, M.H.; Anthony, K.K.; Gil, K.M.; Schanberg, L.E. Use of smartphones to prospectively evaluate predictors and outcomes of caregiver responses to pain in youth with chronic disease. *Pain* **2016**, *158*, 629–636. [CrossRef] [PubMed]
90. Smith, K.; Iversen, C.; Kossowsky, J.; O'Dell, S.; Gambhir, R.; Coakley, R. Apple apps for the management of pediatric pain and pain-related stress. *Clin. Pract. Pediatr. Psychol.* **2015**, *3*, 93–107. [CrossRef]
91. Children's Hospitals and Clinics of Minnesota, Ridgeview Medical Center, and DesignWise Medical. Healing Buddies Comfort Kit. Available online: http://www.Healingbuddiescomfort.org/ (accessed on 26 March 2018).
92. Holgersen, P. Mindful-app. Available online: www.mindful-app.com (accessed on 26 March 2018).
93. Price, S. Positive Penguins. Available online: www.positivepenguins.com (accessed on 26 March 2018).
94. Kiche, M.T.; de Amorim Almeida, F. Therapeutic toy: Strategy for pain management and tension relief during dressing change in children. *Acta Paul. Enferm.* **2009**, *22*, 125–130. [CrossRef]
95. Sproutel, Inc. Jerry the Bear. Available online: www.jerrythebear.com (accessed on 26 March 2018).

96. Schmidt, P.; Otto, M.; Hechler, T.; Metzing, S.; Wolfe, J.; Zernikow, B. Did increased availability of pediatric palliative care lead to improved palliative care outcomes in children with cancer? *J. Palliat. Med.* **2013**, *16*, 1034–1039. [CrossRef] [PubMed]
97. Snaman, J.M.; Kaye, E.C.; Lu, J.J.; Sykes, A.; Baker, J.N. Palliative Care Involvement Is Associated with Less Intensive End-of-Life Care in Adolescent and Young Adult Oncology Patients. *J. Palliat. Med.* **2017**, *20*, 509–516. [CrossRef] [PubMed]
98. Levine, D.R.; Johnson, L.M.; Snyder, A.; Wiser, R.K.; Gibson, D.; Kane, J.R.; Baker, J.N. Integrating Palliative Care in Pediatric Oncology: Evidence for an Evolving Paradigm for Comprehensive Cancer Care. *J. Natl. Compr. Cancer Netw.* **2016**, *14*, 741–748. [CrossRef]
99. Levine, D.R.; Mandrell, B.N.; Sykes, A.; Pritchard, M.; Gibson, D.; Symons, H.J.; Wendler, D.; Baker, J.N. Patients' and Parents' Needs, Attitudes, and Perceptions About Early Palliative Care Integration in Pediatric Oncology. *JAMA Oncol.* **2017**, *3*, 1214–1220. [CrossRef] [PubMed]
100. Waldman, E.; Wolfe, J. Palliative care for children with cancer. *Nat. Rev. Clin. Oncol.* **2013**, *10*, 100–107. [CrossRef] [PubMed]
101. Weaver, M.S.; Heinze, K.E.; Bell, C.J.; Wiener, L.; Garee, A.M.; Kelly, K.P.; Casey, R.L.; Watson, A.; Hinds, P.S. Establishing psychosocial palliative care standards for children and adolescents with cancer and their families: An integrative review. *Palliat. Med.* **2016**, *30*, 212–223. [CrossRef] [PubMed]
102. Wolfe, J.; Friebert, S.; Hilden, J. Caring for children with advanced cancer integrating palliative care. *Pediatr. Clin. N. Am.* **2002**, *49*, 1043–1062. [CrossRef]
103. Kaye, E.C.; Rubenstein, J.; Levine, D.; Baker, J.N.; Dabbs, D.; Friebert, S.E. Pediatric palliative care in the community. *Cancer J. Clin.* **2015**, *65*, 316–333. [CrossRef] [PubMed]
104. Yennurajalingam, S.; Urbauer, D.L.; Casper, K.L.; Reyes-Gibby, C.C.; Chacko, R.; Poulter, V.; Bruera, E. Impact of a palliative care consultation team on cancer-related symptoms in advanced cancer patients referred to an outpatient supportive care clinic. *J. Pain Symptom Manag.* **2011**, *41*, 49–56. [CrossRef] [PubMed]
105. Muir, J.C.; Daly, F.; Davis, M.S.; Weinberg, R.; Heintz, J.S.; Paivanas, T.A.; Beveridge, R. Integrating palliative care into the outpatient, private practice oncology setting. *J. Pain Symptom Manag.* **2010**, *40*, 126–135. [CrossRef] [PubMed]
106. Kaye, E.C.; Snaman, J.M.; Baker, J.N. Pediatric Palliative oncology: Bridging Silos of care through an embedded model. *J. Clin. Oncol. Off. J. Am. Soc. Clin. Oncol.* **2017**, *35*, 2740–2744. [CrossRef] [PubMed]
107. Wu, W.W.; Johnson, R.; Schepp, K.G.; Berry, D.L. Electronic self-report symptom and quality of life for adolescent patients with cancer: A feasibility study. *Cancer Nurs.* **2011**, *34*, 479–486. [CrossRef] [PubMed]
108. Cagle, J.G.; Osteen, P.; Sacco, P.; Jacobson Frey, J. Psychosocial Assessment by Hospice Social Workers: A Content Review of Instruments From a National Sample. *J. Pain Symptom Manag.* **2017**, *53*, 40–48. [CrossRef] [PubMed]
109. McSherry, M.; Kehoe, K.; Carroll, J.M.; Kang, T.I.; Rourke, M.T. Psychosocial and spiritual needs of children living with a life-limiting illness. *Pediatr. Clin. N. Am.* **2007**, *54*, 609–629. [CrossRef] [PubMed]
110. Edlynn, E.; Kaur, H. The role of psychology in pediatric palliative care. *J. Palliat. Med.* **2016**, *19*, 760–762. [CrossRef] [PubMed]
111. DiScala, S.L.; Onofrio, S.; Miller, M.; Nazario, M.; Silverman, M. Integration of a clinical pharmacist into an interdisciplinary palliative care outpatient clinic. *Am. J. Hosp. Palliat. Care* **2017**, *34*, 814–819. [CrossRef] [PubMed]
112. Estacio, C.F.; Butow, P.N.; Lovell, M.R.; Dong, S.T.; Clayton, J.M. What is symptom meaning? A framework analysis of communication in palliative care consultations. *Patient Educ. Couns.* **2017**, *100*, 2088–2094. [CrossRef] [PubMed]

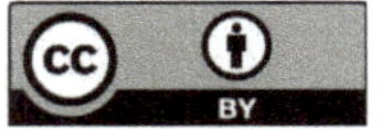

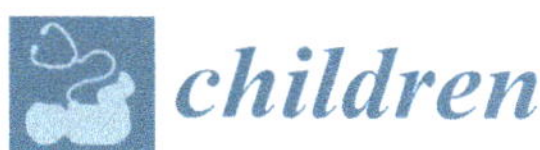
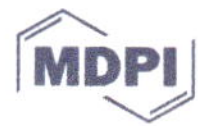

Review

Risk and Resilience Factors Related to Parental Bereavement Following the Death of a Child with a Life-Limiting Condition

Tiina Jaaniste [1,2,*], Sandra Coombs [1], Theresa J. Donnelly [1], Norm Kelk [1] and Danielle Beston [1]

1 Department of Pain and Palliative Care, Sydney Children's Hospital, Randwick NSW 2031, Australia; Sandra.Coombs@health.nsw.gov.au (S.C.); TheresaJDonnelly@gmail.com (T.J.D.); Norm.Kelk@health.nsw.gov.au (N.K.); Danielle.Beston@health.nsw.gov.au (D.B.)

2 School of Women's and Children's Health, University of New South Wales, Kensington NSW 2052, Australia

* Correspondence: Tiina.Jaaniste@health.nsw.gov.au; Tel.: +61-2-9382-5422

Received: 7 August 2017; Accepted: 31 October 2017; Published: 9 November 2017

Abstract: This paper reviews the theoretical and empirical literature on risk and resilience factors impacting on parental bereavement outcomes following the death of a child with a life-limiting condition. Over the past few decades, bereavement research has focussed primarily on a risk-based approach. In light of advances in the literature on resilience, the authors propose a Risk and Resilience Model of Parental Bereavement, thus endeavouring to give more holistic consideration to a range of potential influences on parental bereavement outcomes. The literature will be reviewed with regard to the role of: (i) loss-oriented stressors (e.g., circumstances surrounding the death and multiple losses); (ii) inter-personal factors (e.g., marital factors, social support, and religious practices); (iii) intra-personal factors (e.g., neuroticism, trait optimism, psychological flexibility, attachment style, and gender); and (iv) coping and appraisal, on parental bereavement outcomes. Challenges facing this area of research are discussed, and research and clinical implications considered.

Keywords: bereavement; palliative care; parents; risk factors; resilience factors

---

1. Introduction

Bereavement, or the loss of a loved one through death, results in a process of adaptation to living following the death of the loved one [1]. The grief, or distress resulting from bereavement experienced by a parent following the death of a child is widely recognized as one of the most intense and persistent types of bereavement [2]. Although the main cause of death in childhood is trauma (unexpected accidents and injuries), a much smaller proportion of childhood deaths is due to life-limiting conditions, i.e., conditions which may significantly reduce the child's life-span, with no reasonable hope of cure. Parental bereavement that follows weeks, months or years of caring for a child with a life-limiting condition is a particular context that is likely to have a unique set of factors associated with parental bereavement outcomes. Following a brief overview of some of the unique aspects of the bereavement experience associated with the death of a child due to a life-limiting condition, the current narrative review will consider a range of factors that may influence parental adjustment in this context. The Integrative Risk Factor Framework of Bereavement by Stroebe et al. [3] provides a good structure for considering a broad array of possible risk factors that may impact on the ability of parents to resume functioning with valued activities following the death of their child. The current paper extends the framework of Stroebe et al. [3] to also incorporate a consideration of protective or resilience factors. Thus, the literature pertaining to a broad range of possible risk and resilience factors will be reviewed from within the context of our newly proposed Risk and Resilience Model of Parental Bereavement, with particular focus on the bereavement context following the death of a child with a life-limiting condition. The current narrative review is based on an extensive (though not systematic) review of the literature. Where possible, the associations between risk and resilience factors with bereavement outcomes have been considered in terms of the levels of evidence. Some of the challenges and limitations of carrying out research in this area will be discussed, and implications for further research and clinical practice considered.

2. Parental Bereavement Following the Death of a Child with a Life-Limiting Condition

There are a number of key differences between parental bereavement processes associated with the death of a child with a prolonged, life-limiting condition, relative to an unexpected death due to an injury or acute illness [4,5]. Parents looking after a child with a life-limiting condition commonly experience prolonged suffering in the weeks, months, and years before the death of the child. In some cases, they may have learnt about their child's diagnosis around the time of their birth. The child's death may occur at a point when a parent's coping resources have been tested to the limit across a range of possible areas (e.g., physical, emotional, marital, financial, spiritual, and inter-personal), often for a long period of time. On the one hand, the draining nature of a prolonged period of caring may leave an individual vulnerable to poorer bereavement outcomes. Conversely, however, the stress reduction theory holds that the child's death coincides with a reduction in stressors that had been associated with the long-term care of the child, thus potentially facilitating post-bereavement adjustment [6]. It is extremely difficult to compare bereavement outcomes for expected and unexpected child deaths in a methodologically rigorous way, and results have been mixed. One study found lower levels of parental depression following an unexpected death relative to a long-term illnesses [7], whereas another study found poorer parental bereavement outcomes following a child's violent death (e.g., resulting from accident, homicide, and suicide) relative to a long-term illness [8].

In the context of caring for a child with a life-limiting condition, parental grief processes may have started well before the child's actual death, with similarities (albeit also some differences) between anticipatory mourning/grief reactions and conventional grief reactions [9]. Upon learning of a child's diagnosis and/or prognosis, the parents of a child with a life-limiting condition may start to readjust their cognitive schemas, to accommodate the recognition that their child might not experience a "normal" childhood, nor live to adulthood. However, this recognition does not necessarily equate with preparedness. Indeed, this realization may be associated with such a burden to parents that some authors have described the potential for the draining and debilitating experience of "chronic sorrow" [10].

The parents of children with a life-limiting condition may be more likely than the parents of children following an injury or acute illness to be aware if their child's impending death is imminent. Parents commonly report that the knowledge of their child's impending death enabled them to make appropriate choices, engage in tasks they deemed most important prior to their child's death, and to say goodbye to their child [11]. These actions are likely to help minimize regrets that the parent may feel after their child's death. Nevertheless, in the context of caring for a child with a life-limiting condition, it is not uncommon for parents to experience several occasions when they believe their child's death to be imminent, thus making it difficult for them to know when it is really time to say a final goodbye.

It is important to acknowledge differences in parental bereavement processes following the death of a child due to cancer, relative to the death of a child due to a non-cancer, life-limiting illness. In the context of many life-limiting, non-cancer conditions, parents typically learn at the time of diagnosis that, although there may be uncertainty regarding how long their child is likely to live, they as parents are likely to outlive their child. This information is likely to gradually reshape their cognitive schemas. In contrast, parents whose child has been diagnosed with cancer, may recognize the possibility of their child's death, however, they typically retain hope that their child will make a full recovery and enjoy a full life expectancy. These parents are therefore more inclined to cling to their existing schemas for as long as possible, hoping that the treatments will enable a return to health and normality.

3. The Role of Risk and Resilience Factors in Parental Bereavement

Over the past decade the Integrative Risk Factor Framework of Bereavement [3] has been valuable in drawing attention to a broad array of risk factors that may adversely impact on parental bereavement. This framework grouped potential risk factors as: (i) loss-oriented and restoration-oriented stressors; (ii) intra-personal factors, which are stable factors that are intrinsic to the bereaved individual; (iii) inter-personal factors, which are stable factors external to the individual (e.g., social support and culture); and (iv) coping and appraisal. These factors, alone and in combination, have the potential to impact on the ability of bereaved parents to resume functioning with necessary and valued activities. However, advances in the resilience literature suggest that intra-personal factors and inter-personal factors should not only be considered as potential risk factors for poorer bereavement outcomes, but that they should also be considered as possible resilience factors [12,13]. Although a risk-focussed approach has been useful in some fields of medicine, such as investigating infectious diseases, when investigating more complex conditions with biopsychosocial components, a more comprehensive consideration of both risk and resilience factors is likely to be beneficial [14].

Resilience may be regarded as an individual's ability to respond effectively to challenges or adversity. In some cases, resilience factors may be the opposite end of the spectrum of risk factors, for example, good marital communication may be considered a resilience factor, whereas poor marital communication may be a risk factor. However, risk and resilience factors are not always at opposite ends of the same continuum. For example, substance abuse confers a risk, but it cannot be said that its absence confers any protective value.

Some definitions of resilience highlight an individual's sustainability of purpose in the face of stress [13]. In recent years, the concept of resilience has been applied to the health psychology literature to identify why some individuals adjust to chronic health stressors more readily than others [15,16]. Resilience has been identified as being of importance in the bereavement literature, with the potential to help account for why some individuals are able to resume functioning more readily than others, despite experiencing painful and life-changing losses [17,18]. From a theoretical perspective, resilience factors may operate in a number of ways. Firstly, they may buffer or serve to compensate or minimize the effect of the stressor or loss in some way. For example, having other children in the family may prevent a parent from facing a childless existence, thus enabling, indeed requiring, them to maintain their role as parent. Secondly, resilience factors may facilitate the individual's process of recovery. In this case, the stressor or loss may be experienced just as acutely, but the resilience mechanisms may facilitate coping and accelerate the process of recovery [19,20]. For example, good marital communication may enable the bereaved parents to assist each other with more effective problem-solving.

The current paper draws from the multi-faceted risk framework of bereavement outlined by Stroebe et al. [3] and integrates this framework with a more comprehensive consideration of resilience factors. Thus, we have proposed a new model, namely the Risk and Resilience Model of Parental Bereavement (see Figure 1). Like the Stroebe et al. [3] framework of risk factors, this model groups loss-oriented factors, intra-personal factors, inter-personal factors, and appraisal and coping, separately. However, each of these classes of factors is considered in terms of potential risk and resilience influences on parental bereavement outcomes. This more comprehensive and holistic framework for considering how multiple risk and resilience factors interact is paramount to an improved understanding of parental bereavement outcomes, promoting theoretically-driven research, and guiding evidence-based clinical practice. The specific factors outlined in Figure 1 have been included based on available empirical or theoretical justification. Following a brief discussion of the varied nature of parental bereavement outcomes, the literature on each of the four classes of bereavement risk and resilience factors will be reviewed, where possible with a particular focus on parental bereavement associated with the death of a child following a life-limiting condition.

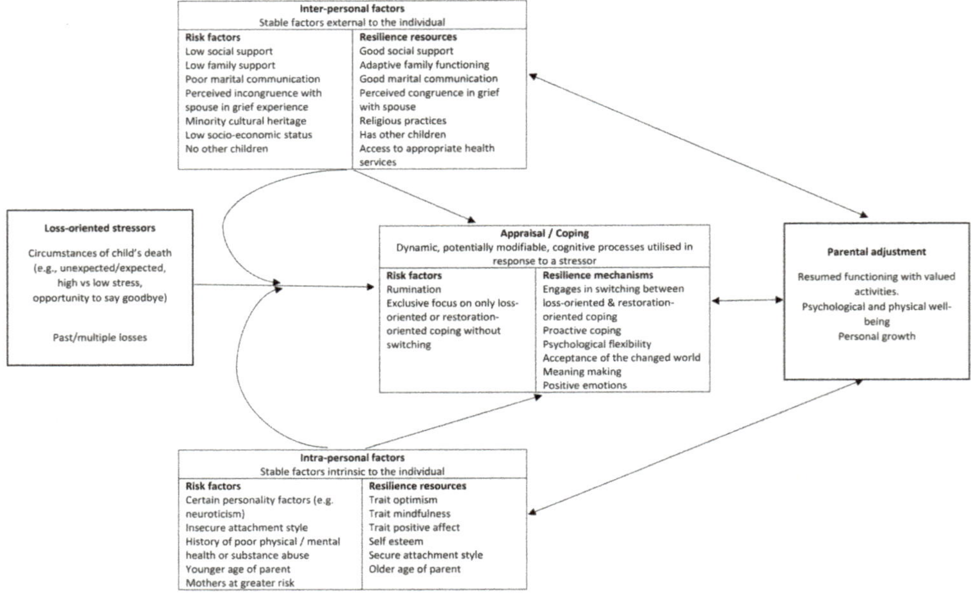

Figure 1. Risk and Resilience Model of Parental Bereavement.

4. Parental Bereavement Outcomes

Whilst there is consensus that grief is a normal experience following a major loss, it is difficult to define the process of normal grief. It is generally recognized that the grief response is dynamic, pervasive and highly individualized [21]. The process of grief is not linear and does not fit neatly into predetermined categories. The death of a child commonly results in detrimental effects on the psychological and physical well-being of parents [22,23]. Psychological responses to parental bereavement may include heightened anxiety, depression, suicidal ideation, and reduced quality of life [22,24–26]. Increased risk of psychiatric hospitalization has also been reported, especially in mothers [27]. Detrimental physical outcomes that have been reported in response to parental bereavement include a greater risk of cardiovascular problems [28], cancer [26], and higher rates of mortality due to natural and unnatural causes [26]. A wide range of detrimental social [29], marital [30], occupational and financial consequences [31] have also been reported amongst bereaved parents.

The adverse outcomes listed above are certainly not experienced by all individuals, with there being considerable variability in symptoms experienced. Moreover, there is also much variability in the duration of intense grief reactions [22]. Most bereaved individuals return to relatively normal functioning, as judged by external standards, within a relatively short time-frame [1], even if their experience of life is now different.

Over the years, various terms and classifications have been used to describe intense and debilitating grief reactions, including persistent complex bereavement disorder, prolonged grief disorder, bereavement-related major depression, complicated grief, pathological grief. Although there remain differences in opinion as to how best to classify these individuals [32,33], it is generally recognized that 5–10% of bereaved individuals experience significant and prolonged impairment of functioning [34]. It is not clear what these figures are for parental bereavement following the loss of a child due to a life-limiting condition, however it has been found that the context of an expected death poses lower risk than unexpected deaths [35]. Where data are available, the current paper will consider risk and resilience factors associated with such intense and debilitating grief reactions;

however, the paper will primarily encompass discussion of risk and resilience factors associated with the full spectrum of grief reactions.

5. Loss-Oriented Stressors

5.1. Circumstances Surrounding the Death

Once parents recognize that their child has a life-limiting condition and may die in the foreseeable future, they may begin to consider and plan for the circumstances surrounding their child's impending death. Palliative care teams often discuss with parents issues such as: (i) whether they have a preference for where the child dies (e.g., at home or at hospital); (ii) who they would like to be present; (iii) what medical interventions are to be used and when these should be ceased; (iv) what will happen to the body immediately after the death; and (v) what psychological support is available to the family regarding this decision-making. Many of the above choices are not always open to the parents, but often there is some scope for parental preferences. It is generally assumed by clinicians that the parents' choices should be respected wherever possible.

Although there is some evidence that different causes of death (illness versus injury/accident) may be associated with different parental bereavement outcomes [7,8], there is little evidence on whether specific circumstances surrounding the death are associated with more favourable bereavement outcomes than others. A study by Grande et al. [36] considered whether the location of the child's death was associated with parental bereavement outcomes six weeks and six months later. They found that parents had better outcomes six weeks following a home death rather than a hospital death, but that there was no difference at six months. Another study also found that fathers reported higher levels of depression, anxiety and stress when their child with cancer died in hospital rather than home [37]. However, given the complex nature of circumstances, and that location of death was not a matter of chance, one cannot infer causality from such associations. For example, the above results may have been due to families who were not coping well in the lead up to the death, being more likely to choose a hospital-based, rather than home-based, death. It should also be noted that another study found that the circumstances associated with a child's death were found to have a lesser impact on parental bereavement outcomes than parental coping styles [38].

Anecdotally, parents report valuing the opportunity to say a final goodbye to their child [11]. This is more likely to be possible when there is a recognition that the child's death is imminent, enabling parents to participate in tasks, processes and rituals that they deemed important prior to their child's death [11].

5.2. Multiple Losses

The way in which parents have responded to, and coped with, previous losses may give some indication of how they are likely to respond to an impending death of a child with a life-limiting condition. Parents who have had a child die from a life-limiting genetic disorder may have another child with the same genetic disorder, which may result in more than one grief experience. It may be clinically useful to ask parents about previous losses, as it can provide useful information about their ability to access and utilize their intra-personal and inter-personal resources when faced with bereavement. Moreover, it is possible that a history of multiple losses may also render individuals more vulnerable to poorer adjustment outcomes. There are relatively few data about the effects of multiple losses and previous grief experiences on the subsequent experience of loss. A study with 190 adult participants found that a history of more than two losses was associated with a higher probability of developing complicated grief, with the number of losses having a cumulative effect [39]. In contrast, another study with gay men found no association between number of losses and grief intensity [40]. Simply considering the number of losses may not be as informative as considering other factors associated with earlier losses, such as coping style and social support. The time period between bereavement experiences may also be a relevant factor, with suggestions that if a subsequent loss occurs soon after an earlier loss, it can "interrupt" a normal bereavement process, leading to poorer adjustment [39,41].

Bereaved individuals experiencing other concurrent losses, such as loss of employment, divorce, and significant financial setbacks, are likely to be at greater risk of poor bereavement outcomes [42,43]. Their coping resources may already be stretched to capacity prior to the bereavement, thus leaving them with few remaining adaptive resources. Moreover, concurrent stressors, such as marital tension or work difficulties, are likely to continue into the bereavement phase, and may therefore exceed the parent's coping resources making it more difficult for them to transition into the new reality of their environment.

6. Inter-Personal Resources

Inter-personal resources are those that originate within the social or environmental context within which the bereaved parent is functioning and include things like marital factors, social support and religious practices.

6.1. Marital Factors

Not only do spouses need to grapple with their own loss following the death of a child, they also need to cope with their partner's grief reaction [44]. Spouses commonly experience and respond to the death of a child differently, which, in the absence of good communication, may result in marital tension. Differences may occur in any number of areas including: patterns of continuing bonds with the deceased child [45], willingness to express emotions [46], timing of readiness to resume usual roles and activities, and readiness to resume sexual intimacy [47]. A recent study of 229 bereaved couples found that bereaved parents who perceived that they had dissimilar levels of grief to their spouse (less or more grief), whilst controlling for actual differences in grief, reported lower relationship satisfaction, compared with bereaved parents who perceived more similar levels of grief [48]. Moreover, the negative effects of the perceived dissimilarity were found to increase over time. Teaching couples about sources of incongruence in their grief has been suggested as an intervention to enhance marital cohesion and relationship quality [49]. Good communication between spouses may serve as a protective buffer to minimize the impact of spousal differences in their grief. Notably, when assessed within the first two years of the loss of their infant, bereaved wives who perceived a lack of opportunity to share their thoughts and feelings with their husbands were found to experience more intense grief reactions two years later than wives who reported more opportunity to share thoughts and feelings with their husbands [50].

In light of the stress that individuals and couples experience following the death of a child, marital disruption is a common, though not inevitable, consequence [51]. Pre-existing marital difficulties, especially following the prolonged illness of a child, may manifest in more overt discord following the death of a child. A study comparing the divorce rates of bereaved parents with a control group of non-bereaved parents found somewhat higher divorce rates among bereaved parents in the first 6 months following the death (5–6%), relative to non-bereaved parents (0.5–1.5%) [30]. However, marital discord is not inevitable following the death of a child, and in some cases parental relationships may even strengthen following the death of a child [51].

It has been suggested that marital disruption may be greater if the bereavement occurs early in married life relative to mid-to-later life [7]. Consistent with this premise, bereavement following neonatal death has been associated with particularly high levels of subsequent marital disruption [30]. Marital disruption has been found to be less if there are other children in the family at the time of the death [28], presumably giving the parents a unified purpose in caring for their other child/children.

6.2. Social Support

Social support, particularly an individual's perception of social support [52], is recognized as being beneficial to all individuals, irrespective of whether or not they currently face bereavement [20].

Nevertheless, social support warrants particular attention in the context of bereavement. Social networks are known to alter in the context of caring for someone with a long-term illness. While some individuals report that their social network galvanized around them to provide support and care, others describe increasing social isolation [53,54], particularly if their child had a long illness. It is well accepted that individuals and families who report having good social support cope with stressors more effectively [55]. These findings have also been found to hold true within the context of bereavement following the death of a child [4].

This leads to the question about whether social support-based interventions are able to improve bereavement outcomes. Social support interventions have been developed across a broad range of contexts, and have differed widely in terms of efficacy (for a review see Hogan et al.) [56]. Despite general acceptance of the importance of social support when faced with bereavement, there has been relatively little research investigating the efficacy of social support interventions in the bereavement context, with the available evidence being mixed. Support groups in the context of parental bereavement have been frequently recommended [57,58], however, the evidence base for such interventions remains relatively weak. An extensive review of the literature [20] found there to be limited evidence to support the widely held view that social support serves as a buffer against the impact of bereavement or facilitates recovery. Many of the studies to report positive effects of social support intervention have either had low numbers or utilized a qualitative research design [59].

More recently, however, a noteworthy randomized control trial [60], albeit using block randomization according to the hospital site at which the child died, with 103 bereaved Finnish fathers, evaluated a social support intervention for bereaved fathers. The intervention consisted of an information support package, peer contact, and health care personnel contact, aimed at showing compassion and care for fathers and providing concrete aid. When assessed six months post-bereavement, fathers in the intervention condition (n = 62) reported stronger personal growth and some lower grief reaction scores (e.g., blame and anger) relative to fathers in the control condition (n = 41). A similar study, with essentially the same intervention program, was carried out with 136 bereaved Finnish mothers [61]. Although mothers who reported greater perceived social support also reported lower grief reactions, there were no significant differences in maternal grief reactions between mothers in the intervention condition (n = 83) and those in the control condition (n = 53).

A cross-sectional study with bereaved mothers found that mothers who endorsed having attended a bereavement support group reported significantly fewer traumatic stress symptoms than women who did not participate [62]. However, the women were not randomly allocated to whether they participated in a support group or not, and therefore other factors may account for these results—for example, the support group participants may have been engaging in more active coping strategies in the first place prompting them to join the support groups.

A Swedish population-based study with 449 parents who had lost a child to cancer 4–9 years earlier found that parents who reported having access to "psychological support" in the last month of the child's life, were more likely to report that they had worked through their grief at the time of the assessment [63]. However, given the retrospective nature of the study, the possible role of memory bias should be acknowledged. Individuals coping better at the time of the assessment may have had a more favourable recall of the psychological support available to them in the month prior to their child's death.

Not all bereaved parents are likely to express the same desire for social support groups. For example, there is some suggestion that social support groups are more desired by parents who did not have adequate forewarning about their child's death [64]. One study found that 80% of bereaved parents who opted to participate in a support group had lost their child without adequate forewarning. In contrast, 76% of parents who opted not to participate in a support group had lost their child after a period of anticipatory grief [64]. Gender differences may also impact on social support group preferences. Males have been found to be less likely to seek emotional support than females, and to be more likely to seek instrumental support rather than emotional support [65]. Moreover, one study found that fathers may be more likely to participate in electronic support groups than face-to-face support groups [66], which is an area that may warrant future research in the bereavement context.

The considerable variability in the efficacy of social support interventions with bereaved parents is, in part, likely to be related to the very varied nature of social support interventions. Some such interventions aim to provide support directly, whereas others aim to establish skills or make changes that are likely to enhance naturally occurring social support. Some interventions offer social support from peers (e.g., family, friends, or other individuals in a similar situation) whereas other interventions offer support from a health professional, some may be parent-driven discussions and others highly structured groups led by a health professional. Moreover, intervention formats may differ in terms of whether they are individually-based versus group-based, or whether they are face-to-face versus electronic. More research is needed into the possibility of matching types of social support interventions to the individual.

Acknowledging some exceptions (as listed above), much of the research investigating social support in the bereavement context has focused on marital bereavement [20]. It is important to recognize some important differences in these contexts. The losses commonly associated with marital bereavement, such as loss of instrumental, emotional and validational support [67], may be partially compensated by effective social support from family and friends [20]. However, the losses associated with the death of a child are somewhat less tangible, and arguably more difficult for family and friends to compensate for in any significant way.

Anecdotally, migrant families commonly report longing for the support of their parents, but may be practically or financially unable to make the necessary travel arrangements.

Cultural heritage may shape and define the way in which individuals express their grief [68,69], such as "culturally approved" somatization [70]. Consequently, first generation immigrants may experience a more challenging bereavement experience if they are cut off from their traditional cultural groups, but have not assimilated into adopting the grief cultural practices of the society in which they now reside [71,72]. The published scientific bereavement literature is very much from a western cultural perspective, leaving health professionals reliant on whatever training is available to them about immigrant cultural practices.

6.3. Religious Practices

The literature on whether parental religious practices are related to bereavement outcomes is mixed. There is some literature on the benefits of religion when coping with stressful life events [73,74]. Walsh et al. [74] found that individuals who professed stronger spiritual beliefs of any religious persuasion (and distinct from religious observance) seemed to have better and more rapid resolution of their grief than individuals who reported no spiritual beliefs. Other researchers have found variable, and at times worse, adjustment among the more religious in a bereavement context [75]. One study found that, when 102 newly bereaved individuals were assessed, frequent church attenders responded with higher optimism and social desirability, but more repression of grief responses than less frequent church attenders [76].

7. Intra-Personal Resources

Intra-personal resources refer to characteristics that are stable and intrinsic to the bereaved individual (e.g., personality, attachment style, gender, predisposing personal vulnerabilities such as substance abuse, physical or mental health problems).

7.1. Personality

Personality variables are stable intrapersonal constructs that are predictive of behavioural responses across both time and situations, and are therefore likely to impact how individuals respond to adverse life events, such as bereavement. They may serve as either risk or resilience factors. Personality variables may impact bereavement outcomes due to their influence on an individual's approach to coping. Some personality variables have been found to be associated with less adaptive approaches to coping, poorer inter-personal interactions, and poorer adjustment to stressors. Other personality variables have been found to be associated with greater resilience in the face of life stressors. Within the bereavement context, neuroticism has been consistently identified as a significant risk factor of poorer outcomes [77], whereas possible personality resilience factors include trait optimism [78,79], psychological flexibility [80], and trait mindfulness [81]. The literature on these factors will be reviewed.

Neuroticism may be defined as the tendency to respond to threat, frustration or loss with negative emotions. Hence it is not surprising that elevated scores on measures of neuroticism have been found to be associated with poorer bereavement outcomes [77]. This may be due the coping responses that individuals high in neuroticism engage in. In a study of 325 bereaved individuals, individuals scoring higher on a measure of neuroticism were found to be less likely to engage in strategies that contribute to meaning-making, or finding understanding in the situation [82]. Another study found that individuals who were high in neuroticism provided narratives about their loss that were more self-focused [83]. The investigators suggested that this served the purpose of obtaining emotional validation and was reminiscent of ruminative coping.

It is important, however, to acknowledge the overlapping conceptual nature of poorer bereavement outcomes, such as elevated anxiety and distress, and behavioural characteristics commonly found in individuals high in neuroticism [77,84]. Similarly, individuals who are high in extraversion are more likely to demonstrate a tendency to be more sociable, active and assertive, characteristics typically associated with better behavioural outcomes. These characteristic similarities may make it difficult to accurately determine the impact of personality variables on measured outcomes, particularly as measures of personality prior to bereavement are often not available.

As growing attention in the literature is being devoted to factors that may make some individuals more resilient in the face of adverse life events [15,17], consideration should be given to which personality factors are likely to be associated with better adjustment following parental bereavement. Trait optimism has been defined as the tendency to adopt favourable expectancies for the future [85]. In the context of parental bereavement, this may manifest as the parent's capacity to envisage engaging in valued activities again in the future, in a world altered by the death of their child. Although depression scores in the clinical range are common in bereavement, trait optimism has been found to predict a shorter duration of elevated depression scores [79]. Moreover, individuals with high trait optimism one month post-bereavement have been found to have significantly better psychological adjustment at 6, 12 and 18 months post-bereavement relative to pessimists [86], even when controlling for differential coping strategies.

Trait optimism is a relatively stable individual difference variable that reflects a predisposition to expect favourable expectancies for one's future [87]. It has been shown to be associated with favourable adjustment outcomes across a wide range of contexts, including surgery, cardiovascular disease, respiratory failure, in vitro fertilization, cancer, AIDS progression, caregiving, and academic examinations (for reviews see [87–89]). One can speculate numerous possible mechanisms by which trait optimism can lead to more favourable outcomes: (i) optimism has been found to be associated with greater approach-based coping responses and fewer avoidance-based coping [89]; (ii) optimism is generally regarded as socially desirable, and may therefore be associated with the availability of greater social support [90]; (iii) optimists are more confident about eventually attaining desired outcomes, which in the context of bereavement may be the ability to re-engage in valued activities, and are therefore more likely to keep trying in the face of difficulties encountered [87]; (iv) optimism is by definition the opposite of hopelessness, the latter being associated with depression and poorer psychological adjustment [91]; and (v) optimism is associated with positive affect, which is likely to confer direct benefits across a range of contexts [92]. Although most bereaved parents would find it difficult to recognize any feelings of optimism following their child's death, and may find the term difficult or even offensive, there is likely to be considerable variability with regard to their ability to conceive of engaging in valued activities again some time in the future. To date there have been relatively few studies investigating the relationship between trait optimism and bereavement outcomes. Nevertheless, a longitudinal study with individuals in the first year after their loss, and then 6 months, and 15 months later, found that trait optimism was inversely associated with concurrent and future levels of depression and prolonged grief [78].

Although psychological flexibility is not a new concept, interest in its application as a personality resilience factor in the health psychology context has emerged relatively recently [80,93]. The term psychological flexibility (also sometimes referred to as regulatory control, executive control or response modulation) has been used to refer to an individual's capacity to efficiently regulate one's behaviour, emotions and coping, based on an awareness of contextual demands, repertoire of coping skills, and responsivity to internal and external feedback [80]. Psychological flexibility has been consistently found to be associated with better overall health and adjustment [94]. Within the context of bereavement, psychological flexibility is likely to have a particularly important role. The dual-process theory of bereavement highlights the importance of shifting attention between a loss-oriented focus (namely a focus on appraising and processing some aspect of the loss experience) and a restoration-oriented focus (namely a focus on reorienting oneself in a changed world without the deceased person) [95]. Arguably, individuals with a greater capacity for psychological flexibility may be able to engage in this shifting more effectively. There has been little empirical investigation into the concept of psychological flexibility and bereavement. A related concept of emotional expressive flexibility has been examined in the context of bereaved spouses (a subset of whom had complicated grief) and non-bereaved married adults [96]. Adults experiencing complicated grief were found to display deficits in expressive flexibility relative to asymptomatic bereaved adults and married controls. In the absence of longitudinal studies it is not possible to infer any causal direction.

Trait mindfulness is the tendency to purposefully and non-judgmentally attend to the present moment. It has been found to be associated with psychological well-being across a range of domains [97]. Within the bereavement context, greater mindfulness may enable individuals to allow themselves to experience the many emotions of grief in a non-judgmental way. Clinical approaches have been developed to facilitate greater mindfulness in bereaved individuals [81,98], though few data have thus far been reported on the efficacy of such approaches.

7.2. Attachment Style

An individual's attachment style influences their behavioural, emotional and cognitive patterns of responding, impacting on their appraisal and coping with life stressors. The theoretical and empirical literature regarding the relationship between parental attachment variables and the paediatric palliative care context has been comprehensively reviewed by Kearney and Byrne [99]. Notably insecure attachment styles (e.g., anxious or avoidant patterns) have been found to be associated with decreased resilience, complicated grief reactions, poorer psychological outcomes, and marital distress [44,84,100–103]. In contrast, secure parental attachment styles have been found to be associated with more effective distress management, active support seeking, better engagement with healthcare providers, and better coping responses [99,104,105], which are likely to contribute to better bereavement outcomes [99]. Notably, there has been little empirical work investigating potential differences in the attachment style of parents of a child with a life-limiting condition, relative to the attachment style of parents of a child with normal life expectancy.

In addition to considering established parental attachment styles, attachment theory holds that bereavement outcomes are also contingent on an individual revising their internal working model of attachment to the deceased individual in accord with the changes in the external world brought about by the loss [106]. Failure to make such revision is what prominent attachment theorists such as Bowlby [107] consider to be at the heart of complicated grief.

7.3. Gender

Gender differences in relation to bereavement outcomes have mostly been considered in the context of the death of a spouse, with greater rates of depression and mortality documented in men relative to women, and gender differences in coping responses (for reviews see [23,108]). However, the issues related to bereavement following the death of child relative to the death of a spouse differ in a number of key ways, making it difficult to generalize across contexts. Research examining parental bereavement typically considers a younger cohort of bereaved individuals, with most fathers and some mothers likely to be employed. Bereaved parents are also more likely to have other family members living in the household, such as their spouse and/or other children for whom they continue to be responsible.

Mothers have been found to rate their grief feelings higher than fathers following the death of an infant [109]. It is not clear, though, whether women experience these reactions more intensely or whether men experience bereavement in a way that is not measured by the assessment instruments commonly used.

A number of specific variables have been identified that differ for bereaved men and women that may impact on bereavement outcomes. Women tend to talk more about their feelings to others, while men tend to minimize the expression of painful emotions and cope with negative emotions in a more solitary way [46], immersing themselves in practical tasks and in their work [110]. Women commonly have additional confidants outside their marriage, whereas men are more likely to rely exclusively on their wives as confidants [108]. Discordant coping styles between husbands and wives are likely to add to the stress of each individual, with feelings that their spouse does not understand them.

7.4. Predisposing Personal Vulnerabilities

There are numerous pre-existing intrapersonal factors, such as substance abuse, mental health problems, and poor physical health, which are widely recognized to compromise an individual's coping resources and place them at greater risk of poor bereavement outcomes [43,111]. Excessive use of alcohol has been widely documented among bereaved individuals, especially males [112]. The use of alcohol as a maladaptive avoidance strategy during the stressful period of caring for a child with a life-limiting condition is likely to place the parent at significant risk of substance abuse problems in the bereavement period. Unfortunately, only a relatively small proportion of the bereavement literature has utilized information collected from carers before the death of a spouse or child, making it difficult to gain a clear understanding of predisposing factors.

Psychological problems are relatively more common among long-term carers than in the general population [113], largely related to the high levels of stress which they experience. The intense stress associated with bereavement is likely to further exacerbate any pre-existing psychological or physical conditions [43]. An early study found that 60 per cent of individuals who committed suicide following bereavement had undergone psychiatric treatment prior to bereavement [114].

Pre-existing physical problems may be more common prior to bereavement following the death of a spouse than the death of a child, given that the loss of a spouse generally occurs at an older age. Nevertheless, anecdotally, parents caring for a seriously unwell child over an extended period of time commonly overlook their own physical healthcare needs, and therefore place their own health at greater risk. Any physical problems may be further exacerbated when faced with the intense stress of bereavement.

Despite the paucity of research to date which has utilized information collected from carers before the death of a child, such research is more feasible in the context of caring for a child with a life-limiting condition. In this context, clinicians (and researchers) may have contact with parents in the weeks and months prior to a child's death. At a minimum, this should allow for a thorough investigation of possible predisposing risk factors, and ideally may provide the opportunity for appropriate supports and interventions to be implemented to address the relevant risk factors.

8. Coping and Appraisal

Coping may broadly be considered as the process by which an individual appraises the personal significance of a situation or event and the options that they have for responding to that situation or event [3]. Over the years, individuals typically develop a tendency to utilize certain coping styles. However, when faced with specific challenges, the individual must appraise the situation and their capacity to respond to it, and apply particular coping strategies accordingly.

Coping is known to be associated with, and likely to mediate, the relationship between interpersonal and intrapersonal variables with adjustment [3,77,115]. Within the context of bereavement, the coping process is of particular importance because it offers possible targets for effective intervention, given that these constructs may be amenable to change [3,116]. In an early paper addressing intervention strategies for coping with transitions, a useful list of coping competencies was outlined [117]. These coping competencies included skills for assessing, developing and utilizing internal and external resources, skills for managing emotional and physiological distress, and skills associated with planning and implementing change. Despite these transition-based coping competencies being articulated more than 35 years ago, more research is needed to investigate the role of coping interventions in the context of parental bereavement.

The majority of the literature on coping pertains to situations that have occurred and present a current challenge or threat to the individual. However, a small body of literature addresses what has been referred to as proactive coping, pertaining to anticipated threats or stressors [118]. The literature regarding bereavement following the death of a child due to a life-limiting condition would benefit from a consideration of both types of coping, given that parents face many ongoing stressors whilst caring for a child with a life-limiting condition, whilst also being mindful that they will one day need to face their child's death. In other contexts, proactive coping has been found to be beneficial, and indeed teachable, heightening an individual's awareness of their personal and social resources, so that they are better placed to make effective coping decisions [119]. However, the concept of proactive coping has, to date, not been well applied to parental bereavement following a child's death due to a life-limiting condition, and warrants further research.

It is generally recognized that specific coping strategies are not uniformly effective (or ineffective) across all contexts and situations. Instead, an individual's coping efficacy is dependent on an efficient process of self-regulation, which requires an awareness of contextual demands, availability of a range of coping skills to select from, and responsivity to internal and external feedback [80]. A small-scale study investigating the coping of bereaved parents found that the coping strategies used by those bereaved for 18 months or less differed considerably from non-bereaved normative samples, whereas those bereaved for more than 18 months engaged in coping strategies similar to normative samples [120]. The efficacy of the coping strategies, however, was not examined.

Within the bereavement literature, Stroebe and Schut [95] made a distinction between loss-oriented coping (namely a focus on appraising and processing some aspect of the loss experience) and restoration-oriented coping (namely a focus on reorienting oneself in a changed world without the deceased person). The dual process theory of bereavement holds that oscillation between these different types of cognitive processing is essential for adaptive bereavement outcomes and that over time more focus is placed on a restoration orientation and less on a loss orientation [121,122]. In a study of 219 couples following the death of their child, Wijngaards-de Meij et al. investigated parental use of restoration-coping and loss-oriented coping [123]. Although utilizing quite a limited set of items to assess coping, Wijngaards-de Meij et al. found that a greater focus on future-oriented, restoration-coping, irrespective of the amount of loss-oriented coping that was used, was associated with more beneficial outcomes [123]. Moreover, when women made greater use of restoration coping, their husbands also benefited, showing lower levels of depression.

Although psychological flexibility is sometimes regarded as a personality dimension, it may also be considered as a more malleable, cognitive coping process. Within the Acceptance and Commitment Therapy (ACT) framework, psychological flexibility has been taken to refer to an ability to be present-focussed, acting in a manner consistent with one's values, even in the presence of interfering thoughts and emotions [93]. ACT interventions with the parents of children with a life-limiting condition have successfully increased aspects of parental psychological flexibility [124]. However, to our knowledge, studies have not investigated parental psychological flexibility following the death of a child following a life-limiting condition.

Similarly, within the body of literature on mindfulness, the concept of acceptance has emerged as being of importance in the face of life stressors [125]. Within the trauma literature, acceptance has been found to be associated with greater psychological adjustment following exposure to trauma (for review, see [125]). Within the context of bereavement, the concept of acceptance has been integral to clinical mindfulness interventions that have been developed, such as based on the ATTEND (attunement, trust, touch, egalitarianism, nuance, and death education) framework [81]. However, evaluations of these interventions have thus far been limited [126].

Meaning-making is a term that has emerged and proliferated in the literature over the past decade, referring to the restoration of meaning following a highly stressful situation [127]. Meaning-making requires the integration of the meaning given to a stressful event with one's global orienting system or cognitive framework [127]. Highly stressful situations have the potential to challenge one's global cognitive systems. The extent to which the meaning that an individual attributes to a stressful event is discrepant with their global cognitive system is likely to determine the extent to which they experience distress. It has been found that the degree to which parents have made sense or meaning out of their child's unexpected death was inversely related to their degree of distress [128], albeit one study found this relationship was only significant in the first year of bereavement [129].

The nature of a child's death has been found to impact on the ability of parents to find meaning in the situation. Parents whose child died a violent death (i.e., accident, homicide or suicide) found it more challenging to make-meaning of the situation relative to parents whose child died a non-violent death (perinatal, natural anticipated, or natural sudden) [130]. There has been little work investigating the process of meaning-making specifically among parents of children who died from a life-limiting disorder.

Positive emotions have been suggested to serve a restorative role in bereavement, and as a catalyst for meaning finding and benefit finding [92]. Moskowitz, Folkman and Acree [79] noted a positive association between positive affect and bereavement outcomes, which they attributed to an increased likelihood to engage in positive reappraisal. Moreover, a positive affect renders individuals more able to seek social support. However, the overlapping nature of measures of positive emotions and of bereavement outcomes makes it difficult to disentangle these constructs or to consider issues of causality.

Rumination is a coping style characterized by recurrent, self-focused negative thinking. It is widely regarded as a normal part of grieving. However, more extreme rumination is likely to be problematic and a predictor of poorer bereavement outcomes [131]. In a study with 55 bereaved individuals (following the death of a first degree relative within the previous three years), greater rumination was associated with symptoms of psychopathology over a 12-month period [132]. It has been suggested that the repeated focus of attention on negative emotions associated with rumination interferes with problem solving capabilities, and impedes instrumental behaviour and the utilization of social support [131]. Females and individuals with lower social support have been found to engage in more ruminating behaviour following the death of a loved one [116].

Rumination used to be considered a confrontational strategy, requiring individuals to confront and experience distress and negative emotions. More recently, though, rumination has been appraised as an avoidance strategy [133], whereby an individual focuses disproportionately on loss-oriented coping with little attention to restoration-oriented coping. According to this view, individuals engage in ruminative thinking, dwelling on negative aspects of their personal loss, and in so doing avoid confronting the new realities of their life and fail to restructure their cognitive schemata accordingly.

The nature of the cognitive appraisal that an individual engages in may be influenced by their cultural beliefs. For example, individuals holding traditional Chinese beliefs are more likely than individuals holding Western beliefs to adopt an external locus of control and attribute the cause of a death to predestined rules or higher powers such as sick *qi* (negative energy that could pass to the unlucky) or evil spirits [134]. This remains an under-researched area.

9. Challenges to Carrying Out Bereavement Research

Studying the bereavement process and factors associated with parental bereavement outcomes is fraught with challenges [135]. Key areas of difficulty relate to participant recruitment, inter-relatedness of variables, and the selection and use of multiple outcome measures. Each of these areas of difficulty will be briefly described.

Research participation is voluntary; hence self-selection is likely to influence who participates in bereavement research [136]. Individuals may decline to participate due to: depressed mood, feeling they are too upset to answer questions about their bereavement, fear that participation may increase their grief, or greater use of avoidant coping strategies. It is therefore possible that individuals who are most disabled by grief, perhaps meeting the Diagnostic and Statistical Manual of Mental Disorders—5th Edition (DSM-5) criteria of persistent complex bereavement disorder, may commonly not participate in bereavement research. Individuals who agree to participate in bereavement research may be more willing to talk about their experience, and therefore may already be engaging in more adaptive coping strategies. Notably, given that women are more likely to seek social support and talk about their feelings and experiences [46], they may be more likely to engage in bereavement research. This issue is likely to be magnified if recruitment occurs through bereavement support services, which may predominantly be utilized by individuals who are willing to talk about their experiences. Alternatively, it is conceivable that individuals who are more distressed may be more likely to take up the opportunity to talk with someone about their feelings [136]. Moreover, there is evidence of a selective invitation bias in paediatric palliative care research, whereby not all eligible families are invited to participate due to non-random factors [137].

Factors that potentially render parents at greater or lower risk of poor bereavement outcomes are often difficult to disentangle from complex, inter-related circumstances and attitudes. For example, decisions regarding the preferred location of the child's death may be related to the family's coping efficacy, their perceptions of how well their child's symptoms are able to be managed outside of hospital, the supports and services available to the family, and considerations regarding the presence of other siblings. Randomization is rarely appropriate to study such factors in a methodologically rigorous way. A multivariate statistical approach would also be useful in minimizing the reporting of spurious associations, but requires an adequate sample size.

When carrying out research with bereaved individuals it is difficult to find the right balance between assessing multiple outcome domains of possible interest and not wanting to over-burden bereaved parents. Many studies have considered only a single measure of bereavement outcome, failing to acknowledge the complex and varied ways in which different individuals respond to the death of a child. For example, it is increasingly recognized that mothers and fathers experience the loss of a child differently [108]. Some outcome measures may be more sensitive to identifying the responses of women rather than men, or vice versa.

10. Future Directions for Research and Clinical Practice

It is important to achieve better alignment between quality research in the area of parental bereavement, particularly in the context of a death following life-limiting condition, and clinical practice. Although the natural trajectory of bereavement has been documented in the context of bereaved older spouses [138], at present the natural history of bereavement in parents following the death of a child has not been well studied. Prospective studies in this area are needed, though challenging due to the relatively small numbers of children known to be approaching death and the difficulty of engaging parents at this time. Multi-centre collaboration would be useful to achieve sufficient sample sizes. Alternatively, the use of large-scale, longitudinal databases (i.e., Big Data) would not only provide useful longitudinal data, but, importantly, also avoid many self-selection and recruitment biases common in this area of research, given that participation is not specific to their bereavement status.

The evidence for clinical interventions with bereaved parents is currently poor [139]. In a systematic review by Endo et al. [139], nine articles were retrieved, describing eight randomized controlled trials of clinical interventions with bereaved parents or siblings following a child's death. The interventions were varied, and included support groups, counselling, psychotherapy and crisis intervention. However, the authors of the systematic review concluded that there was limited evidence of sufficient quality to support the intervention techniques used. Similarly, the literature in other areas of bereavement suggests that most individuals regain their pre-loss levels of functioning after a transitory period of distress (e.g., 6–12 months) irrespective of whether they receive any intervention [140]. The authors of an earlier meta-analysis evaluating the efficacy of psychotherapeutic interventions for bereavement concluded that more favourable outcomes were obtained for programs that specifically targeted bereaved individuals experiencing most marked difficulties [141].

Within the context of the Risk and Resilience Model of Parental Bereavement proposed in this paper, the current review has identified various inter-personal and intra-personal factors that may positively or detrimentally impact parental bereavement outcomes. These risk and resilience factors may be identified in the weeks, months, or even years prior to a child's death within the supportive context of a relationship with a palliative healthcare provider. Many risk factors, such as low social support, previous losses, predisposing personal vulnerabilities (such as psychiatric history or history of substance abuse), are likely to be identifiable through clinical interview. Other factors, such as attachment style, trait mindfulness and psychological flexibility, may warrant the use of brief, validated questionnaires. A clearer identification of which parents are at greatest risk of adverse bereavement outcomes will help pave the way for the development and evaluation of targeted interventions. Consideration should be given to the possibility of enhancing the resilience of parents, arguably even prior to their child's death, such as by enhancing mindfulness, acceptance and psychological flexibility. Importantly, the Risk and Resilience Model of Parental Bereavement highlights the importance of considering both risk and resilience factors, and how these may, in combination, impact on bereavement outcomes.

A number of key issues warrant further research in order to better inform the development of evidence-based clinical interventions. If factors such as psychological flexibility and mindfulness are indeed associated with more favourable parental bereavement outcomes, how can these coping styles be taught? At what point should they be taught—before or after a child's death? Would all parents facing bereavement benefit from these approaches, or is there a subset of parents who would receive most benefit? Notably, Bonanno [17] cautioned against assuming that there is a single resilience pathway. It may be that individuals with certain risk factors receive particular benefit from specific resilience factors that serve to compensate for the risk. More research is needed to address these questions.

11. Conclusions

The death of a child following a life-limiting illness is an incredibly stressful experience for parents, which may render these parents vulnerable to a range of adverse bereavement outcomes. The current paper sought to enhance understanding of a wide range of factors potentially impacting on parental bereavement outcomes following the death of a child due to a life-limiting condition. Studies have commonly focused on single risk factors and/or have been compromised by recruitment limitations and very small sample sizes, consequently resulting in some conflicting findings. These limitations are further heightened if the research lacks a theoretical framework. The Risk and Resilience Model of Parental Bereavement was proposed to enable consideration of a range of factors from within a broader theoretical framework. A better understanding of the complex interplay between various risk and resilience factors may allow health professionals to carry out comprehensive, holistic assessments prior to a child's death, enabling them to identify parents who may be vulnerable to poorer bereavement outcomes. Further research is needed into interventions that heighten or promote resilience, particularly amongst parents identified as being at high risk of poor bereavement outcomes.

Acknowledgments: The authors are grateful for the feedback provided by Maria Heaton, who generously shared insights from the perspective of a bereaved parent as well as a pediatric palliative care nurse. The constructive comments of Susan Trethewie are acknowledged. The assistance of Sara Sarraf with referencing is gratefully acknowledged. Tiina Jaaniste's position is supported by the Sydney Children's Hospital Foundation.

Author Contributions: T.J., S.C., T.J.D., N.K. and D.B. each contributed to the research, drafting and reviewing of the paper.

Conflicts of Interest: The authors declare no conflict of interest.

References

1. Genevro, J.L.; Marshall, T.; Miller, T.; Center for the Advancement of Health. Report on bereavement and grief research. *Death Stud.* **2004**, *28*, 491–575. [PubMed]
2. Middleton, W.; Raphael, B.; Burnett, P.; Martinek, N. A longitudinal study comparing bereavement phenomena in recently bereaved spouses, adult children and parents. *Aust. N. Z. J. Psychiatry* **1998**, *32*, 235–241. [CrossRef] [PubMed]
3. Stroebe, M.S.; Folkman, S.; Hansson, R.O.; Schut, H. The prediction of bereavement outcome: Development of an integrative risk factor framework. *Soc. Sci. Med.* **2006**, *63*, 2440–2451. [CrossRef] [PubMed]
4. Hazzard, A.; Weston, J.; Gutterres, C. After a child's death: Factors related to parental bereavement. *J. Dev. Behav. Pediatr.* **1992**, *13*, 24–30. [PubMed]
5. Lundin, T. Long-term outcome of bereavement. *Br. J. Psychiatry* **1984**, *145*, 424–428. [CrossRef] [PubMed]
6. Breen, L.J. The effect of caring on post-bereavement outcome: Research gaps and practice priorities. *Prog. Palliat. Care* **2012**, *20*, 27–30. [CrossRef]
7. Floyd, F.J.; Mailick Seltzer, M.; Greenberg, J.S.; Song, J. Parental bereavement during mid-to-later life: Pre-to postbereavement functioning and intrapersonal resources for coping. *Psychol. Aging* **2013**, *28*, 402–413. [CrossRef] [PubMed]
8. Song, J.; Floyd, F.J.; Seltzer, M.M.; Greenberg, J.S.; Hong, J. Long-term effects of child death on parents' health-related quality of life: A dyadic analysis. *Fam. Relat.* **2010**, *59*, 269–282. [CrossRef] [PubMed]
9. Gilliland, G.; Fleming, S. A comparison of spousal anticipatory grief and conventional grief. *Death Stud.* **1998**, *22*, 541–569. [PubMed]
10. Eakes, G.G.; Burke, M.L.; Hainsworth, M.A. Middle-range theory of chronic sorrow. *J. Nurs. Scholarsh.* **1998**, *30*, 179–184. [CrossRef]
11. Rini, A.; Loriz, L. Anticipatory mourning in parents with a child who dies while hospitalized. *J. Pediatr. Nurs.* **2007**, *22*, 272–282. [CrossRef] [PubMed]
12. Stewart, D.E.; Yuen, T. A systematic review of resilience in the physically Ill. *Psychosomatics* **2011**, *52*, 199–209. [CrossRef] [PubMed]
13. Zautra, A.J.; Hall, J.S.; Murray, K.E.; Resilience Solutions Group 1. Resilience: A new integrative approach to health and mental health research. *Health Psychol. Rev.* **2008**, *2*, 41–64. [CrossRef]
14. Kumpfer, K.L. Factors and Processes Contributing to Resilience. In *Resilience and Development*; Glantz, M.D., Johnson, J.L., Eds.; Springer: New York, NY, USA, 2002; pp. 179–224.
15. Cousins, L.A.; Kalapurakkel, S.; Cohen, L.L.; Simons, L.E. Topical review: Resilience resources and mechanisms in pediatric chronic pain. *J. Pediatr. Psychol.* **2015**, *40*, 840–845. [CrossRef] [PubMed]
16. Yi, J.P.; Vitaliano, P.P.; Smith, R.E.; Yi, J.C.; Weinger, K. The role of resilience on psychological adjustment and physical health in patients with diabetes. *Br. J. Health Psychol.* **2008**, *13*, 311–325. [CrossRef] [PubMed]
17. Bonanno, G.A. Loss, trauma, and human resilience: Have we underestimated the human capacity to thrive after extremely aversive events? *Am. Psychol.* **2004**, *59*, 20–28. [CrossRef] [PubMed]
18. Bonanno, G.A.; Papa, A.; O'Neill, K. Loss and human resilience. *Appl. Prev. Psychol.* **2001**, *10*, 193–206. [CrossRef]

19. Cohen, S.; Wills, T.A. Stress, social support, and the buffering hypothesis. *Psychol. Bull.* **1985**, *98*, 310–357. [CrossRef] [PubMed]
20. Stroebe, W.; Zech, E.; Stroebe, M.S.; Abakoumkin, G. Does social support help in bereavement? *J. Soc. Clin. Psychol.* **2005**, *24*, 1030–1050. [CrossRef]
21. Cowles, K.V. Cultural perspectives of grief: An expanded concept analysis. *J. Adv. Nurs.* **1996**, *23*, 287–294. [CrossRef] [PubMed]
22. Hendrickson, K.C. Morbidity, mortality, and parental grief: A review of the literature on the relationship between the death of a child and the subsequent health of parents. *Palliat. Support. Care* **2009**, *7*, 109–119. [CrossRef] [PubMed]
23. Stroebe, M.; Schut, H.; Stroebe, W. Health outcomes of bereavement. *Lancet* **2007**, *370*, 1960–1973. [CrossRef]
24. Cacciatore, J.; Lacasse, J.R.; Lietz, C.A.; McPherson, J. A parent's tears: Primary results from the traumatic experiences and resiliency study. *Omega (Westport)* **2014**, *68*, 183–205. [CrossRef]
25. Rosenberg, A.R.; Baker, K.S.; Syrjala, K.; Wolfe, J. Systematic review of psychosocial morbidities among bereaved parents of children with cancer. *Pediatr. Blood Cancer* **2012**, *58*, 503–512. [CrossRef] [PubMed]
26. Li, J.; Precht, D.H.; Mortensen, P.B.; Olsen, J. Mortality in parents after death of a child in Denmark: A nationwide follow-up study. *Lancet* **2003**, *361*, 363–367. [CrossRef]
27. Li, J.; Laursen, T.M.; Precht, D.H.; Olsen, J.; Mortensen, P.B. Hospitalization for mental illness among parents after the death of a child. *N. Engl. J. Med.* **2005**, *352*, 1190–1196. [CrossRef] [PubMed]
28. Rogers, C.H.; Floyd, F.J.; Seltzer, M.M.; Greenberg, J.; Hong, J. Long-term effects of the death of a child on parents' adjustment in midlife. *J. Fam. Psychol.* **2008**, *22*, 203–211. [CrossRef] [PubMed]
29. Prigerson, H.G.; Maciejewski, P.K. Grief and acceptance as opposite sides of the same coin: Setting a research agenda to study peaceful acceptance of loss. *Br. J. Psychiatry* **2008**, *193*, 435–437. [CrossRef] [PubMed]
30. Najman, J.M.; Vance, J.C.; Boyle, F.; Embleton, G.; Foster, B.; Thearle, J. The impact of a child death on marital adjustment. *Soc. Sci. Med.* **1993**, *37*, 1005–1010. [CrossRef]
31. Corden, A.; Sloper, P.; Sainsbury, R. Financial effects for families after the death of a disabled or chronically ill child: A neglected dimension of bereavement. *Child Care Health Dev.* **2002**, *28*, 199–204. [CrossRef] [PubMed]
32. Bryant, R.A. Prolonged grief: Where to after diagnostic and statistical manual of mental disorders, 5th edition? *Curr. Opin. Psychiatry* **2014**, *27*, 21–26. [CrossRef] [PubMed]
33. Wakefield, J.C. The DSM-5 debate over the bereavement exclusion: Psychiatric diagnosis and the future of empirically supported treatment. *Clin. Psychol. Rev.* **2013**, *33*, 825–845. [CrossRef] [PubMed]
34. Boelen, P.A.; Smid, G.E. The traumatic grief inventory self-report version (TGI-SR): Introduction and preliminary psychometric evaluation. *J. Loss Trauma* **2017**, *22*, 196–212. [CrossRef]
35. Valdimarsdottir, U.; Helgason, A.R.; Furst, C.J.; Adolfsson, J.; Steineck, G. Awareness of husband's impending death from cancer and long-term anxiety in widowhood: A nationwide follow-up. *Palliat. Med.* **2004**, *18*, 432–443. [CrossRef] [PubMed]
36. Grande, G.E.; Farquhar, M.C.; Barclay, S.I.; Todd, C.J. Caregiver bereavement outcome: relationship with hospice at home, satisfaction with care, and home death. *J. Palliat. Care* **2004**, *20*, 69–77. [PubMed]
37. Goodenough, B.; Drew, D.; Higgins, S.; Trethewie, S. Bereavement outcomes for parents who lose a child to cancer: Are place of death and sex of parent associated with differences in psychological functioning? *Psycho-Oncology* **2004**, *13*, 779–791. [CrossRef] [PubMed]
38. Harper, M.; O'Connor, R.C.; O'Carroll, R.E. Factors associated with grief and depression following the loss of a child: A multivariate analysis. *Psychol. Health. Med.* **2014**, *19*, 247–252. [CrossRef] [PubMed]
39. Castro, S.I.; Rocha, J.C. The moderating effects of previous losses and emotional clarity on bereavement outcome. *J. Loss Trauma* **2013**, *18*, 248–259. [CrossRef]
40. Cherney, P.M.; Verhey, M.P. Grief among gay men associated with muitiple losses from aids. *Death Stud.* **1996**, *20*, 115–132. [CrossRef] [PubMed]
41. Mercer, D.L.; Evans, J.M. The impact of multiple losses on the grieving process: An exploratory study. *J. Loss Trauma* **2006**, *11*, 219–227. [CrossRef]
42. Parkes, C.M. Determinants of outcome following bereavement. *Omega (Westport)* **1976**, *6*, 303–323. [CrossRef]
43. Sanders, C.M. Risk factors in bereavement outcome. *J. Soc. Issues* **1988**, *44*, 97–111. [CrossRef]
44. Wijngaards-de Meij, L.; Stroebe, M.; Schut, H.; Stroebe, W.; Van den Bout, J.; Van der Heijden, P.G.; Dijkstra, I. Patterns of attachment and parents' adjustment to the death of their child. *Personal. Soc. Psychol. Bull.* **2007**, *33*, 537–548. [CrossRef] [PubMed]

45. Root, B.L.; Exline, J.J. The role of continuing bonds in coping with grief: Overview and future directions. *Death Stud.* **2014**, *38*, 1–8. [CrossRef] [PubMed]
46. Wing, D.G.; Burge-Callaway, K.; Rose Clance, P.; Armistead, L. Understanding gender differences in bereavement following the death of an infant: Implications of or treatment. *Psychotherapy* **2001**, *38*, 60–73. [CrossRef]
47. Dyregrov, A.; Gjestad, R. Sexuality following the loss of a child. *Death Stud.* **2011**, *35*, 289–315. [CrossRef] [PubMed]
48. Buyukcan-Tetik, A.; Finkenauer, C.; Schut, H.; Stroebe, M.; Stroebe, W. The impact of bereaved parents' perceived grief similarity on relationship satisfaction. *J. Fam. Psychol.* **2017**, *31*, 409–419. [CrossRef] [PubMed]
49. Stroebe, M.; Schut, H. Family matters in bereavement: Toward an integrative intra-interpersonal coping model. *Perspect. Psychol. Sci.* **2015**, *10*, 873–879. [CrossRef] [PubMed]
50. Lang, A.; Gottlieb, L.N.; Amsel, R. Predictors of husbands' and wives' grief reactions following infant death: The role of marital intimacy. *Death Stud.* **1996**, *20*, 33–57. [CrossRef] [PubMed]
51. Kamm, S.; Vandenberg, B. Grief communication, grief reactions and marital satisfaction in bereaved parents. *Death Stud.* **2001**, *25*, 569–582. [CrossRef] [PubMed]
52. Sloper, P. Predictors of distress in parents of children with cancer: A prospective study. *J. Pediatr. Psychol.* **2000**, *25*, 79–91. [CrossRef] [PubMed]
53. Waldrop, D.P. Caregiver grief in terminal illness and bereavement: A mixed-methods study. *Health Soc. Work* **2007**, *32*, 197–206. [CrossRef] [PubMed]
54. Collins, A.; Hennessy-Anderson, N.; Hosking, S.; Hynson, J.; Remedios, C.; Thomas, K. Lived experiences of parents caring for a child with a life-limiting condition in Australia: A qualitative study. *Palliat. Med.* **2016**, *30*, 950–959. [CrossRef] [PubMed]
55. Cohen, S.; Hoberman, H.M. Positive events and social supports as buffers of life change stress. *J. Appl. Soc. Psychol.* **1983**, *13*, 99–125. [CrossRef]
56. Hogan, B.E.; Linden, W.; Najarian, B. Social support interventions: Do they work? *Clin. Psychol. Rev.* **2002**, *22*, 381–440. [CrossRef]
57. Decinque, N.; Monterosso, L.; Dadd, G.; Sidhu, R.; Macpherson, R.; Aoun, S. Bereavement support for families following the death of a child from cancer: experience of bereaved parents. *J. Psychosoc. Oncol.* **2006**, *24*, 65–83. [CrossRef] [PubMed]
58. Klass, D. *The Spiritual Lives of Bereaved Parents*; Psychology Press: Hove, UK, 1999.
59. Reilly-Smorawski, B.; Armstrong, A.V.; Catlin, E.A. Bereavement support for couples following death of a baby: Program development and 14-year exit analysis. *Death Stud.* **2002**, *26*, 21–37. [CrossRef] [PubMed]
60. Aho, A.L.; Tarkka, M.-T.; Åstedt-Kurki, P.; Sorvari, L.; Kaunonen, M. Evaluating a bereavement follow-up intervention for grieving fathers and their experiences of support after the death of a child—A pilot study. *Death Stud.* **2011**, *35*, 879–904. [CrossRef] [PubMed]
61. Raitio, K.; Kaunonen, M.; Aho, A.L. Evaluating a bereavement follow-up intervention for grieving mothers after the death of a child. *Scand. J. Caring Sci.* **2015**, *29*, 510–520. [CrossRef] [PubMed]
62. Cacciatore, J. Effects of support groups on post traumatic stress responses in women experiencing stillbirth. *Omega (Westport)* **2007**, *55*, 71–90. [CrossRef] [PubMed]
63. Kreicbergs, U.C.; Lannen, P.; Onelov, E.; Wolfe, J. Parental grief after losing a child to cancer: Impact of professional and social support on long-term outcomes. *J. Clin. Oncol.* **2007**, *25*, 3307–3312. [CrossRef] [PubMed]
64. Schwab, R. Bereaved parents and support group participation. *Omega (Westport)* **1996**, *32*, 49–61. [CrossRef]
65. Ashton, W.A.; Fuehrer, A. Effects of gender and gender role identification of participant and type of social support resource on support seeking. *Sex Roles* **1993**, *28*, 461–476. [CrossRef]
66. Mickelson, K.D. *Seeking Social Support: Parents in Electronic Support Groups*; Lawrence Erbaum Associates, Inc.: Mahwah, NJ, USA, 1997; pp. 157–178.
67. Stroebe, W.; Stroebe, M.S. *Bereavement and Health: The Psychological and Physical Consequences of Partner Loss*; Cambridge University Press: Cambridge, UK, 1987.
68. Cook, A.S.; Oltjenbruns, K.A. *Dying and Grieving: Life Span and Family Perspectives*; Holt, Rinehart, and Winston: New York, NY, USA, 1989; p. 491.

69. Rosenblatt, P.C. Grief across Cultures: A Review and Research Agenda. In *Handbook of Bereavement Research and Practice: Advances in Theory and Intervention*; Stroebe, M.S., Hansson, R.O., Schut, H., Stroebe, W., Eds.; American Psychological Association: Washington, DC, USA, 2008; pp. 207–222.
70. Katon, W.; Kleinman, A.; Rosen, G. Depression and somatization: A review: Part I. *Am. J. Med.* **1982**, *72*, 127–135. [CrossRef]
71. Institute of Medicine (US) Committee for the Study of Health Consequences of the Stress of Bereavement. *Bereavement: Reactions, Consequences, and Care*; Osterweis, M., Solomon, F., Green, M., Eds.; National Academies Press (US): Washington, DC, USA, 1984.
72. Rider, J.; Hayslip, B. *Ambiguity of Loss, Anticipatory Grief, and Boundary Ambiguity in Caregiver Spouses and Parents*; University of Texas: Denton, TX, USA, 1993.
73. Pargament, K.I. *The Psychology of Religion and Coping: Theory, Research, Practice*; Guilford Press: New York, NY, USA, 2001.
74. Walsh, K.; King, M.; Jones, L.; Tookman, A.; Blizard, R. Spiritual beliefs may affect outcome of bereavement: Prospective study. *BMJ* **2002**, *324*, 1551. [CrossRef] [PubMed]
75. Stroebe, M.S. Commentary: Religion in coping with bereavement: Confidence of convictions or scientific scrutiny? *Int. J. Psychol. Relig.* **2004**, *14*, 23–36. [CrossRef]
76. Sanders, C.M. A comparison of adult bereavement in the death of a spouse, child, and parent. *Omega (Westport)* **1980**, *10*, 303–322. [CrossRef]
77. Robinson, T.; Marwit, S.J. An investigation of the relationship of personality, coping, and grief intensity among bereaved mothers. *Death Stud.* **2006**, *30*, 677–696. [CrossRef] [PubMed]
78. Boelen, P.A. Optimism in prolonged grief and depression following loss: A three-wave longitudinal study. *Psychiatry Res.* **2015**, *227*, 313–317. [CrossRef] [PubMed]
79. Moskowitz, J.T.; Folkman, S.; Acree, M. Do positive psychological states shed light on recovery from bereavement? Findings from a 3-year longitudinal study. *Death Stud.* **2003**, *27*, 471–500. [CrossRef] [PubMed]
80. Bonanno, G.A.; Burton, C.L. Regulatory flexibility: An individual differences perspective on coping and emotion regulation. *Perspect. Psychol. Sci.* **2013**, *8*, 591–612. [CrossRef] [PubMed]
81. Cacciatore, J.; Flint, M. ATTEND: Toward a mindfulness-based bereavement care model. *Death Stud.* **2012**, *36*, 61–82. [CrossRef] [PubMed]
82. Boyraz, G.; Horne, S.G.; Sayger, T.V. Finding meaning in loss: The mediating role of social support between personality and two construals of meaning. *Death Stud.* **2012**, *36*, 519–540. [CrossRef] [PubMed]
83. Baddeley, J.L.; Singer, J.A. Telling losses: Personality correlates and functions of bereavement narratives. *J. Res. Personal.* **2008**, *42*, 421–438. [CrossRef]
84. Wijngaards-de Meij, L.; Stroebe, M.; Schut, H.; Stroebe, W.; Van den Bout, J.; Van der Heijden, P.; Dijkstra, I. Neuroticism and attachment insecurity as predictors of bereavement outcome. *J. Res. Personal.* **2007**, *41*, 498–505. [CrossRef]
85. Scheier, M.F.; Carver, C.S. Optimism, coping, and health: Assessment and implications of generalized outcome expectancies. *Health Psychol.* **1985**, *4*, 219–247. [CrossRef] [PubMed]
86. Nolen-Hoeksema, S.; Larson, J. *Coping with Loss*; Lawrence Erlbaum Associates, Inc.: Mahwah, NJ, USA, 1999.
87. Carver, C.S.; Scheier, M.F.; Segerstrom, S.C. Optimism. *Clin. Psychol. Rev.* **2010**, *30*, 879–889. [CrossRef] [PubMed]
88. Avvenuti, G.; Baiardini, I.; Giardini, A. Optimism's explicative role for chronic diseases. *Front. Psychol.* **2016**, *7*, 295. [CrossRef] [PubMed]
89. Nes, L.S.; Segerstrom, S.C. Dispositional optimism and coping: A meta-analytic review. *Personal. Soc. Psychol. Rev.* **2006**, *10*, 235–251. [CrossRef] [PubMed]
90. Brissette, I.; Scheier, M.F.; Carver, C.S. The role of optimism in social network development, coping, and psychological adjustment during a life transition. *J. Personal. Soc. Psychol.* **2002**, *82*, 102–111. [CrossRef] [PubMed]
91. Tanaka, E.; Sakamoto, S.; Ono, Y.; Fujihara, S.; Kitamura, T. Hopelessness in a community population: Factorial structure and psychosocial correlates. *J. Soc. Psychol.* **1998**, *138*, 581–590. [CrossRef] [PubMed]
92. Folkman, S. The case for positive emotions in the stress process. *Anxiety Stress Coping* **2008**, *21*, 3–14. [CrossRef] [PubMed]
93. McCracken, L.M.; Morley, S. The psychological flexibility model: A basis for integration and progress in psychological approaches to chronic pain management. *J. Pain* **2014**, *15*, 221–234. [CrossRef] [PubMed]

94. Kashdan, T.B.; Rottenberg, J. Psychological flexibility as a fundamental aspect of health. *Clin. Psychol. Rev.* **2010**, *30*, 865–878. [CrossRef] [PubMed]
95. Stroebe, M.; Schut, H. The dual process model of coping with bereavement: Rationale and description. *Death Stud.* **1999**, *23*, 197–224. [PubMed]
96. Gupta, S.; Bonanno, G.A. Complicated grief and deficits in emotional expressive flexibility. *J. Abnorm. Psychol.* **2011**, *120*, 635–643. [CrossRef] [PubMed]
97. Brown, K.W.; Ryan, R.M. The benefits of being present: Mindfulness and its role in psychological well-being. *J. Personal. Soc. Psychol.* **2003**, *84*, 822–848. [CrossRef] [PubMed]
98. Cacciatore, J.; Thieleman, K.; Osborn, J.; Orlowski, K. Of the soul and suffering: Mindfulness-based interventions and bereavement. *Clin. Soc. Work J.* **2014**, *42*, 269–281. [CrossRef]
99. Kearney, J.A.; Byrne, M.W. Understanding parental behavior in pediatric palliative care: Attachment theory as a paradigm. *Palliat. Support. Care* **2015**, *13*, 1559–1568. [CrossRef] [PubMed]
100. Berant, E.; Mikulincer, M.; Florian, V. The association of mothers' attachment style and their psychological reactions to the diagnosis of infant's congenital heart disease. *J. Soc. Clin. Psychol.* **2001**, *20*, 208–232. [CrossRef]
101. Berant, E.; Mikulincer, M.; Florian, V. Attachment style and mental health: A 1-year follow-up study of mothers of infants with congenital heart disease. *Personal. Soc. Psychol. Bull.* **2001**, *27*, 956–968. [CrossRef]
102. Berant, E.; Mikulincer, M.; Shaver, P.R. Mothers' attachment style, their mental health, and their children's emotional vulnerabilities: A 7-year study of children with congenital heart disease. *J. Personal.* **2008**, *76*, 31–66. [CrossRef] [PubMed]
103. Meert, K.L.; Donaldson, A.E.; Newth, C.J.; Harrison, R.; Berger, J.; Zimmerman, J.; Anand, K.; Carcillo, J.; Dean, J.M.; Willson, D.F. Complicated grief and associated risk factors among parents following a child's death in the pediatric intensive care unit. *Arch. Pediatr. Adolesc. Med.* **2010**, *164*, 1045–1051. [CrossRef] [PubMed]
104. Mikulincer, M.; Shaver, P. Mental representations and attachment security. In *Interpersonal Cognition*; Guilford Press: New York, NY, USA, 2005; pp. 233–266.
105. Mikulincer, M.; Shaver, P.R. *Attachment in Adulthood: Structure, Dynamics, and Change*; Guilford Press: New York, NY, USA, 2007.
106. Field, N.P.; Gao, B.; Paderna, L. Continuing bonds in bereavement: An attachment theory based perspective. *Death Stud.* **2005**, *29*, 277–299. [CrossRef] [PubMed]
107. Bowlby, E.J.M. *Attachment and Loss: Sadness and Depression*; Basic Books: New York, NY, USA, 1980; Volume 3.
108. Stroebe, M. Gender differences in adjustment to bereavement: An empirical and theoretical review. *Rev. Gen. Psychol.* **2001**, *5*, 62–83. [CrossRef]
109. Lang, A.; Gottlieb, L. Parental grief reactions and marital intimacy following infant death. *Death Stud.* **1993**, *17*, 233–255. [CrossRef]
110. Alam, R.; Barrera, M.; D'Agostino, N.; Nicholas, D.B.; Schneiderman, G. Bereavement experiences of mothers and fathers over time after the death of a child due to cancer. *Death Stud.* **2012**, *36*, 1–22. [CrossRef] [PubMed]
111. Lobb, E.A.; Kristjanson, L.J.; Aoun, S.M.; Monterosso, L.; Halkett, G.K.; Davies, A. Predictors of complicated grief: A systematic review of empirical studies. *Death Stud.* **2010**, *34*, 673–698. [CrossRef] [PubMed]
112. Pilling, J.; Thege, B.K.; Demetrovics, Z.; Kopp, M.S. Alcohol use in the first three years of bereavement: A national representative survey. *Subst. Abuse Treat. Prev. Policy* **2012**, *7*, 3. [CrossRef] [PubMed]
113. Pinquart, M.; Sörensen, S. Differences between caregivers and noncaregivers in psychological health and physical health: A meta-analysis. *Psychol. Aging* **2003**, *18*, 250–267. [CrossRef] [PubMed]
114. Bunch, J. Recent bereavement in relation to suicide. *J. Psychosom. Res.* **1972**, *16*, 361–366. [CrossRef]
115. Folkman, S. Revised coping theory and the process of bereavement. In *Handbook of Bereavement Research: Consequences, Coping, and Care*; Stroebe, M.S., Hansson, R.O., Stroebe, W., Schut, H., Eds.; American Psychological Association: Washington, DC, USA, 2001; pp. 563–584.
116. Van der Houwen, K.; Stroebe, M.; Schut, H.; Stroebe, W.; Van den Bout, J. Mediating processes in bereavement: The role of rumination, threatening grief interpretations, and deliberate grief avoidance. *Soc. Sci. Med.* **2010**, *71*, 1669–1676. [CrossRef] [PubMed]
117. Brammer, L.M.; Abrego, P.J. Intervention strategies for coping with transitions. *J. Couns. Psychol.* **1981**, *9*, 19–36. [CrossRef]

118. Sohl, S.J.; Moyer, A. Refining the conceptualization of a future-oriented self-regulatory behavior: Proactive coping. *Personal. Individ. Differ.* **2009**, *47*, 139–144. [CrossRef] [PubMed]
119. Aspinwall, L.G. Future-oriented thinking, proactive coping, and the management of potential threats to health and well-being. In *The Oxford Handbook of Stress, Health and Coping*; Folkman, S., Nathan, P.E., Eds.; Oxford University Press: Oxford, UK, 2011; pp. 334–365.
120. Littlewood, J.L.; Cramer, D.; Hoekstra, J.; Humphrey, G. Gender differences in parental coping following their child's death. *Br. J. Guid. Couns.* **1991**, *19*, 139–148. [CrossRef]
121. Caserta, M.S.; Lund, D.A. Toward the development of an Inventory of Daily Widowed Life (IDWL): Guided by the dual process model of coping with bereavement. *Death Stud.* **2007**, *31*, 505–535. [CrossRef] [PubMed]
122. Stroebe, M.S.; Schut, H. The dual process model of coping and bereavement: Overview and update. *Grief Matters* **2008**, *11*, 4.
123. Wijngaards-de Meij, L.; Stroebe, M.; Schut, H.; Stroebe, W.; Bout, J.; Heijden, P.G.; Dijkstra, I. Parents grieving the loss of their child: Interdependence in coping. *Br. J. Clin. Psychol.* **2008**, *47*, 31–42. [CrossRef] [PubMed]
124. Burke, K.; Muscara, F.; McCarthy, M.; Dimovski, A.; Hearps, S.; Anderson, V.; Walser, R. Adapting acceptance and commitment therapy for parents of children with life-threatening illness: Pilot study. *Fam. Syst. Health* **2014**, *32*, 122–127. [CrossRef] [PubMed]
125. Thompson, R.W.; Arnkoff, D.B.; Glass, C.R. Conceptualizing mindfulness and acceptance as components of psychological resilience to trauma. *Trauma Violence Abuse* **2011**, *12*, 220–235. [CrossRef] [PubMed]
126. Thieleman, K.; Cacciatore, J.; Hill, P.W. Traumatic bereavement and mindfulness: A preliminary study of mental health outcomes using the ATTEND Model. *Clin. Soc. Work J.* **2014**, *42*, 260–268. [CrossRef]
127. Park, C.L. Making sense of the meaning literature: an integrative review of meaning making and its effects on adjustment to stressful life events. *Psychol. Bull.* **2010**, *136*, 257–301. [CrossRef] [PubMed]
128. Keesee, N.J.; Currier, J.M.; Neimeyer, R.A. Predictors of grief following the death of one's child: The contribution of finding meaning. *J. Clin. Psychol.* **2008**, *64*, 1145–1163. [CrossRef] [PubMed]
129. Davis, C.G.; Nolen-Hoeksema, S.; Larson, J. Making sense of loss and benefiting from the experience: Two construals of meaning. *J. Personal. Soc. Psychol.* **1998**, *75*, 561–574. [CrossRef] [PubMed]
130. Lichtenthal, W.G.; Neimeyer, R.A.; Currier, J.M.; Roberts, K.; Jordan, N. Cause of death and the quest for meaning after the loss of a child. *Death Stud.* **2013**, *37*, 311–342. [CrossRef] [PubMed]
131. Nolen-Hoeksema, S. Ruminative coping and adjustment to bereavement. In *Handbook of Bereavement Research: Consequences, Coping, and Care*; Stroebe, M.S., Hansson, R.O., Stroebe, W., Schut, H., Eds.; American Psychological Association: Washington, DC, USA, 2001.
132. Eisma, M.C.; Stroebe, M.S.; Schut, H.A.; Stroebe, W.; Boelen, P.A.; Van den Bout, J. Avoidance processes mediate the relationship between rumination and symptoms of complicated grief and depression following loss. *J. Abnorm. Psychol.* **2013**, *122*, 961–970. [CrossRef] [PubMed]
133. Nolen-Hoeksema, S.; Wisco, B.E.; Lyubomirsky, S. Rethinking rumination. *Perspect. Psychol. Sci.* **2008**, *3*, 400–424. [CrossRef] [PubMed]
134. Chan, C.L.; Chow, A.Y.; Ho, S.M.; Tsui, Y.K.; Tin, A.F.; Koo, B.W.; Koo, E.W. The experience of Chinese bereaved persons: A preliminary study of meaning making and continuing bonds. *Death Stud.* **2005**, *29*, 923–947. [CrossRef] [PubMed]
135. Stroebe, M.; Stroebe, W.; Schut, H. Bereavement research: Methodological issues and ethical concerns. *Palliat. Med.* **2003**, *17*, 235–240. [CrossRef] [PubMed]
136. Stroebe, M.S.; Stroebe, W. Who participates in bereavement research? A review and empirical study. *Omega (Westport)* **1990**, *20*, 1–29. [CrossRef]
137. Crocker, J.C.; Beecham, E.; Kelly, P.; Dinsdale, A.P.; Hemsley, J.; Jones, L.; Bluebond-Langner, M. Inviting parents to take part in paediatric palliative care research: a mixed-methods examination of selection bias. *Palliat. Med.* **2015**, *29*, 231–240. [CrossRef] [PubMed]
138. Bonnano, G.; Boerner, K.; Wortman, C.B. Trajectories of grieving. In *Handbook of Bereavement Research and Practice: Advances in Theory and Intervention*; Stroebe, M.S., Hansson, R.O., Schut, H., Stroebe, W., Eds.; American Psychological Association: Washington, DC, USA, 2008.
139. Endo, K.; Yonemoto, N.; Yamada, M. Interventions for bereaved parents following a child's death: A systematic review. *Palliat. Med.* **2015**, *29*, 590–604. [CrossRef] [PubMed]

140. Neimeyer, R.A.; Currier, J.M. Bereavement interventions: Present status and future horizons. *Grief Matters* **2008**, *11*, 18–22.
141. Currier, J.M.; Neimeyer, R.A.; Berman, J.S. The effectiveness of psychotherapeutic interventions for bereaved persons: A comprehensive quantitative review. *Psychol. Bull.* **2008**, *134*, 648–661. [CrossRef] [PubMed]

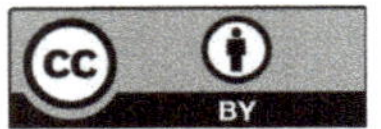

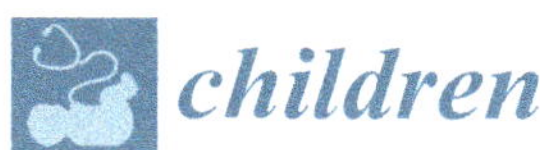

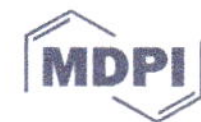

Brief Report

Trending Longitudinal Agreement between Parent and Child Perceptions of Quality of Life for Pediatric Palliative Care Patients

Meaghann S. Weaver [1,*], Cheryl Darnall [1], Sue Bace [1], Catherine Vail [1], Andrew MacFadyen [1] and Christopher Wichman [2]

1. Children's Hospital and Medical Center Omaha, Division of Palliative Care, 8200 Dodge Street, Omaha, NE 68114, USA; meahcloud@yahoo.com (C.D.); sbace@childrensomaha.org (S.B.); cvail@childrensomaha.org (C.V.); amacfadyen@childrensomaha.org (A.M.)
2. University of Nebraska Medical Center, Department of Biostatistics, Omaha, NE 68198, USA; Wichmchristopher.wichman@unmc.edu

* Correspondence: MeWeaver@childrensomaha.org

Academic Editor: Stefan J. Friedrichsdorf
Received: 27 April 2017; Accepted: 28 July 2017; Published: 1 August 2017

Abstract: Pediatric palliative care studies often rely on proxy-reported instead of direct child-reported quality of life metrics. The purpose of this study was to longitudinally evaluate quality of life for pediatric patients receiving palliative care consultations and to compare patient-reported quality of life with parent perception of the child's quality of life across wellness domains. The 23-item PedsQL™ V4.0 Measurement Model was utilized for ten child and parent dyads at time of initial palliative care consultation, Month 6, and Month 12 to assess for physical, emotional, social, and cognitive dimensions of quality of life as reported independently by the child and by the parent for the child. Findings were analyzed using Bland–Altman plots to compare observed differences to limits of agreement. This study revealed overall consistency between parent- and child-reported quality of life across domains. Physical health was noted to be in closest agreement. At the time of initial palliative care consult, children collectively scored their social quality of life higher than parental perception of the child's social quality of life; whereas, emotional and cognitive quality of life domains were scored lower by children than by the parental report. At the one year survey time point, the physical, emotional, and social domains trended toward more positive patient perception than proxy perception with congruence between quality of life scores for the cognitive domain. Findings reveal the importance of eliciting a child report in addition to a parent report when measuring and longitudinally trending perceptions on quality of life.

Keywords: quality of life; pediatric palliative care; patient reported outcomes

---

1. Introduction

The vast majority of symptom burden and quality of life metrics from children receiving palliative care are obtained from a proxy report rather than the voice of the child. In a systematic review of research papers measuring outcomes for children with cancer, only four out of 26 papers (15.4%) included actual patient-reported outcomes while six (23.1%) included parent-reported outcomes, and five (19.2%) included nursing reported outcomes [1]. In another review of pediatric palliative care peer-reviewed publications specific to child outcomes, only nine out of 72 (13%) papers provided direct patient perspectives [2]. Reasons for exclusion of the child's voice in quality of life (QOL) reporting includes that children may be unwilling or unable to respond for themselves due to developmental stage or illness impact or because of cognitive impairment. The reason may also be that providers and researchers are not routinely pursuing direct child-reported metrics as part of the gold standard approach to care and research [3]. Studies coordinating caregiver and pediatric child quality of life metrics in pediatric palliative care are meaningful but few [4].

It cannot be assumed that clinician or even parent report accurately reflects the burden of illness or treatments as perceived by the child. A growing body of adult literature reminds clinicians that the clinician report of symptoms relevant to overall quality of life systematically under-reports both the prevalence and the severity of these symptoms [5,6]. Comparisons of a child report versus a parental proxy report of symptoms has revealed varied levels of agreement with higher correlation for observable symptoms such as nausea (the observation being presumed change in eating pattern or even emesis) and pain (the observation being activity level or nonverbal/verbal signs of discomfort) and poorer level agreement for less observable symptom profiles [7,8]. Agreement between the child report and parent report of symptom burden varies with child age, with poorer agreement for adolescent patients than for younger children [9,10]. Agreement is further confounded by a parent's personal physical and mental health status impacting parental perception of his/her own child's quality of life [11].

The translation of symptom burden into perceived quality of life warrants a direct patient report with supplemental, informative parental insight to place the child's experience into the family interpretation of the child's experience.

2. Methods

2.1. Patients

This prospective study followed a total of ten patients (four males and six females) aged 5 years through 18 years (mean 12.4 years) from time of initial palliative care consultation through one full year of palliative care integrated service. Only ten out of 87 total consulted patients were able to provide patient voice due to medical fragility (neuro-cognitive participatory or development level). Of these ten participants, three utilized the 5–7-year-old tool; three used the 8–12-year old tool; and four completed the 13–18-year old tool based on age at time of study participation. Primary diagnoses included four children with neurodegenerative conditions, three with cardiac conditions, two with pulmonary conditions, and one with a genetic condition. Two families completed the quality of life scales in Spanish, all others were completed in English.

2.2. Study Design

This study was approved as a Quality Improvement Process Study by the Institutional Review Board. Child and parent demographic information was collected at baseline. QOL questionnaires were administered at baseline (defined as time of initial palliative care consultation), Month 6, and Month 12 of integrated palliative care services. Integrated palliative care services meant longitudinal inclusion of a palliative care team and palliative care case management with established needs assessment/goals of care guiding interventions across outpatient and inpatient medical settings. The questionnaire was completed separately by each participating child and parent during scheduled palliative care visits either as an inpatient or outpatient. Each child had the option for the questionnaire items to be read out loud if the child preferred audible scale administration.

2.3. Measures

Quality of life was assessed using the Pediatric Quality of Life Inventory (PedsQL™ Copyright © 1998 JW Varni, Ph.D. All rights reserved), a 23-item Likert-type scale measuring: physical, social, cognitive, and emotional domains [12]. The validated pediatric scale has parallel instruments for child and parent administration [13]. The Likert scale scores are converted to a 0-, 25-, 50-, and 100-point scale, with higher scores reflecting a higher perceived quality of life for that domain.

2.4. Statistical Analysis for Parent–Child Quality of Life Agreement

Bland–Altman plots and absolute agreement (scatter) plots were used to assess the agreement between parent and child when scoring the QOL questionnaire on the Physical, Social, Cognitive, and Emotional Scales [14]. Bland-Altman plots are used to compare observed differences to limits of agreement which are based on the mean of all differences +/− $z_{1-\alpha/2}$ times the standard deviation of the differences. The Bland–Altman plot offers visual appeal since the solid black horizontal line represents the average of the difference between scores across all child–parent combinations. This graphical format enables convenient visualization of collective analyses of quality of life agreement between patient–proxy reports (Figure 1). The outlier marks then revealed moments in which a parent or child differed significantly in perception of quality of life.

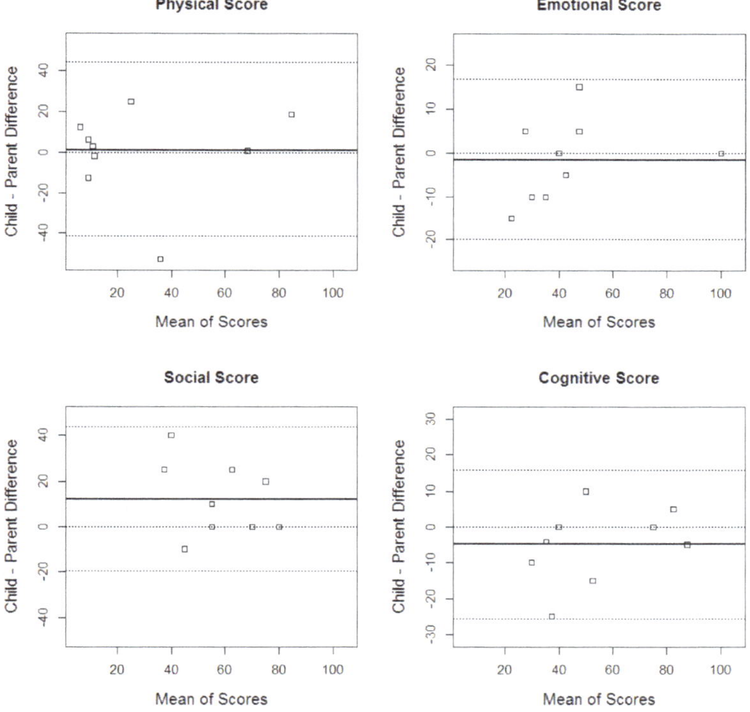

Figure 1. Bland–Altman agreement plots for the four domains at baseline. The solid black line represents the mean of the child–parent differences. The two extreme dotted gray lines mark the upper and lower agreement boundaries.

3. Results

At baseline, Month 6, and Month 12 there were 10, 6, and 5 parent–child pairings that scored the QOL assessment, respectively. Three of these parent–child pairings scored the assessment at all three time points. Reason for loss of dyad-based date was death in four cases and loss of ability for child to interact in the other cases (intubated, sedate, or decline in conversational ability).

Figure 1 reveals overall good agreement between parent and child across domains at time of initial palliative care consultation. Agreement was judged as good based on 10 out of 10 child–parent differences lying within the agreement boundaries for the emotional, social and cognitive domains and 9 out of 10 lying within the agreement boundaries for the physical domain. For physical health quality of life domains, the parent and child report on quality of life were not far off zero at baseline (the average difference between child and parent scores was 1.2, revealing agreement between patient and proxy report). However, for the social domain the child tended to score himself/herself higher than parental perception of social quality of life by an average of 12.2. For emotional domain and cognitive interaction, the children collectively scored themselves lower than parental perception of quality of life in these domains, 1.7 and 4.9 on average, respectively.

At six months, the parent–child assessment of physical and social quality of life measures were consistent between parent–child with children still scoring their own emotional and cognitive domains lower than the parental report. At a year, the children began to score their physical, emotional, and social domains collectively higher than parental perception.

4. Discussion

Inquiring into quality of life fosters insight into the effect of disease trajectory on a child and overall perception of lived experience. This novel study serves as a pilot model of feasibility which could next be utilized in an earlier palliative integration model for larger and longer data points. Although there is an increasing call for pediatric providers to foster patient voice, pediatric care teams often grade symptoms and report quality of life or for the parent to report such as proxy. The graded symptoms which lead to patient-interpretation of quality of life often include subjective symptoms such as nausea, dyspnea, fatigue, insomnia, anxiety, depression, and pain. Eliciting a patient report not just for symptom report but for collective translation into perceived quality of life fosters the overall child perception of lived experience.

The finding that parents and children had the closest agreement in physical quality of life assessment may hint that the physical symptomatology is more objectively measured based on observed behavior changes or biomedical changes. Parent trend toward over-elevating a child's emotional and cognitive wellness at time of diagnosis may imply that children are experiencing more psychosocial and mental toll than is readily recognized within families. This speaks to opportunity for palliative care teams to proactively screen for total pain dimensions and not just physical evaluations in pediatric palliative care intake.

The finding that children viewed their social wellness as higher than parental perception may be a reflection of generational differences regarding the perceived relational aspects of social media or peer support. We observe many pre-teens and adolescent children who text or video-engage with peers as still feeling socially supported/connected with these friendships, while parents may perceive less in-person engagement in playdates as social alienation.

We were fascinated to note the trend of decreased agreement between child–parent quality of life report over time with children trending toward self-reporting higher total quality of life than parent perception. This may be an area of future inquiry, particularly to study whether ego-resiliency may help patients adapt to the changes associated with the illness [15]. This raises thoughts as to how this trend may differ for patients who are not followed by a palliative care team.

A limitation of the study is the lack of direct questioning on spiritual dimensions of wellness in the instrument, as we recognize that spirituality and sense of meaning weigh heavily on quality of life perceptions. Our study was further limited by small sample size, although the progressive morbidity due to disease progression (loosing ability to self-report) and eventual mortality are inevitable in our study sampling. Loss of participants longitudinally is a reality when caring for a pediatric palliative care population toward natural end of life. While it is possible to monitor scores over twelve months, the large reduction in the number of patients who were able to complete quality of life scores represents a reality of our patient population.

Our clinical team adapts this plot approach to guide our understanding of collective quality of life trends for children receiving palliative care consultations. This plot approach enables monitoring for congruence or discongruence between child and proxy perspectives. Quality of life metrics foster a meaningful opportunity to honor patient voice, while also attending to family interpretation of child experience.

5. Disclosures

This research did not receive any specific grant from funding agencies in the public, commercial, or not-for-profit sectors.

Acknowledgments: The study team wishes to thank Gregory Snyder, Sara Woodworth, and the Hand in Hand Team at Children's Hospital and Medical Center in Omaha, Nebraska. Gratitude to participating patients and families. We recognize Mapi Research Trust, Lyon, France (https://eprovide.mapi-trust.org and www.pedsql.org) for permission to use the study scales.

Author Contributions: CD, SB, and AM conceived and designed the experiments; CD, SB, AM performed the experiments; MW and CW analyzed the data; CV contributed analysis perspective; MW wrote the paper.

Conflicts of Interest: The authors declare no conflict of interest.

References

1. Hinds, P.S.; Brandon, J.; Allen, C. Patient-reported outcomes in end-of-life research in pediatric oncology. *J. Pediatr. Psychol.* **2007**, *32*, 1079–1088. [CrossRef] [PubMed]
2. Weaver, M.S.; Heinze, K.E.; Bell, C.J.; Heinze, K.E.; Bell, C.J.; Wiener, L.; Garee, A.M.; Kelly, K.P.; Casey, R.L.; Watson, A.; et al. Establishing psychosocial palliative care standards for children and adolescents with cancer and their families: An integrative review. *Palliat. Med.* **2016**, *30*, 212–223. [CrossRef] [PubMed]
3. Cremeens, J.; Eiser, C.; Blades, M. Factors influencing agreement between child self-report and parent proxy-reports on the Pediatric Quality of life Inventory 4.0 (PedsQL™) generic core scales. *Health Qual. Life Outcomes* **2006**, *30*, 58. [CrossRef] [PubMed]
4. Rosenberg, A.R.; Oreliana, L.; Ullrich, C.; Kang, T.; Geyer, J.R.; Feudtner, C.; Dussel, V.; Wolfe, J. Quality of life in children with advanced cancer: A Report from the PediQUEST Study. *J. Pain Symptom Manag.* **2016**, *52*, 243–253. [CrossRef] [PubMed]
5. Fromme, E.K.; Eilers, K.M.; Mori, M.; Hsieh, Y.C.; Beer, T.M. How accurate is clinician reporting of chemotherapy adverse effects? A comparison with patient-reported symptoms from the Quality-of-Life Questionnaire C30. *J. Clin. Oncol.* **2004**, *22*, 3485–3490. [CrossRef] [PubMed]
6. Basch, E. The missing voice of patients in drug-safety reporting. *N. Engl. J. Med.* **2010**, *362*, 865–869. [CrossRef] [PubMed]
7. Eiser, C.; Morse, R. Can parents rate their child's health-related quality of life? Results of a systematic review. *Qual. Life Res.* **2001**, *10*, 347–357. [CrossRef] [PubMed]
8. Collins, J.J.; Devine, T.D.; Dick, G.S.; Johnson, E.A.; Kilham, H.A.; Pinkerton, C.R.; Stevens, M.M.; Thaler, H.T.; Portenoy, R.K. The measurement of symptoms in young children with cancer: The validation of the Memorial Symptom Assessment Scale in children aged 7–12. *J. Pain Symptom Manag.* **2002**, *23*, 10–16. [CrossRef]
9. Chang, P.C.; Yeh, C.H. Agreement between child self-report and parent proxy-report to evaluate quality of life in children with cancer. *Psycho-Oncology* **2005**, *14*, 125–134. [CrossRef] [PubMed]
10. Waters, E.; Stewart-Brown, S.; Fitzpatrick, R. Agreement between adolescent self-report and parent reports of health and well-being: Results of an epidemiological study. *Child Care Health Dev.* **2003**, *29*, 501–509. [CrossRef] [PubMed]
11. Panepinto, J.A.; Hoffmann, R.G.; Pajewski, N.M. The effect of parental mental health on proxy reports of health-related qualify of life in children with sickle cell disease. *Pediatr. Blood Cancer* **2010**, *55*, 714–721. [CrossRef] [PubMed]
12. Varni, J.W.; Seid, M.; Rode, C.A. The PedsQL™: Measurement Model for the Pediatric Quality of Life Inventory. *Med. Care* **1999**, *37*, 126–139. [CrossRef] [PubMed]
13. Varni, J.W.; Burwinkle, T.M.; Seid, M.; Skarr, D. The PedsQL™ 4.0 as a pediatric population health measure: Feasibility, reliability, and validity. *Ambul. Pediatr.* **2003**, *3*, 329–341. [CrossRef]

14. Bland, J.M.; Altman, D.G. Measuring agreement in method of comparison studies. *Stat. Methods Med. Res.* **1999**, *8*, 135–160. [CrossRef] [PubMed]
15. Mandrell, B.; Baker, J.; Levine, D.; Gattuso, J.; West, N.; Sykes, A.; Gajjar, A.; Broniscer, A. Children with minimal chance for cure: Parent proxy of the child's health-related quality of life and the effect on parental physical and mental health during treatment. *J. Neurooncol.* **2016**, *129*, 373–381. [CrossRef] [PubMed]

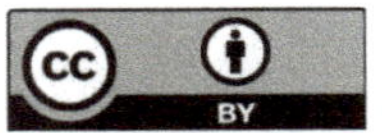

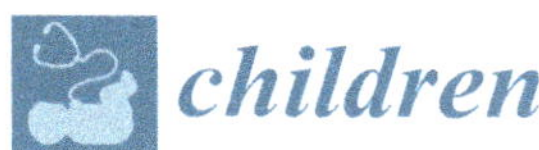
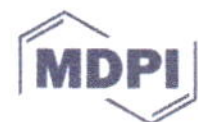

Review

Enhancing Pediatric Palliative Care for Latino Children and Their Families: A Review of the Literature and Recommendations for Research and Practice in the United States

Sara Muñoz-Blanco [1], Jessica C. Raisanen [2], Pamela K. Donohue [1,3] and Renee D. Boss [1,2,*]

1 Department of Pediatrics, Johns Hopkins University School of Medicine, Baltimore, MD 21205, USA; smunozb1@jhmi.edu (S.M.-B.); pdonohue@jhmi.edu (P.K.D.)
2 Clinical Ethics, Johns Hopkins Berman Institute of Bioethics, Baltimore, MD 21205, USA; jraisan1@jhu.edu
3 Department of Population, Family and Reproductive Health, Johns Hopkins Bloomberg School of Public Health, Baltimore, MD 21205, USA
* Correspondence: rboss1@jhmi.edu; Tel.: +1-410-614-5635

Received: 17 November 2017; Accepted: 20 December 2017; Published: 22 December 2017

Abstract: As the demand for pediatric palliative care (PC) increases, data suggest that Latino children are less likely to receive services than non-Latino children. Evidence on how to best provide PC to Latino children is sparse. We conducted a narrative review of literature related to PC for Latino children and their families in the United States. In the United States, Latinos face multiple barriers that affect their receipt of PC, including poverty, lack of access to health insurance, language barriers, discrimination, and cultural differences. Pediatric PC research and clinical initiatives that target the needs of Latino families are sparse, underfunded, but essential. Education of providers on Latino cultural values is necessary. Additionally, advocacy efforts with a focus on equitable care and policy reform are essential to improving the health of this vulnerable population.

Keywords: pediatric palliative care; Latino health; chronic illness; children with medical complexity

---

1. Introduction

Medical advancements and technology have decreased the number of deaths for medically fragile children over time [1–3]. With the increased life expectancy of this population, the demand for pediatric palliative care (PC) and end-of-life (EOL) care is also on the rise. In the United States, pediatric PC services are rapidly developing with the goal of improving quality of life for children with serious illness and their families [4]. However, research exposes disparities in pediatric PC use in the US by race/ethnicity such that European Americans are more likely to use pediatric PC services than Latinos living in the US [5]. It has also been shown that Latino children incur lower expenditures in hospice care than non-Latino children suggesting that there may be delays in admission to care or persistent barriers to pediatric PC services for Latino families in the US [6]. For the purposes of this paper, we use the term "Latino" to represent people of all genders that emigrated to the United States from Latin America and/or have strong cultural ties to this region. Individuals within this population might use other labels such as Latino/a, Latina, Latinx, Latin American, and Hispanic to identify their ethnicity. Furthermore, data suggest that minority pediatric cancer patients receive more intensive care at the EOL and are more likely to die in the hospital [7]. This is especially concerning given the growing body of work suggesting that early integration of pediatric PC services results in improved outcomes [8,9]. The objective of this paper is to review existing theory and research relating to PC services for Latino children and their families. We analyze the findings within current cultural and political contexts and present recommendations for future clinical care, research, and policy related to pediatric PC for Latino populations in the US.

2. Methods

We searched MEDLINE and Pubmed from inception to August 2017 for English language articles relevant to palliative care in the Latino population, particularly of pediatric patients using the terms: palliative care, Latino, Hispanic, pediatric palliative care. We then reviewed bibliographies of relevant studies to broaden our search. At a later stage, we also searched for references related to the current political context and its effect on the Latino US population. Two authors made the final selections and critically reviewed the existing data and models of care to identify current state of pediatric palliative care services for Latino children in the US.

3. Review of the Literature

3.1. Cultural Considerations Relevant to Palliative Care for Latino Pediatric Populations

Latino individuals make up the largest ethnic minority group in the US, and it is estimated that the number of Latino people will reach 28.6% of the total US population by the year 2060 [10]. People of Latino ethnicity are often treated as one monolithic group when interacting with health care systems and participating in research, but this perception of Latinos as homogeneous is flawed; many Latinos that reside in the US have roots in different countries and have different cultural backgrounds. Therefore, clinicians providing care to Latino patients in the US are likely to encounter an array of beliefs, values, and languages. However, shared experiences among Latinos, such as Spanish colonization of indigenous people in Latin America and the Caribbean [11], language [11,12], and ethnic discrimination [12] contribute to a sense of unity and community. These experiences foster cultural connections in ways that influence medical care. Here, we review common Latino cultural values surrounding family, gender roles, religion, spirituality, and decision-making preferences that may influence the availability, acceptability, and receipt of pediatric PC services within this ethnic group.

The role of the extended Latino family in making decisions for children with serious illness may be of particular importance. *Familismo*, a value of commitment and loyalty to immediate and extended family [11], is important for many Latinos [13–20]. Latino families are often tight-knit and large, which can lead to increased support and pooling of resources [16]. However, it can also complicate discussions around care, as it may lead to high levels of family involvement in decision-making [17]. It may be difficult to arrange large family meetings or reach consensus and understanding of the dying process [17], especially if there are language barriers between families and providers. This additional consultation with extended family may lead to delays in care [20,21].

Cultural perceptions of masculinity and femininity within the Latino community, often referred to as *machismo* and *marianismo/hembrismo*, may also shape care and decision-making for children with serious illness. Specifically, gender roles influence health-seeking behavior, medical decision-making, and caretaking such that mothers are often expected to act as caretakers and facilitators of health-seeking behavior. In contrast, fathers are often conditioned not to engage in daily caretaking for children, yet they are expected to lead decision-making surrounding health care, while mothers may feel obligated to obtain the father's permission to participate [14,16]. Gender norms within Latino populations may contribute to the reasons why some male family members deny engagement with PC services, because sharing feelings or concerns about illness may not be acceptable to some Latino men; they may prefer that their female family members be the focus of any support services and efforts [13].

While spirituality, religious community, and belief systems may be a source of support for families and children [22,23], it has also been suggested that spirituality and/or religiosity can create a barrier to care for some Latino families [17,24]. For example, strong religious beliefs, such as belief in miracles, may lead families to deny the dying process [13,17] or to view pain and suffering as a test of faith [24,25].

Religious values around the sanctity of human life and life as a gift from God may also influence EOL care in that for some Latinos, brain death may not be sufficient to justify withdrawal of life support [26]. Finally, *fatalismo*, or a belief in fate that one's future is predetermined, may also play a role in deterring Latinos from seeking care [14,16]. Abraído-Lanza et al. [27] posit that inaccessibility and discrimination within the healthcare system may reinforce feelings about *fatalismo* in Latino populations because of the lack of access to adequate and appropriate services. Structural barriers like racial bias, poverty, health insurance inaccessibility, and immigration barriers may reaffirm fatalistic ideology among people that experience oppression, undermining access to care even further [27]. These beliefs may influence some Latinos to postpone or refuse pediatric PC services. Multiple studies demonstrate that health care providers rarely engage patients in discussions of how religion/spirituality impact their health and health decisions [28,29]; this failure may have added significance for Latino families where reasons for delaying or refusing care may be misunderstood and inadequately addressed.

Respeto refers to the way Latinos interact with each other according to a person's age, gender, socioeconomic status, and authority [15,21]. This can be especially influential to the parent-physician relationship. For example, deference to authority figures may hinder families from questioning recommendations given by healthcare providers, even when those recommendations are incongruent with families' wishes, beliefs, and cultural norms [15,21,24]. Unfortunately, this can lead to misunderstandings and non-compliance with care [15]. In turn, providers are expected to behave according to Latino hierarchical norms by showing *respeto* and including extended family members in decision-making [15,21,24].

Because PC providers commonly engage with parents of children with serious illness in making medical decisions, it is also important to be aware of potential cultural variability in preferred decision-making roles. It is common for clinicians to assume that Latino patients prefer passive roles in medical decision-making [18,30–32]. However, there is little empirical data supporting this passive role preference. On the contrary, research suggests that people of Latino ethnicity living in the US may prefer more active or shared decision-making roles [21,33], especially when compared to Latinos living in Latin America [33]. Regardless of decisional-control preferences, Latino patients report that they want to know their diagnosis and prognosis [34]. Clinicians in the US are tasked with developing an understanding of how cultural contexts influence individual preferences for care within this heterogeneous population.

This previous research on the influence of cultural beliefs on health-seeking behavior lays a foundation for contextualizing the inequity observed in pediatric PC of Latino populations (Figure 1).

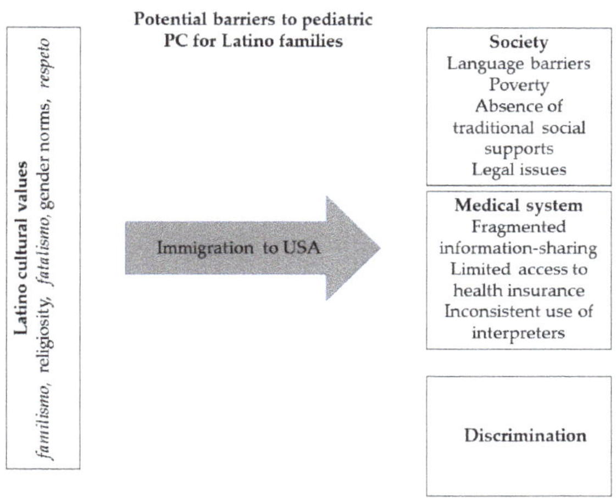

Figure 1. Mediators of the pediatric palliative care (PC) experience for latino families.

3.2. Insights from Latin America

Overall, PC is underdeveloped in Latin America [35–37]. Because of this, Latino patients in the US may have a limited understanding of the role of PC. However, PC services vary greatly from region to region in Latin America [35,38]. Therefore, understanding and acceptance of pediatric PC by Latino families in the US may also depend on where the family's roots are situated. Literature on pediatric PC in Latin America could inform care of Latino children in the US. However, research on best practices in PC is sparse and underfunded in Latin America [35,39,40], and while children and their families have unique PC needs, Latin American literature does not explicitly discuss considerations for PC in pediatric populations. International collaboration may be helpful to advance the research agenda in this topic and inform US practice. In the meantime, clinicians are encouraged to inquire families' understanding of and prior experience with pediatric PC.

3.3. Pediatric Palliative Care Experiences of Latino Families in the US

Over the past decade, literature focusing on PC in the US Latino population, which is not robust, has expanded to include the adult and pediatric PC and hospice experience, barriers to quality care, and suggestions for clinical care and research. There remain substantial gaps in the evidence base regarding PC for Latino children. In this section, we will review what is known about PC delivery in the US for Latino children and their families.

Poverty, absence of traditional social supports, and difficulties with the healthcare system are important mediators of PC experiences for Latino families [41]. Poverty can interfere with cultural practices around death and the bereavement process, as when some families are forced to opt for cremation [41]. Furthermore, the high cost of healthcare is an added source of burden for poor families [19,42]. In addition, geographic separation from family and traditional social supports can lead to feelings of isolation, as expected given the cultural value of *familismo* [16,41,43]. Despite this, however, Latino families also report a sense of trade-off that being in the US allows their child to receive the best care possible [41]. Lastly, some families also struggle with the complexity of the US healthcare system. For example, having multiple doctors, an experience different than in many countries in Latin America, can lead to fragmented information-sharing and thus affect communication and trust [41,44].

The importance of honest communication, direct communication by medical providers, emotional, financial, and physical strains associated with caregiving, and anxieties felt around time of the child's death are important mediators of the pediatric hospice experience [43]. Latino families, in particular, value the opportunity that hospice provides for their loved one to be home [42,43]. In addition, compared to English-speaking counterparts, Spanish-speaking families are less distressed by issues of symptom management at the end of life, report difficulties with doing bedside nursing care [43], and express desire to reduce caregiver burden [19], suggesting differences in the hospice experience between Latinos and other racial/ethnic groups.

Limited English proficiency is a barrier to quality pediatric PC [41,43]. Most Latino immigrants speak Spanish and only a fourth report fluency in English [45]. However, most medical care in the US is delivered in English. While there are health care providers in the US that report being fluent in Spanish, a majority of these providers are non-Latino and are not native Spanish speakers. Thus, even for these providers, communication may still be difficult [46]. The meaning of the word hospice, for example, is not easily translated into Spanish and patients often think that it refers to a place and not a service [17].

Language barriers, which often lead to miscommunication, can be a source of mistrust between Latino families and PC providers [19,44]. An uncertain understanding of their child's condition can leave these families feeling isolated, confused, and distrustful of the healthcare system [44]. Due to the inability to speak English, some families fear not being able to do what is needed to care for their child [43], others report difficulty with reaching out for help [41]. Some parents also report dissatisfaction with communication; for example, when interpreter-facilitated family meetings are held in the child's room and parents and children hear difficult news at the same time [43].

Furthermore, parents with limited English proficiency report feeling distressed when they do not understand the implications of the information they receive, which leads to dissatisfaction with care and long-term psychosocial stress [47]. This can be especially detrimental when discussing EOL issues.

Discrimination based on race/ethnicity remains a problem in US health care systems across a broad range of care sites and is more difficult to address than the language barriers [19,41,48]. Discrimination has also been reported in the delivery of PC services. Davies et al reported that Mexican-American families felt discriminated against based on race, language, socio-economic status, and appearance [48]. They also reported feeling confused, angry, and hurt by these experiences. However, few families spoke up about their concerns with care; most assumed a passive/submissive role, as dictated by cultural norms of *respeto* of authority figures, or for fear of recrimination against their child [48].

Documented disparities in rates of advance directives for pediatric Latino patients are sparse. However, research among adult patients may have implications for families of children with serious illness. In a study of older Latino adults, 84% reported that they would want comfort-focused care if seriously ill, a proportion that contradicts the high rates of aggressive treatments at the EOL observed in this population. However, over three quarters of these participants reported that they did not have an advanced care directive and almost half had not discussed their preferences with their family or doctor [18]. Kelley et al., argue that these missed opportunities put patients at risk of receiving aggressive and unwanted treatment at the EOL [18]. This could also be true for children. A study in which a majority of the participants were Latino parents found that 62% had never heard of advance directives and that 82% had never discussed advance directives. However, after being educated, 49% of parents expressed interest in creating an advance directive for their chronically ill child. Of note, Spanish-speaking Latino participants were less likely to have knowledge on advance directives than English-speaking participants [49]. Though there are global difficulties with expanding advance directives overall, health system policies which work to address these may still miss those patient populations—like Latino patients—that experience discrimination within the health care system or have difficulty communicating their desires with providers.

Barriers in access to health insurance for Latino children have historically presented issues for care [50–53]. Additionally, chronically ill children that are Latino have the lowest rates of insurance coverage when compared to chronically ill children of other ethnic or racial groups in the US [52,54]. While health care reform in the US, namely the Affordable Care Act (ACA), increased insurance rates across the board, Latinos still have the highest probability of being uninsured compared to White and African American populations [55]. Additionally, the recent challenges to the ACA, such as the Senate Tax Cuts and Jobs Act, may reverse initiatives directed at equity in health insurance access. These policy changes have implications for medically complex Latino children in that they may be underinsured, leading to decreased access to pediatric PC services.

Poverty and political turmoil have led many people from Latin America to migrate to the US or other areas of the world [21], and the vast majority of undocumented immigrants residing in the US are from Latin America [56]. These undocumented immigrants with life-limiting illness face additional barriers to care such as fear of deportation, lack of insurance, and limited access to services, including PC and hospice. While some children who are undocumented are able to access medical coverage due to state-based policies in a small number of states (i.e., California, New York, Illinois, Massachusetts, Washington, and the District of Columbia), in a majority of states, undocumented immigrants are unable to access health insurance through Medicaid, Medicare, or the Insurance Marketplace established by the ACA [57]. These restrictions contribute to many Latino people being denied access to necessary medical care, which some consider to be a violation of their human rights. Jaramillo and Hui describe the difficult experience of an undocumented young adult immigrant with advanced cancer at the EOL [42]. Language and cultural barriers, delayed diagnosis, limited social support, increased financial burden, limited access to EOL care, and fear of deportation are just a handful of issues that undocumented immigrants face that may impede care [42]; undocumented children with chronic illness and their families face these hardships as well. US anti-immigration legislation poses a threat to the health and well-being of many Latinos, including medically complex children and their families. For example, elimination of the Deferred Action for Childhood Arrivals (DACA) Program will leave some Latinos unable to work or continue their education in the US and at risk of deportation, which will likely increase poverty among this population, decrease educational attainment and employer-based health insurance coverage, and contribute to increasing inequity in access to pediatric PC services [52]. To our knowledge there are no studies that focus directly on the pediatric PC experience for immigrant, uninsured children in the US.

As illustrated in this review, the literature on the pediatric PC experience for Latino children and their families is sparse. The growing body of evidence on the delivery, experience, and gaps in PC drawn from the adult literature can serve as a starting point and guide for pediatric PC providers and researchers who serve Latino families. Absence of traditional social supports, language barriers, difficulties with navigating and understanding the US healthcare system, and discrimination are important mediators of the pediatric PC experience of Latino families, though this is likely just the tip of the iceberg.

4. Discussion

4.1. Improving Clinical Care

Latinos are often thought of and treated as one group in the US; however, the heterogeneity of this population cannot be ignored. Even though language is a common bond between Latino populations, culture, beliefs, and attitudes that shape their experience and understanding of pediatric PC may differ by country of origin.

4.1.1. Becoming Patient Advocates

Vulnerability of Latino patients framed by language barriers, access to healthcare, socioeconomic hardship, and cultural differences is accentuated in serious illness and at the EOL. Thus, providers are encouraged to become avid patient advocates when caring for Latino children. Close attention to socioeconomic particularities of each family is recommended. This includes being aware of competing agendas between hospital administration and patient discharge planning and outpatient care, increasingly important for those patients who are uninsured [58]. In addition, proactively but empathetically assessing the economic situation and home environment of a family can help determine the kind of care the family can provide at home [41]. This is particularly important when discussing medical technology with families, for example.

4.1.2. Bridging the Language Barrier

Language barriers have long been recognized as a limitation to receiving quality care. It is also important to recognize that language fluency does not equal cultural competency. Thus, it is best to use simple and clear language when discussing terminal illness issues and avoid using euphemisms that are likely to be lost in translation [24]. In addition, not using interpreters consistently has been perceived by parents as discriminatory [48], a cause of poor information-sharing, and lack of acknowledgement regarding their emotions and concerns [47]. Increasing access to interpretation services and increasing the number of native Spanish-speaking staff and providers will assist in bridging the communication gaps. Even among providers that are highly proficient and fluent in Spanish, it may still be best to use an interpreter. Children and relatives should not be used as interpreters, especially when discussing EOL care and decision making due to the sensitive nature of the conversation and confidentiality issues.

4.1.3. Cultural Humility

Cultural humility centered around common Latino cultural values and strategies on how to overcome language barriers should be a priority to everyone who provides pediatric PC to Latino children [15,47]. Employing universal strategies for communication (i.e., ask-tell-ask model or teach-back method); assessing acculturation with open-ended, respectful questions; and, practicing strategies for establishing trust (i.e., naming the emotion or asking about discrimination experiences) are also encouraged [16]. Latino cultural values need to be recognized, taught, and integrated into a culture-centered model of PC [15]. This model is a framework in which to weigh the influence of acculturation and ethnic identity on a Latino patient's and family's experience of PC. However, one must be conscious that given the variability in decisional-control and information-sharing preferences among Latinos, individual assessment of each patient and family is equally important.

4.1.4. Continuity of Care

The stratification of care characteristic of the US healthcare system can be confusing for some Latino families since in many Latin American countries, one physician is in charge of directing care and communicating with the family. As such, Latino families may not be familiar with a multi-disciplinary approach to care. Assigning a continuity provider, preferably one who speaks Spanish and has established rapport with the family, may help with trust building and comprehension of information [41,44].

4.2. Implications for Research

As highlighted in this narrative review, data on how to best provide quality pediatric PC to Latino children are scarce. We found two studies that focused on the experiences of Mexican American families with pediatric PC [41] and perceived discrimination during interaction with pediatric healthcare providers [48]. While these are pioneer studies, they have limited generalizability. One other study explored English- and Spanish-speaking families' perceptions of pediatric hospice [43]. Although exploratory in nature, and limited by a small sample size, the study provides insight on how language, and likely culture, can shape families' experience with hospice. Language is often the first perceived barrier to care. Thus, studying the barriers to consistent use of interpreters may help decrease communication gaps.

Palliative care services in Latin America vary by region. As such, Latino families' experience with PC can vary widely. Thus, educating Latino communities on PC, and developing evidence-based ways to do so, should be a primary goal of research. Community outreach programs [59] and media utilization, such as videos [60], specifically designed for pediatric PC are potential interventions to be studied. Likewise, culturally-competent patient navigators that address education and patient activation through home visits could serve to increase baseline knowledge of pediatric PC and facilitate care delivery [61].

Latino families often have socioeconomic realities that are different from those of white or black families [17,53,55,62]; these socioeconomic characteristics contribute to health inequity. Correspondingly, studies that explore Latino caregiver burden and search for ways in which allocation of pediatric PC resources can help ameliorate burden are also needed [43]. Lastly, more population-based studies are needed to explore potential causes for disparities in intensive care at the EOL for minority pediatric patients like those observed by Johnston et al. [7]. In particular, it will be important to elucidate if these disparities are due to healthcare system issues (i.e., access to PC) or to family preference/goals [7,63].

Pediatric PC research is limited in Latin America; financial and educational barriers hinder its development. Given the heterogeneity of the US immigrant Latino population, collaboration between US and Latin American researchers is imperative for the advancement of pediatric PC for Latino children. Limited resources and minimal expertise and training in research [37,40] are some reasons to advocate for international collaboration with developed countries. In addition, translating published literature to Spanish may help with dissemination of evidence in Latin America.

4.3. Policy, Advocacy and Education

Vulnerable populations, such as Latino children, depend on advocacy efforts from those who are passionate, as much as those who are in power. Advocacy can occur at many levels: individual patient, single institution, community, state, and federal. Current need is at all levels and providers are encouraged to take action.

Advocating for immigration reform that supports legal pathways to immigration and health care reform that expands health insurance coverage is important to improving access to PC for medically complex Latino children and decreasing inequity. While a small number of states have assisted undocumented immigrants in accessing health insurance, we are unaware of protections or allocation of funds to assist this population at the federal level.

Unfortunately, no official legislation exists to support parents in making advance medical directives. In the United States, at least one state, Maryland, mandates consideration of advance directives for hospitalized children through use of Medical Orders for Life-Sustaining Treatment (MOLST) [64]. This document, however, is not pediatric specific. Pediatric advanced care planning programs, nonetheless, can be successfully implemented [65]. In addition, data shows parents favor a MOLST for hospitalized children, though providers as well as parents recognize conversations about pediatric advance care planning are challenging and require good communication skills [66,67]. Communication training for providers and pediatric advance directive education for parents can help de-stigmatize conversations around advance care planning [65,66]. Furthermore, state and federal legislation is needed to implement a structured system to address pediatric advance directives [49]. Families whose children have chronic medical conditions or life-limiting illnesses would likely benefit from such a system.

Action can feel like a daunting task, and avidly advocating for patients on a day-to-day basis can lead to feelings of frustration and burnout among providers who lack necessary skills for advocacy [58]. However, the clinician's role has inherent potential for advocacy that could be utilized. One way that this might be able to take place is through encouraging partnerships between hospitals, medical schools, community hospices, home care agencies, and Latino community resources, such as outreach programs, volunteers, or churches [41,60]. These partnerships may increase educational opportunities for providers and elicit organizational-level changes to assist with provision of care to Latino children.

Without doubt, change in clinical practice and more research are needed to determine the best way to deliver pediatric PC to Latino children (Figure 2). With more data, advocacy at the state and federal levels is likely to be more effective.

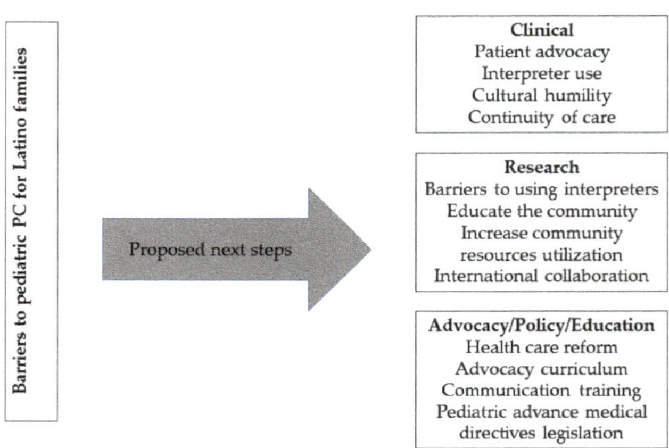

Figure 2. Proposed next steps to enhance the pediatric palliative care experience for Latino families.

5. Conclusions

While the demand for pediatric PC is increasing with medical advancements, care is not universally available. Moreover, political, economic, and social injustices can systematically undermine access to care for Latino populations. Additionally, cultural values, clinical experiences with discrimination, and health-related policy influence Latinos' access to care. Integrating Latino cultural values into clinical practice is key to the delivery of culturally sensitive pediatric PC for Latino children. Research focusing on provision of pediatric PC services to this population is essential in order to move forward and improve the quality of life of Latino children with serious illness and their families. Partnerships between lower-resourced countries in Latin America and higher-resourced entities, such as academic institutions in the US, would likely benefit the research agenda and lead to improvements in care for this vulnerable population. Finally, advocacy will play a large role in enhancing the availability of pediatric PC for Latino children and their families.

Author Contributions: S.M.-B. conducted literature search and review, wrote manuscript, created figures, critically revised manuscript, and approved final manuscript version to be published. J.C.R. conducted literature search and review, wrote manuscript, critically revised manuscript, and approved final manuscript version to be published. P.K.D. and R.D.B. critically revised manuscript and approved of final version to be published.

Conflicts of Interest: The authors declare no conflict of interest.

References

1. Feudtner, C.; Hays, R.M.; Haynes, G.; Geyer, J.R.; Neff, J.M.; Koepsell, T.D. Deaths attributed to pediatric complex chronic conditions: National trends and implications for supportive care services. *Pediatrics* **2001**, *107*, e99–e104. [CrossRef] [PubMed]
2. Palta, M.; Weinstein, M.R.; McGuinness, G.; Gabbert, D.; Brady, W.; Peters, M.E. A Population Study: Mortality and Morbidity after Availability of Surfactant Therapy. *Arch. Pediatr. Adolesc. Med.* **1994**, *148*, 1295–1301. [CrossRef] [PubMed]
3. Tennant, P.W.G.; Pearce, M.S.; Bythell, M.; Rankin, J. 20-year survival of children born with congenital anomalies: A population-based study. *Lancet* **2010**, *375*, 649–656. [CrossRef]
4. Morrison, R.S.; Maroney-Galin, C.; Kralovec, P.D.; Meier, D.E. The Growth of Palliative Care Programs in United States Hospitals. *J. Palliat. Med.* **2005**, *8*, 1127–1134. [CrossRef] [PubMed]
5. Colon, M.; Lyke, J. Comparison of hospice use by European Americans, African Americans, and Latinos: A follow-up study. *Am. J. Hosp. Palliat. Care* **2015**, *32*, 205–209. [CrossRef] [PubMed]
6. Knapp, C.A.; Shenkman, E.A.; Marcu, M.I.; Madden, V.L.; Terza, J.V. Pediatric Palliative Care: Describing Hospice Users and Identifying Factors that Affect Hospice Expenditures. *J. Palliat. Med.* **2009**, *12*, 223–229. [CrossRef] [PubMed]
7. Johnston, E.E.; Alvarez, E.; Saynina, O.; Sanders, L.; Bhatia, S.; Chamberlain, L.J. Disparities in the Intensity of End-of-Life Care for Children with Cancer. *Pediatrics* **2017**, *140*, e20170671. [CrossRef] [PubMed]
8. Temel, J.S.; Greer, J.A.; Muzikansky, A.; Gallagher, E.R.; Admane, S.; Jackson, V.A.; Dahlin, C.M.; Blinderman, C.D.; Jacobsen, J.; Pirl, W.F.; et al. Early Palliative Care for Patients with Metastatic Non-Small-Cell Lung Cancer. *N. Engl. J. Med.* **2010**, *363*, 733–742. [CrossRef] [PubMed]
9. Mack, J.W.; Wolfe, J. Early integration of pediatric palliative care: For some children, palliative care starts at diagnosis. *Curr. Opin. Pediatr.* **2006**, *18*, 10–14. [CrossRef] [PubMed]
10. U.S. Census Bureau. *Table 10. Projections of the Population by Sex, Hispanic Origin, and Race for the United States: 2015 to 2060 (NP2014-T10)*; U.S. Census Bureau: Suitland, MD, USA, 2014.
11. Campesino, M.; Schwartz, G.E. Spirituality among Latinas/os: Implications of culture in conceptualization and measurement. *Adv. Nurs. Sci.* **2006**, *29*, 69–81. [CrossRef]
12. Flores Niemann, Y.; Romero, A.J.; Arredondo, J.; Rodriguez, V. What does it mean to be 'Mexican'? Social Construction of an Ethnic Identity. *Hisp. J. Behav. Sci.* **1999**, *21*, 47–60. [CrossRef]
13. Del Gaudio, F.; Hichenberg, S.; Eisenberg, M.; Zaider, T.I.; Kissane, D.W. Latino Values in the Context of Palliative Care: Illustrative Cases from the Family Focused Grief Therapy Trial. *Am. J. Hosp. Palliat. Med.* **2012**, *30*, 271–278. [CrossRef] [PubMed]

14. Wiener, L.; McConnell, D.G.; Latella, L.; Ludi, E. Cultural and religious considerations in pediatric palliative care. *Palliat. Support. Care* **2013**, *11*, 47–67. [CrossRef] [PubMed]
15. Adames, H.Y.; Chavez-Dueñas, N.Y.; Fuentes, M.A.; Salas, S.P.; Perez-Chavez, J.G. Integration of Latino/a cultural values into palliative health care: A culture centered model. *Palliat. Support. Care* **2014**, *12*, 149–157. [CrossRef] [PubMed]
16. Smith, A.K.; Sudore, R.L.; Pérez-Stable, E.J. Palliative care for Latino patients and their families: Whenever we prayed, she wept. *JAMA* **2009**, *301*, 1047–1057. [CrossRef] [PubMed]
17. Cruz-Oliver, D.M.; Sanchez-Reilly, S. Barriers to Quality End-of-Life Care for Latinos. *J. Hosp. Palliat. Nurs.* **2016**, *18*, 505–511. [CrossRef]
18. Kelley, A.S.; Wenger, N.S.; Sarkisian, C.A. Opiniones: End-of-life care preferences and planning of older Latinos. *J. Am. Geriatr. Soc.* **2010**, *58*, 1109–1116. [CrossRef] [PubMed]
19. Born, W.; Greiner, A.; Sylvia, E.; Butler, J.; Ahluwalia, J.S. Knowledge, Attitudes, and Beliefs about End-of-life Care among Inner-City African Americans and Latinos. *J. Palliat. Med.* **2004**, *7*, 247–257. [CrossRef] [PubMed]
20. Flores, G.; Abreu, M.; Schwartz, I.; Hill, M. The importance of language and culture in pediatric care: Case studies from the Latino community. *J. Pediatr.* **2000**, *137*, 842–848. [CrossRef] [PubMed]
21. Del Río, N. The influence of Latino ethnocultural factors on decision making at the end of life: Withholding and withdrawing artificial nutrition and hydration. *J. Soc. Work End Life Palliat. Care* **2010**, *6*, 125–149. [CrossRef] [PubMed]
22. Jim, H.S.; Pustejovsky, J.E.; Park, C.L.; Danhauer, S.C.; Sherman, A.C.; Fitchett, G.; Merluzzi, T.V.; Munoz, A.R.; George, L.; Snyder, M.A.; et al. Religion, spirituality, and physical health in cancer patients: A meta-analysis. *Cancer* **2015**, *121*, 3760–3768. [CrossRef] [PubMed]
23. Li, L.; Sloan, D.H.; Mehta, A.K.; Willis, G.; Weaver, M.S.; Berger, A.C. Life perceptions of patients receiving palliative care and experiencing psycho-social-spiritual healing. *Ann. Palliat. Med.* **2017**, *6*, 211–219. [CrossRef] [PubMed]
24. O'Mara, S.K.; Zborovskaya, Y. End-of-Life Care in the Hispanic Community. *J. Hosp. Palliat. Nurs.* **2016**, *18*, 53–59. [CrossRef]
25. Braun, U.K.; Beyth, R.J.; Ford, M.E.; McCullough, L.B. Voices of African American, Caucasian, and Hispanic surrogates on the burdens of end-of-life decision making. *J. Gen. Intern. Med.* **2008**, *23*, 267–274. [CrossRef] [PubMed]
26. Althabe, M.; Cardigni, G.; Vassallo, J.C.; Allende, D.; Berrueta, M.; Codermatz, M.; Córdoba, J.; Castellano, S.; Jabornisky, R.; Marrone, Y.; et al. Dying in the intensive care unit: Collaborative multicenter study about forgoing life-sustaining treatment in Argentine pediatric intensive care units. *Pediatr. Crit. Care Med.* **2003**, *4*, 164–169. [CrossRef] [PubMed]
27. Abraído-Lanza, A.F.; Viladrich, A.; Flórez, K.R.; Céspedes, A.; Aguirre, A.N.; De La Cruz, A.A. Commentary: Fatalismo reconsidered: A cautionary note for health-related research and practice with Latino populations. *Ethn. Dis.* **2007**, *17*, 153–158. [PubMed]
28. Phelps, A.C.; Lauderdale, K.E.; Alcorn, S.; Dillinger, J.; Balboni, M.T.; Van Wert, M.; Vanderweele, T.J.; Balboni, T.A. Addressing spirituality within the care of patients at the end of life: Perspectives of patients with advanced cancer, oncologists, and oncology nurses. *J. Clin. Oncol.* **2012**, *30*, 2538–2544. [CrossRef] [PubMed]
29. Ernecoff, N.C.; Curlin, F.A.; Buddadhumaruk, P.; White, D.B. Health Care Professionals' Responses to Religious or Spiritual Statements by Surrogate Decision Makers during Goals-of-Care Discussions. *JAMA Intern. Med.* **2015**, *175*, 1662–1669. [CrossRef] [PubMed]
30. Caralis, P.; Davis, B.; Wright, K.; Marcial, E. The influence of ethnicity and race on attitudes toward advance directives, life-prolonging treatments, and euthanasia. *J. Clin. Ethics* **1993**, *4*, 155–165. [PubMed]
31. Wallace, L.S.; DeVoe, J.E.; Rogers, E.S.; Malagon-Rogers, M.; Fryer, G.E. The medical dialogue: Disentangling differences between Hispanic and non-Hispanic whites. *J. Gen. Intern. Med.* **2007**, *22*, 1538–1543. [CrossRef] [PubMed]
32. Katz, J.N.; Lyons, N.; Wolff, L.S.; Silverman, J.; Emrani, P.; Holt, H.L.; Corbett, K.L.; Escalante, A.; Losina, E. Medical decision-making among Hispanics and non-Hispanic Whites with chronic back and knee pain: A qualitative study. *BMC Musculoskelet. Disord.* **2011**, *12*, 78. [CrossRef] [PubMed]

33. Yennurajalingam, S.; Parsons, H.A.; Duarte, E.R.; Palma, A.; Bunge, S.; Palmer, J.L.; Delgado-Guay, M.O.; Allo, J.; Bruera, E. Decisional control preferences of Hispanic patients with advanced cancer from the United States and Latin America. *J. Pain Symptom Manag.* **2013**, *46*, 376–385. [CrossRef] [PubMed]
34. Noguera, A.; Yennurajalingam, S.; Torres-Vigil, I.; Parsons, H.A.; Duarte, E.R.; Palma, A.; Bunge, S.; Palmer, J.L.; Bruera, E. Decisional control preferences, disclosure of information preferences, and satisfaction among Hispanic patients with advanced cancer. *J. Pain Symptom Manag.* **2014**, *47*, 896–905. [CrossRef] [PubMed]
35. Pastrana, T.; Centeno, C.; De Lima, L. Palliative Care in Latin America from the Professional Perspective: A SWOT Analysis. *J. Palliat. Med.* **2015**, *18*, 429–437. [CrossRef] [PubMed]
36. Basu, A.; Mittag-Leffler, B.N.; Miller, K. Palliative care in low- and medium-resource countries. *Cancer J.* **2013**, *19*, 410–413. [CrossRef] [PubMed]
37. Wenk, R.; Bertolino, M. Palliative Care Development in South America: A Focus on Argentina. *J. Pain Symptom Manag.* **2007**, *33*, 645–650. [CrossRef] [PubMed]
38. Pastrana, T.; De Lima, L.; Wenk, R.; Eisenchlas, J.; Monti, C.; Rocafort, J.; Centeno, C. *Atlas of Palliative Care in Latin America ALCP*, 1st ed.; IAHPC Press: Houston, TX, USA, 2012.
39. Wenk, R.; De Lima, L.; Eisenchlas, J. Palliative care research in Latin America: Results of a survey within the scope of the Declaration of Venice. *J. Palliat. Med.* **2008**, *11*, 717–722. [CrossRef] [PubMed]
40. Pastrana, T.; De Lima, L.; Eisenchlas, J.; Wenk, R. Palliative care research in Latin America and the Caribbean: From the beginning to the Declaration of Venice and beyond. *J. Palliat. Med.* **2012**, *15*, 352–358. [PubMed]
41. Contro, N.; Davies, B.; Larson, J.; Sourkes, B. Away from home: Experiences of Mexican American families in pediatric palliative care. *J. Soc. Work End Life Palliat. Care* **2010**, *6*, 185–204. [CrossRef] [PubMed]
42. Jaramillo, S.; Hui, D. End-of-Life Care for Undocumented Immigrants with Advanced Cancer: Documenting the Undocumented. *J. Pain Symptom Manag.* **2016**, *51*, 784–788. [CrossRef] [PubMed]
43. Thienprayoon, R.; Marks, E.; Funes, M.; Martinez-Puente, L.M.; Winick, N.; Lee, S.C. Perceptions of the Pediatric Hospice Experience among English- and Spanish-Speaking Families. *J. Palliat. Med.* **2016**, *19*, 30–41. [CrossRef] [PubMed]
44. Contro, N.; Larson, J.; Scofield, S.; Sourkes, B.; Cohen, H. Family perspectives on the quality of pediatric palliative care. *Arch. Pediatr. Adolesc. Med.* **2002**, *156*, 14–19. [CrossRef] [PubMed]
45. Tienda, M.; Mitchell, F. *Hispanics and the Future of America*; The National Academies Press: Washington, DC, USA, 2006.
46. Moreno, G.; Walker, K.O.; Grumbach, K. Self-reported fluency in Non-English languages among physicians practicing in California. *Fam. Med.* **2010**, *42*, 414–420. [PubMed]
47. Davies, A.B.; Contro, N. Culturally-Sensitive Information-Sharing in Pediatric Palliative Care. *Pediatrics* **2010**, *125*, e859–e865. [CrossRef] [PubMed]
48. Davies, B.; Larson, J.; Contro, N.; Cabrera, A.P. Perceptions of discrimination among Mexican American families of seriously ill children. *J. Palliat. Med.* **2011**, *14*, 71–76. [CrossRef] [PubMed]
49. Liberman, D.B.; Pham, P.K.; Nager, A.L. Pediatric advance directives: Parents' knowledge, experience, and preferences. *Pediatrics* **2014**, *134*, e436–e443. [CrossRef] [PubMed]
50. Kataoka, S.H.; Zhang, L.; Wells, K.B. Unmet need for mental health care among U.S. children: Variation by ethnicity and insurance status. *Am. J. Psychiatry* **2002**, *159*, 1548–1555. [CrossRef] [PubMed]
51. Flores, G.; Abreu, M.A.; Olivar, M.A.; Kastner, B. Access Barriers to Health Care for Latino Children. *Arch. Pediatr. Adolesc. Med.* **1998**, *152*, 1119–1125. [CrossRef] [PubMed]
52. Flores, G.; Vega, L. Barriers to health care access for Latino children: A review. *Fam. Med.* **1998**, *30*, 196–205. [CrossRef] [PubMed]
53. Langellier, B.A.; Chen, J.; Vargas-Bustamante, A.; Inkelas, M.; Ortega, A.N. Understanding health-care access and utilization disparities among Latino children in the United States. *J. Child Health Care* **2016**, *20*, 133–144. [CrossRef] [PubMed]
54. McManus, M.; Newacheck, P. Health Insurance Differentials among Minority children with chronic conditions and the role of federal agencies and private foundations in improving financial access. *Pediatrics* **1993**, *91*, 1040–1047. [PubMed]
55. Chen, J.; Vargas-Bustamante, A.; Mortensen, K.; Ortega, A.N. Racial and Ethnic Disparities in Health Care Access and Utilization under the Affordable Care Act. *Med. Care* **2016**, *54*, 140–146. [CrossRef] [PubMed]

56. Baker, B.; Rytina, N. *Estimates of the Unauthorized Immigrant Population Residing in the United States*; Office of Immigration Statistics: Washington, DC, USA, 2013.
57. Fabi, R.; Saloner, B. Covering Undocumented Immigrants—State Innovation in California. *N. Engl. J. Med.* **2016**, *375*, 1913–1915. [CrossRef] [PubMed]
58. Nedjat-Haiem, F.R.; Carrion, I.V.; Cribbs, K.; Lorenz, K. Advocacy at the end of life: Meeting the needs of vulnerable Latino patients. *Soc. Work Health Care* **2013**, *52*, 558–577. [CrossRef] [PubMed]
59. Quinones-Gonzalez, S. Bridging the communication gap in hospice and palliative care for Hispanics and Latinos. *Omega* **2013**, *67*, 193–200. [CrossRef] [PubMed]
60. Cruz-Oliver, D.M.; Talamantes, M.; Sanchez-Reilly, S. What evidence is available on end-of-life (EOL) care and Latino elders? A literature review. *Am. J. Hosp. Palliat. Care* **2014**, *31*, 87–97. [CrossRef] [PubMed]
61. Fischer, S.M.; Cervantes, L.; Fink, R.M.; Kutner, J.S. Apoyo con Cariño: A pilot randomized controlled trial of a patient navigator intervention to improve palliative care outcomes for Latinos with serious illness. *J. Pain Symptom Manag.* **2015**, *49*, 657–665. [CrossRef] [PubMed]
62. Garrido, M.M.; Harrington, S.T.; Prigerson, H.G. End-of-life treatment preferences: A key to reducing ethnic/racial disparities in advance care planning? *Cancer* **2014**, *120*, 3981–3986. [CrossRef] [PubMed]
63. Bona, K.; Wolfe, J. Disparities in Pediatric Palliative Care: An Opportunity to Strive for Equity. *Pediatrics* **2017**, *140*, e20171662. [CrossRef] [PubMed]
64. *Annotated Code of Maryland—Health General Article, Subtitle 6: Health Care Decisions Act*; Maryland Attorney General's Office: Baltimore, MD, USA, 2010.
65. Lotz, J.D.; Jox, R.J.; Borasio, G.D.; Fuhrer, M. Pediatric Advance Care Planning: A Systematic Review. *Pediatrics* **2013**, *131*, e873–e880. [CrossRef] [PubMed]
66. Boss, R.D.; Hutton, N.; Griffin, P.L.; Wieczorek, B.H.; Donohue, P.K. Novel legislation for pediatric advance directives: Surveys and focus groups capture parent and clinician perspectives. *Palliat. Med.* **2015**, *29*, 346–353. [CrossRef] [PubMed]
67. Lotz, J.D.; Daxer, M.; Jox, R.J.; Borasio, G.D.; Führer, M. 'Hope for the best, prepare for the worst': A qualitative interview study on parents' needs and fears in pediatric advance care planning. *Palliat. Med.* **2017**, *31*, 764–771. [CrossRef] [PubMed]

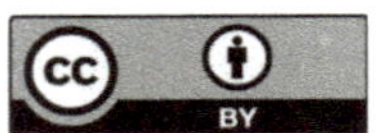

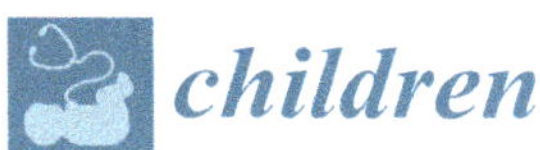

MDPI

Article

A Retrospective Review of Resuscitation Planning at a Children's Hospital

Jean Kelly [1], Jo Ritchie [2], Leigh Donovan [1,3], Carol Graham [4] and Anthony Herbert [1,4,*]

[1] Paediatric Palliative Care Service, Division of Medicine, Children's Health Queensland Hospital and Health Service, South Brisbane, QLD 4101, Australia; jean.kelly@health.qld.gov.au (J.K.); leigh.donovan@health.qld.gov.au (L.D.)

[2] Bone Marrow and Transplant Service, Children's Health Queensland Hospital and Health Service, South Brisbane, QLD 4101, Australia; jo.ritchie@health.qld.gov.au

[3] Behavioural Sciences Unit, School of Women's and Children's Health, University of New South Wales, Randwick, NSW 2031, Australia

[4] Children's Health Queensland Clinical Unit, Faculty of Medicine, University of Queensland, South Brisbane, QLD 4101, Australia; carol.graham@uq.net.au

* Correspondence: anthony.herbert@health.qld.gov.au; Tel.: +61-7-3068-3775

Received: 30 November 2017; Accepted: 20 December 2017; Published: 4 January 2018

Abstract: Resuscitation plans (RP) are an important clinical indicator relating to care at the end of life in paediatrics. A retrospective review of the medical records of children who had been referred to the Royal Children's Hospital, Brisbane, Australia who died in the calendar year 2011 was performed. Of 62 records available, 40 patients (65%) had a life limiting condition and 43 medical records (69%) contained a documented RP. This study demonstrated that both the underlying condition (life-limiting or life-threatening) and the setting of care (Pediatric Intensive Care Unit or home) influenced the development of resuscitation plans. Patients referred to the paediatric palliative care (PPC) service had a significantly longer time interval from documentation of a resuscitation plan to death and were more likely to die at home. All of the patients who died in the paediatric intensive care unit (PICU) had a RP that was documented within the last 48 h of life. Most RPs were not easy to locate. Documentation of discussions related to resuscitation planning should accommodate patient and family centered care based on individual needs. With varied diagnoses and settings of care, it is important that there is inter-professional collaboration, particularly involving PICU and PPC services, in developing protocols of how to manage this difficult but inevitable clinical scenario.

Keywords: resuscitation plan; advance care plan; paediatric palliative care; shared decision-making

1. Introduction

There is increasing interest and research around pediatric Advance Care Planning (pACP) [1]. pACP incorporates the wishes of parents or guardians of children with life-limiting or life-threatening conditions. The wishes and preferences of adolescents who have an emerging competence is also important to consider [2]. Advance care planning in children includes consideration of the goals of care at the end of life, including location of care, cultural and spiritual preferences, and organ/tissue donation. It also includes resuscitation planning, which is the focus of this paper [3].

Resuscitation planning refers to the discussions and decisions related to how health care professionals and parents will respond to a child if they deteriorate rapidly. This is often in the context of a cardiac or respiratory arrest. The response at such times would usually include basic life support including cardio-pulmonary resuscitation (e.g., airway support, expired air resuscitation and chest compressions) as well as advance life support (e.g., intubation, mechanical ventilation, administration of medications such as cardiac inotropes, and cardiac defibrillation). In the context of a life limiting condition, particularly if there are concerns the child may not live for longer than 12 months, then it may be appropriate to not provide cardiopulmonary resuscitation (CPR) and to limit or withhold other life sustaining measures such as advance life support. This is particularly in the context of the child's condition being progressive, with no obvious reversible component of the child's underlying illness. When a decision has been made to not provide CPR, it is important that other aspects of care such as pain and symptom management are provided, and the dignity of the child is maintained. The patient's primary pediatrician would usually lead these sensitive discussions around such management with the family often trying to balance hope with reality. Such discussions are becomingly increasingly complex with the emergence of new technologies such as non-invasive ventilation and extracorporeal membrane oxygenation (ECMO) [4,5].

There are a number of barriers to initiating these discussions including time constraints, prognostic uncertainty, disagreement between parents, and clinicians' difficulty accepting that the patient is not going to recover [6]. Despite the uncertainty in determining prognosis in children, discussion around the issues of resuscitation during end of life care can improve the quality of death and dignity for a child and their family at this difficult time [3].

Parental involvement and shared decision-making regarding treatment of their child throughout end of life is critical as this can influence the family's bereavement experience [7]. In some studies, parental experience at the end of life is improved if there is comprehensive and sensitive communication from medical staff and an opportunity to talk to the child about death [8]. Those who could acknowledge that there may be a negative outcome earlier and partake in advanced care planning described less distress and an improvement in the quality of life of the child [8,9].

The development of a resuscitation plan (RP) affords the patient and family choice, empowerment and a sense of clarity in communication between clinicians caring for the child [10,11]. In addition, RPs prevent the initiation of invasive procedures with little perceived benefit [11,12]. RPs can be difficult to locate in a medical record outlining the importance of clear documentation to facilitate communication to all involved in the care of the child [13]. In this context, documentation of resuscitation can serve as a quality indicator of shared decision-making with parents (and children where appropriate), and also serves as a clinical tool that can be used at the time of deterioration of a child.

Practice varies between clinicians and ongoing education and evaluation of the approach to resuscitation planning and end of life care is necessary. This study aimed to review both the documentation of resuscitation planning and the ease of access to documentation of discussions relating to resuscitation planning.

2. Materials and Methods

The Royal Children's Hospital (RCH) was a quaternary referral center for pediatric care serving a large area including Queensland and northern New South Wales, Australia, with 20,418 admissions and 166,865 outpatient visits in 2010. A retrospective chart review was performed of the medical records of all children who had been referred to the RCH who died in 2011. A list of deceased patients was obtained from the Health Information Services department and ethics approval was granted by the RCH Human Research Ethics Committee on 20 November 2012 (Reference Number HREC/12/QRCH/224). An audit tool was developed specifically for the purpose of this study and data was collated using Microsoft Excel (Microsoft Corporation, Redmond, WA, USA) and analysed using GraphPad Prism version 7 (GraphPad Software, La Jolla, CA, USA). The RCH closed operations in November 2014 after it merged with the Mater Children's Hospital to form the Lady Cilento Children's Hospital.

Data for this audit included the paper-based medical records and the database of the paediatric palliative care service (PPCS), reviewed by a single investigator. Information collected regarding patient characteristics included: age; gender; diagnosis; referral to PPCS; and the cause, date and location of death. Patients were defined as having a life-limiting condition (LLC) using the Directory of Life-Limiting conditions [14]. Parental demographic information was recorded (i.e., marital status, education level and ethnic background). If documentation regarding end of life care, or limitations to treatment was found this was recorded as the "resuscitation plan". Also recorded was the timing and location of the RP, the individual treatments specified during the discussion, the parent (or guardian) considered to be the decision-maker and whether the individual was considered to be "Gillick competent" [15]. This standard is based on the 1985 decision of the House of Lords in Gillick vs. West Norfolk and Eisbech Area Health Authority, England. The case is binding in England and Wales, and has been adopted in jurisdictions such as Australia, New Zealand and Canada. The original Gillick case related to the prescription of contraception and whether a minor could consent to such treatment without the knowledge or permission of their parent.

A Gillick-competent child has the legal capacity to consent to the provision of medical treatment if they can demonstrate sufficient maturity and intelligence to understand the nature and implications of the proposed treatment, including the risk and alternative courses of actions. There is no fixed age at which a young person is automatically capable of consenting to medical treatment generally, or to specific types of medical treatment. This right to consent is a developing right as the child gains sufficient maturity to make an informed decision. At the same time, the parents' right to consent decreases, although there will be some overlap.

In some cases, the child's primary institution was not the RCH and records were either not available or inadequate for inclusion in any analysis. Demographics of patients who suffered from acute trauma resulting in death were recorded but these patients were not included in the present analysis regarding RPs.

Sample means and standard deviations were calculated for the time intervals from resuscitation planning to death in each case in which this information was available. Non-parametric testing was applied using the chi square test to determine if there was statistical significance between proportions. Independent *t*-tests were used when comparing means between groups.

3. Results

Seventy-nine deaths were recorded in the calendar year 2011. Sufficient demographic information was available in 71 of these charts and is outlined in Table 1. Twenty-seven per cent of deaths occurred in the first year of life. The condition with the highest prevalence was malignancy ($n = 22$), followed by neurologic conditions ($n = 8$). Sufficient data for analysis was available in the medical records of 62 patients (Figure 1). Variables that were analysed (i.e., presence of a resuscitation plan, life-limiting condition, referral to palliative care and place of death) are presented in Appendix A.

Of the 62 records available, 43 (69%) contained information related to resuscitation planning. Of these 62 patients, an illness with a poor prognosis or a LLC was diagnosed in 65% of cases (40 of 62). A discussion regarding resuscitation planning was found in the records of 63% (27 of 43) of these patients with a LLC (Figure 1).

The wishes of the child were documented as being considered in only two cases and Gillick competency in three cases. Seven children were aged twelve and over at the time of their death. There was no occasion where treatment was administered which was against the wishes of the parent or guardian.

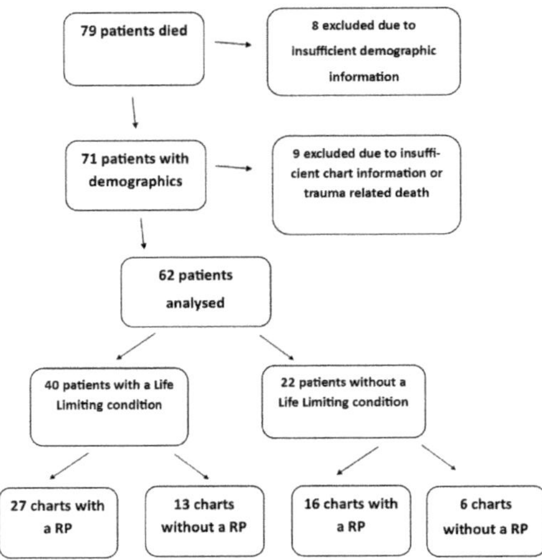

Figure 1. Medical records in which a resuscitation plan (RP) was documented.

Table 1. Patient characteristics.

Gender of Child		$n = 71$
Male		36
Female		35
Age of Child		$n = 71$
0–3 months		8
3–6 months		5
6–12 months		6
1–5 years		12
5–10 years		28
>10 years		12
Diagnosis		$n = 71$
Oncology	Brain Tumour	10
	ALL	4
	PTLD	2
	Other malignancy *	6
Neurological		8
Congenital		7
Chromosomal abnormalities		6
Infection		4
Metabolic		4
Prematurity		4
Unknown		4
Meningitis		3
Accident		3
Other		3

Table 1. *Cont.*

Parent Demographics		$n = 71$
Marital Status	Married	47
	Single	0
	Separated/Divorced	15
	Foster care	2
	Unknown	7
Parent Education	Year 12 or less	12
	Tertiary	8
	Trade	6
	Unknown	45
Parent Ethnicity	Caucasian	43
	Aboriginal or Torres Strait Islander	1
	Other	11
	Unknown	15

ALL: acute lymphoblastic leukaemia; PTLD: post-transplant lymphoproliferative disorder. * Other malignancy includes: sarcoma, ovarian tumour, Wilms tumour, hepatoblastoma, rhabdoid tumour and metastatic adrenocortical carcinoma.

The largest group of patients died in their own home (23, 37%). Sixteen patients (26%) died in a paediatric intensive care unit (PICU) or high dependency unit (HDU), 15 (24%) died in another medical ward (not PICU or HDU) and 8 (13%) died in an unknown location. The location of death was statistically associated with having a RP ($p < 0.005$), with 100% of patients who died in the PICU having a RP (Figure 2).

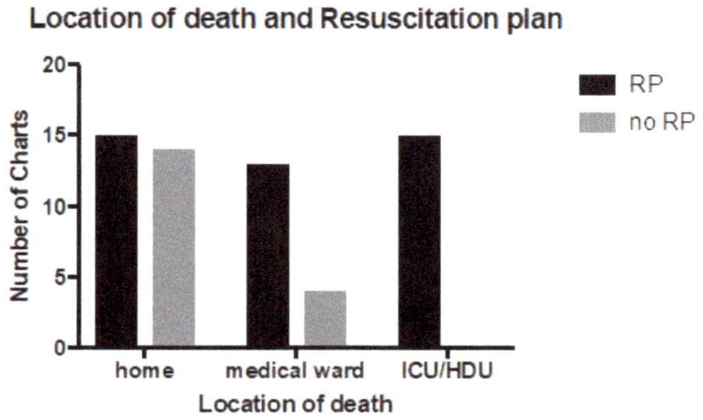

Figure 2. Location of death and presence of a resuscitation plan in 61 patients. ICU: intensive care unit; HDU: high dependency unit.

Thirty-nine patients had been referred to palliative care (63%). Of the 16 children who died on the medical ward, 13 (81%) were referred to the PPCS, and among the 15 children who died in the PICU or HDU, four (27%) had been referred to palliative care. Referral to palliative care was significantly associated with dying at home ($p < 0.05$) and outside of the PICU environment (Figure 3) and with a longer time from resuscitation planning to death ($p < 0.005$) (Figure 4). Of the children with a LLC who died at home, 95% had been referred to the PPCS (19 of 20), and 60% (12 of 20) had a RP. Neither a referral to palliative care nor having a LLC was significantly associated with having a RP.

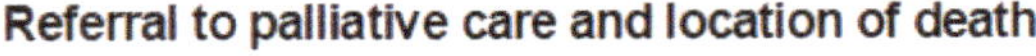

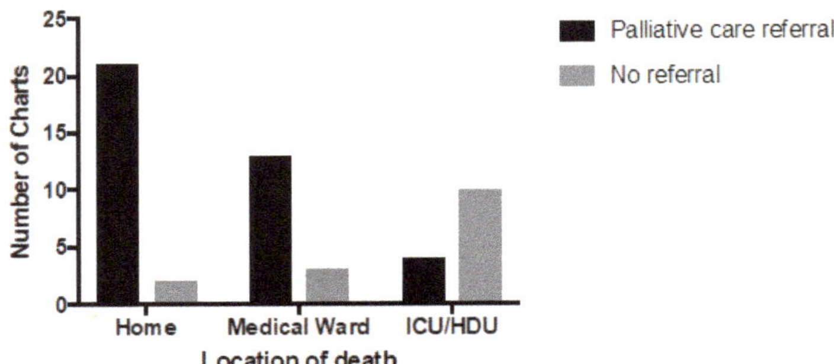

Figure 3. Location of child at time of death and referral to palliative care in 53 patients.

The time from the documentation of a RP to the child's death ranged from less than 24 h to over one year and was on average 51 days (standard deviation (SD) = 101). However, this included three cases where the RP had been made over 200 days prior to the child's death (240, 390 and 425 days from RP until death) and when these values were excluded, the average time in days from RP to the death of the child was 25 days (SD = 39). For those patients who died in the PICU or HDU who had a RP, all were documented in the 48-h period before the child died. Overall, discussions relating to the withholding or withdrawing of life sustaining treatment (WWLST) were documented in the 48-h period before death in 37% of cases (n = 16).

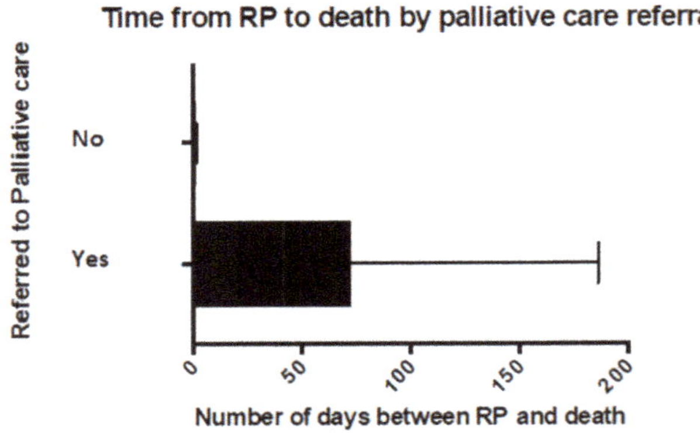

Figure 4. Time from development of RP to death by palliative care referral.

Only four RPs were easily located. The term "easily located" being considered applicable if it was in a prominent position in the paper-based medical record, highlighted by means of a "tag" or if a distinctive colored ink had been used. Most resuscitation plans were found in the final admission (n = 23) with other locations including correspondence (n = 16), and prior admissions and notes (n = 3) (Figure 5).

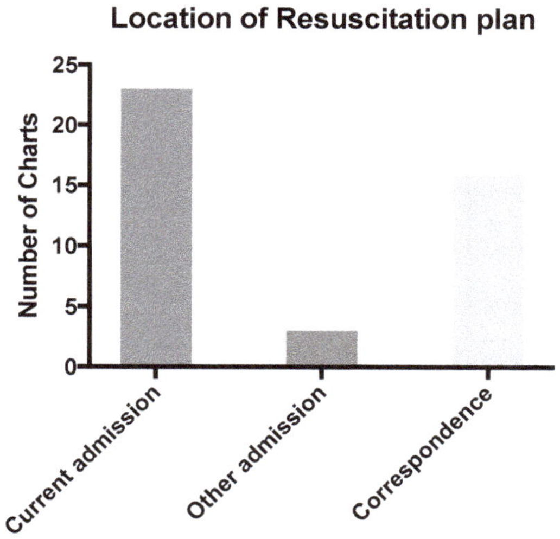

Location of Resuscitation plan

Figure 5. Location of RP.

4. Discussion

4.1. Shared Decision-Making

Some clinicians working within paediatric palliative care argue that a focus on RPs is of limited value [16]. There are significant other components to paediatric palliative care (such as symptom management, practical and emotional support) and appropriate spiritual or cultural care that go beyond resuscitation planning. Further, it is argued that the documentation does not truly capture the series of sensitive conversations that may be required for a child and family to experience a dignified death. Nevertheless, a documented RP is a clinical indicator of an important example of shared decision-making related to a very sensitive and difficult aspect of clinical care.

It has been found that early discussion of resuscitation planning is beneficial in a variety of ways, including perceived reduction in pain and suffering, increased psychological support, decreased invasive interventions and importantly, the opportunity for the patient and family to express their wishes and achieve personal goals [8]. This decision also has long-term ramifications, both positive and negative, for other members of the family [7,17,18].

In the current study, there was no care provided that was not consistent with the RP. Similarly, in a children hospice, RPs were followed in all cases except one case where the child underwent unsuccessful resuscitation by a family member who was not a decision-maker [16].

4.2. Place of Death

In the current study, RPs were documented in 69% of all patients reviewed. All patients receiving care in the PICU or HDU had RPs documented. This may reflect the practice of shared decision-making and its documentation within the Australian context. One study of 50 consecutive inpatient paediatric deaths at a children's hospital in Melbourne, Australia found that life-sustaining treatment were either withdrawn or limited prior to death in 84% of cases. There was documented family involvement in the decision-making process in 98% of these cases [13].

In a study of children dying in five different PICUs in the USA, only 56% of patients with life-threatening illness and 64% of patients with life limiting conditions had a formal DNR (Do Not Resuscitate) order in place at the time of death [19]. It was argued that there was a shared understanding of the plan between the multi-disciplinary team within PICU and the family around the process of withdrawal of mechanical ventilation or other life-sustaining therapies. In such a context, it was felt that discussion and documentation of CPR was distracting or irrelevant [19]. Often, DNR orders are established within PICU in the last day or days of life [13,20].

Only 15 patients (15 of 29, 51%) being cared for at home had a RP. This may be due to perception that there is less of a need for such plan in a non-acute healthcare setting. A smaller number of patients (9%) did not have a Do Not Attempt Resuscitation Plan (DNAR) at the time of their death in a study of 207 deaths over a 15-year period within a children's hospice [16]. It is also possible a RP may have been established in the home by community healthcare professionals (e.g., community nurses or general practitioners) and these had not been communicated back to the hospital. Despite this finding, it is important to develop a RP when home care is being provided, as families may still utilize emergency medical services for various reasons when receiving care at home [21,22].

4.3. Palliative Care Involvement

This study found 39 (63%) of patients were referred to palliative care. Sixteen patients (26%) were not referred to palliative care while it was uncertain from the medial record whether a palliative care referral was made in seven cases (11%)—see Appendix A. There are various reasons why a patient may not be referred to palliative care. This would include the patient having an acute and sudden onset life-threatening condition such as sepsis or trauma where there may not be sufficient time for a palliative care referral to be made. In this context, end of life care would appropriately be provided by the PICU. Some children with chronic LLC may not have been referred to the PPCS because their primary team felt they were able to meet the patient's needs, and a referral to palliative care was not required.

The time between resuscitation planning and death ranged from over one year to less than 24 h, with only two patients having a RP for over one year, and 17 patients having a RP within 24 h of death. The right time to have a RP discussion is influenced by clinical and professional experience, location of care, parental prompts, personal experience, education and religious beliefs [20,23]. As seen with the present study, it appears that when death becomes more of a certainty, discussions regarding WWLST occur more frequently [24]. The development of a RP should ideally occur in a non-crisis environment and afford the family choice, empowerment and a sense of clarity in communication between clinicians caring for their child [10,12].

Patients who were referred to palliative care were more likely to have an earlier documented discussion than patients who were not referred in the current study. The majority of patients who died at home were referred to palliative care. The proportion of patients with a RP who died at home was smaller than that for those who died in hospital. Those who died in hospital, particularly PICU, tended to have their resuscitation plan completed in the final 24 h before the child's death.

The small sample size in the comparison groups are a limitation in this analysis, but the results are both statistically and clinically significant with all patients who were not referred to palliative care having a RP documented within two days of death. Previous studies have reported an increase in RPs and an increase in time interval between RP and deaths with palliative care and advanced care team consults [3,25]. Wolfe et al. have described early referral to palliative care and instigation of resuscitation planning as markers of quality end of life care [3]. It is likely that those who were not referred to palliative care had a more acute presentation or unpredictable trajectory [19]. However, 65% of patients in the current study had a pre-existing diagnosis associated with a poor prognosis. This suggests opportunities to refer to palliative care earlier in the course of the disease trajectory for some children.

In addition to other components of holistic palliative care (such as addressing goals of care, symptom management and psychosocial support), discussions of prognosis and resuscitation discussions are more likely to occur in children who have received a palliative care consultation [26]. Children who receive a palliative care consultation are more likely to have a DNR order in place for a longer time before death (six versus two days) [27]. Death was also more likely to occur outside of the intensive care environment [27]. The current study supports such findings and extends into the non-cancer and homecare context.

4.4. Role of Documentation

Documentation and ease of access of RPs are essential for the health care team to communicate plans to each other and to relieve some stress from the child's caregivers [8]. Locating documentation regarding RPs was a challenge in the current study and has been reported elsewhere [13]. RPs were not filed in a consistent place in the current study. The inclusion in this study of a large number of patients who died at home has highlighted the role of the RP as a tool, which can communicate the patients' and parents' wishes to a variety of service providers [21,22]. The number of clinicians parents encounter during an acute admission to hospital can be overwhelming [11]. In this context, it is helpful if staff can locate a RP readily within the patient's medical record.

A RP template can serve as a helpful clinical tool. Firstly, it can foster a logical sequence of clinical reasoning—see Paediatric Acute Resuscitation Plan (PARP) in supplementary materials (Figure S2). This can include clinical assessment and decisions relating to treatments that will be provided and those that will be withheld or limited. The form can also encourage documentation of discussion with key decision-makers such as the parent. The form can also prompt health professionals to use clear and compassionate language with families, so they feel supported in this process [12]. In this context, the form can allow both a personalized approach to care, whilst at the same time minimizing unhelpful variation in practice and documentation [10,28]. Finally, such a form can serve as an audit tool when examining practices such a resuscitation planning and advance care planning within paediatrics.

With a move to the use of electronic medical records, such a form can be readily scanned into the medical record. It is possible to place an alert that such a plan exists, including on what date the plan was made. The form can also pop-up as an initial key document when, for example, a "clinical notes" tab is clicked. In the future, we hope to establish a clearly marked "Advance Care Planning" tab where both a resuscitation plan and an advance care plan can be found. The form can also be scanned and forwarded on to the Ambulance Service. In Queensland, the ambulance service will use this form as a basis for their own resuscitation plan. When the ambulance is called to the patient's address, the paramedics will be notified that a resuscitation plan is in place for one of the residents at that address. We also encourage the parents to hold a printed version of the form that they can present to emergency staff (both paramedics and those working within the emergency department) at the time of presentation.

A further development would be having the form present within the electronic medical record as a template upon which the health professional can fill in the details by typing rather than handwriting. While the use of the PARP is encouraged, other forms of clear documentation or correspondence are permissible as an alternative. A similar process for establishing an alert and liaison with the ambulance service is still possible in this context.

4.5. Limitations

As with any chart review, data was limited to the information charted by the healthcare professionals. Limitations included incomplete charting, differences in documentation style and procedures, location of documents and missing information. Additionally, some charts had discontinuity in terms of location of care for patients, potentially resulting in incomplete chart information. The current audit identified if the decision-maker (usually the parent) was documented and also whether the young person had the ability to provide consent. Further improvement would be to audit whether there was a documentation of the discussion between the parents and the health professionals as a marker of shared decision-making. Furthermore, it would be helpful to also audit whether young people had Gillick competence, or alternatively if they had developmental disability precluding involvement in medical decision-making.

In addition to observing the place of death of the child, it would also be helpful to determine if the child and family had expressed a wish for where they would die. It would then be possible to determine how many patients died in their preferred location of death. Such information is more likely to be contained in an Advance Care Plan rather than a Resuscitation Plan. Some research suggests that it is not necessarily the location of death, or whether the child died in the preferred location of death, but rather if the family were given the options and choices around where their child could die [29].

5. Conclusions

This study has suggested a number of improvements in practice. This included prominent placement of RP within the medical record and improved documentation of resuscitation plans for those who die at home. Documentation of the shared decision-making process between health professionals and families in relation to RP is also important. This would include assessment of the competency of the older child to be involved in such discussions and decision-making. Setting of care and sub-specialty involvement (e.g., palliative care and/or intensive care) also impacted RPs. Patients who died in PICU were more likely to have a resuscitation plan in place compared to those who died at home. Those patients involved with palliative care were more likely to have their resuscitation plan developed more than 48 h before they died. The use of a template to document resuscitation plans can be an effective clinical and communication tool for families and clinicians at the time of deterioration.

Supplementary Materials: The following are available online at www.mdpi.com/2227-9067/5/1/9/s1, Figure S1: Audit form, Figure S2: Paediatric Acute Resuscitation Plan.

Acknowledgments: This study received no external sources of funding. We would like to thank Shelley Rumble for assistance with graphical presentation and Lesley Pampling for assistance with obtaining medical records. We also thank the End of Life Care Project, Clinical Policy Team, Access Improvement Services, Centre for Healthcare Improvement, Queensland Health who developed the Paediatric Acute Resuscitation Plan (PARP) form in 2011. Wendy Corfield, Aurora Hodges and Julie White were members of this project team. The Palliative Care Working Group of the Statewide Child and Youth Network, Queensland Health, provided guidance on how this retrospective review was undertaken and also in the development of the PARP. Members of this group in 2001–2012 included Elizabeth Chenoweth, Helen Irving (Chair), Anthony Herbert, Will Cairns, Lee-anne Pedersen, Leigh Donovan, Liz Crowe, David Levitt, Nicolette Thornton, David Van Gend and Sue Nancarrow. Professor Ross Pinkerton was Chair of the Statewide Child and Youth Network at this time. Christine Smith assisted with the first draft of the PARP.

Author Contributions: J.K., J.R. and A.H. conceived and designed the study; J.K. performed the review; J.K., J.R., L.D. and C.G. analysed the data; and C.G., J.K. and A.H. wrote the paper.

Conflicts of Interest: The authors declare no conflict of interest.

Appendix A

Table A1. Frequency of analysed variables (62 patients).

Resuscitation Plan	Yes	43 (69%)
	No	19 (31%)
Life Limiting Condition	Yes	40 (65%)
	No	22 (35%)
Palliative Care	Yes	39 (63%)
	No	16 (26%)
	Unknown	7 (11%)
Place of Death	Home	23 (37%)
	Medical ward	16 (26%)
	Paediatric Intensive Care Unit/High Dependency Unit	15 (24%)
	Unknown	8 (13%)

References

1. Lotz, J.D.; Jox, R.J.; Borasio, G.D.; Fuhrer, M. Pediatric advance care planning: A systematic review. *Pediatrics* **2013**, *131*, e873–e880. [CrossRef] [PubMed]
2. Lyon, M.E.; D'Angelo, L.J.; Dallas, R.H.; Hinds, P.S.; Garvie, P.A.; Wilkins, M.L.; Garcia, A.; Briggs, L.; Flynn, P.M.; Rana, S.R.; et al. A randomized clinical trial of adolescents with HIV/AIDS: Pediatric advance care planning. *AIDS Care* **2017**, *29*, 1287–1296. [CrossRef] [PubMed]
3. Wolfe, J.; Hammel, J.F.; Edwards, K.E.; Duncan, J.; Comeau, M.; Breyer, J.; Aldridge, S.A.; Grier, H.E.; Berde, C.; Dussel, V.; et al. Easing of suffering in children with cancer at the end of life: Is care changing? *J. Clin. Oncol.* **2008**, *26*, 1717–1723. [CrossRef] [PubMed]
4. Nava, S.; Ferrer, M.; Esquinas, A.; Scala, R.; Groff, P.; Cosentini, R.; Guido, D.; Lin, C.H.; Cuomo, A.M.; Grassi, M. Palliative use of non-invasive ventilation in end-of-life patients with solid tumours: A randomised feasibility trial. *Lancet Oncol.* **2013**, *14*, 219–227. [CrossRef]
5. Yuerek, M.; Rossano, J.W. ECMO in Resuscitation. *Int. Anesthesiol. Clin.* **2017**, *55*, 19–35. [CrossRef] [PubMed]
6. Forbes, T.; Goeman, E.; Stark, Z.; Hynson, J.; Forrester, M. Discussing withdrawing and withholding of life-sustaining medical treatment in a tertiary paediatric hospital: A survey of clinician attitudes and practices. *J. Paediatr. Child Health* **2008**, *44*, 392–398. [CrossRef] [PubMed]
7. Van der Geest, I.M.; Darlington, A.S.; Streng, I.C.; Michiels, E.M.; Pieters, R.; van den Heuvel-Eibrink, M.M. Parents' experiences of pediatric palliative care and the impact on long-term parental grief. *J. Pain Symptom Manag.* **2014**, *47*, 1043–1053. [CrossRef] [PubMed]
8. McCarthy, M.C.; Clarke, N.E.; Ting, C.L.; Conroy, R.; Anderson, V.A.; Heath, J.A. Prevalence and predictors of parental grief and depression after the death of a child from cancer. *J. Palliat. Med.* **2010**, *13*, 1321–1326. [CrossRef] [PubMed]
9. Tan, J.S.; Docherty, S.L.; Barfield, R.; Brandon, D.H. Addressing parental bereavement support needs at the end of life for infants with complex chronic conditions. *J. Palliat. Med.* **2012**, *15*, 579–584. [CrossRef] [PubMed]
10. Wolff, A.; Browne, J.; Whitehouse, W.P. Personal resuscitation plans and end of life planning for children with disability and life-limiting/life-threatening conditions. *Arch. Dis. Child. Educ. Pract. Ed.* **2011**, *96*, 42–48. [CrossRef] [PubMed]
11. Meert, K.L.; Briller, S.H.; Schim, S.M.; Thurston, C.; Kabel, A. Examining the needs of bereaved parents in the pediatric intensive care unit: A qualitative study. *Death Stud.* **2009**, *33*, 712–740. [CrossRef] [PubMed]
12. Jones, B.L.; Parker-Raley, J.; Higgerson, R.; Christie, L.M.; Legett, S.; Greathouse, J. Finding the right words: Using the terms allow natural death (AND) and do not resuscitate (DNR) in pediatric palliative care. *J. Healthc. Qual.* **2008**, *30*, 55–63. [CrossRef] [PubMed]
13. Stark, Z.; Hynson, J.; Forrester, M. Discussing withholding and withdrawing of life-sustaining medical treatment in paediatric inpatients: Audit of current practice. *J. Paediatr. Child Health* **2008**, *44*, 399–403. [CrossRef] [PubMed]
14. Hain, R.; Devins, M.; Hastings, R.; Noyes, J. Paediatric palliative care: Development and pilot study of a 'Directory' of life-limiting conditions. *BMC Palliat. Care* **2013**, *12*, 43. [CrossRef] [PubMed]
15. Larcher, V.; Hutchinson, A. How should paediatricians assess Gillick competence? *Arch. Dis. Child.* **2010**, *95*, 307–311. [CrossRef] [PubMed]
16. Siden, H.H.; Chavoshi, N. Shifting Focus in Pediatric Advance Care Planning: From Advance Directives to Family Engagement. *J. Pain Symptom Manag.* **2016**, *52*, e1–e3. [CrossRef] [PubMed]
17. Truog, R.D. Is it always wrong to perform futile CPR? *N. Engl. J. Med.* **2010**, *362*, 477–479. [CrossRef] [PubMed]
18. Lovgren, M.; Sveen, J.; Nyberg, T.; Eilegard Wallin, A.; Prigerson, H.G.; Steineck, G.; Kreicbergs, U. Care at End of Life Influences Grief: A Nationwide Long-Term Follow-Up among Young Adults Who Lost a Brother or Sister to Childhood Cancer. *J. Palliat. Med.* **2017**. [CrossRef] [PubMed]
19. Burns, J.P.; Sellers, D.E.; Meyer, E.C.; Lewis-Newby, M.; Truog, R.D. Epidemiology of death in the PICU at five U.S. teaching hospitals. *Crit. Care Med.* **2014**, *42*, 2101–2108. [CrossRef] [PubMed]
20. Drake, R.; Frost, J.; Collins, J.J. The symptoms of dying children. *J. Pain Symptom Manag.* **2003**, *26*, 594–603. [CrossRef]

21. Ananth, P.; Melvin, P.; Berry, J.G.; Wolfe, J. Trends in Hospital Utilization and Costs among Pediatric Palliative Care Recipients. *J. Palliat. Med.* **2017**, *20*, 946–953. [CrossRef] [PubMed]
22. McGinley, J.; Waldrop, D.P.; Clemency, B. Emergency medical services providers' perspective of end-of-life decision-making for people with intellectual disabilities. *J. Appl. Res. Intellect. Disabil.* **2017**, *30*, 1057–1064. [CrossRef] [PubMed]
23. Gillam, L. End of life decision-making in paediatrics. *J. Paediatr. Child Health* **2008**, *44*, 389–391. [PubMed]
24. Detering, K.M.; Hancock, A.D.; Reade, M.C.; Silvester, W. The impact of advance care planning on end of life care in elderly patients: Randomised controlled trial. *BMJ* **2010**, *340*, c1345. [CrossRef] [PubMed]
25. Oberender, F.; Tibballs, J. Withdrawal of life-support in paediatric intensive care—A study of time intervals between discussion, decision and death. *BMC Pediatr.* **2011**, *11*, 39. [CrossRef] [PubMed]
26. Ullrich, C.K.; Lehmann, L.; London, W.B.; Guo, D.; Sridharan, M.; Koch, R.; Wolfe, J. End-of-Life Care Patterns Associated with Pediatric Palliative Care among Children Who Underwent Hematopoietic Stem Cell Transplant. *Biol. Blood Marrow Transplant.* **2016**, *22*, 1049–1055. [CrossRef] [PubMed]
27. Snaman, J.M.; Kaye, E.C.; Lu, J.J.; Sykes, A.; Baker, J.N. Palliative care involvement is associated with less intensive end-of-life care in adolescent and young adult oncology patients. *J. Palliat. Med.* **2017**, *20*, 509–516. [CrossRef] [PubMed]
28. Kennedy, P.J.; Leathley, C.M.; Hughes, C.F. Clinical practice variation. *Med. J. Aust.* **2010**, *193* (Suppl. 8), S97–S99. [PubMed]
29. Dussel, V.; Kreicbergs, U.; Hilden, J.M.; Watterson, J.; Moore, C.; Turner, B.G.; Weeks, J.C.; Wolfe, J. Looking beyond where children die: Determinants and effects of planning a child's location of death. *J. Pain Symptom Manag.* **2009**, *37*, 33–43. [CrossRef] [PubMed]

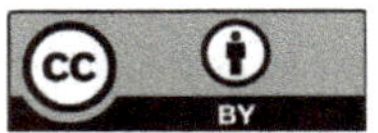

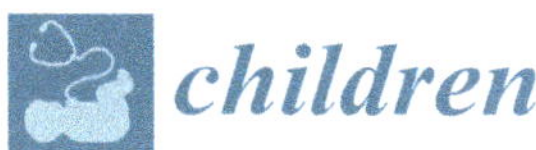

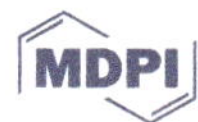

Article

A Sleep Questionnaire for Children with Severe Psychomotor Impairment (SNAKE)—Concordance with a Global Rating of Sleep Quality

Larissa Alice Dreier [1,2], Boris Zernikow [1,2], Markus Blankenburg [2,3] and Julia Wager [1,2,*]

1 Paediatric Palliative Care Centre, Children's and Adolescents' Hospital, 45711 Datteln, Germany; l.dreier@kinderpalliativzentrum.de (L.A.D.); b.zernikow@deutsches-kinderschmerzzentrum.de (B.Z.)

2 Department of Children's Pain Therapy and Paediatric Palliative Care, Faculty of Health, School of Medicine, Witten/Herdecke University, 58448 Witten, Germany; m.blankenburg@klinikum-stuttgart.de

3 Paediatric Neurology, Psychosomatics and Pain Therapy, Center for Child, Youth and Women's Health, Klinikum Stuttgart, Olgahospital/Frauenklinik, 70174 Stuttgart, Germany

* Correspondence: j.wager@deutsches-kinderschmerzzentrum.de; Tel.: +49-2363-975-184

Received: 29 November 2017; Accepted: 30 January 2018; Published: 1 February 2018

Abstract: Sleep problems are a common and serious issue in children with life-limiting conditions (LLCs) and severe psychomotor impairment (SPMI). The "Sleep Questionnaire for Children with Severe Psychomotor Impairment" (Schlaffragebogen für Kinder mit Neurologischen und Anderen Komplexen Erkrankungen, SNAKE) was developed for this unique patient group. In a proxy rating, the SNAKE assesses five different dimensions of sleep(-associated) problems (disturbances going to sleep, disturbances remaining asleep, arousal and breathing disorders, daytime sleepiness, and daytime behavior disorders). It has been tested with respect to construct validity and some aspects of criterion validity. The present study examined whether the five SNAKE scales are consistent with parents' or other caregivers' global ratings of a child's sleep quality. Data from a comprehensive dataset of children and adolescents with LLCs and SPMI were analyzed through correlation coefficients and Mann–Whitney U testing. The results confirmed the consistency of both sources of information. The highest levels of agreements with the global rating were achieved for disturbances in terms of going to sleep and disturbances with respect to remaining asleep. The results demonstrate that the scales and therefore the SNAKE itself is well-suited for gathering information on different sleep(-associated) problems in this vulnerable population.

Keywords: sleep; pediatric; SNAKE; life-limiting; neurological; impairments

1. Introduction

Referring to data from the UK, approximately 32 per 10,000 children and adolescents suffer from life-limiting conditions (LLCs), with a rising trend [1]. Accordingly, genetic, neurological, or metabolic diseases that are accompanied by severe psychomotor impairments (SPMI) constitute the most represented diagnoses [2,3].

With an assumed prevalence of 60–80%, sleep problems are a common issue in these children and adolescents [4]. In accordance with the "International Classification of Sleep disorders" (ICSD-2; [5]), sleep problems can generally be categorized into excessive sleepiness, sleeplessness, and behavioral disturbances [6]. There are several studies that confirm the relationship between severe chronic illnesses and sleep disturbances, such as difficulties in initiating and maintaining sleep [7–10], sleep-associated respiratory problems [4,11,12], daytime sleepiness [13], parasomnia [14,15], and irregular sleep–wake rhythm [16,17]. Pediatric sleep problems burden both the children themselves and their caregivers [18,19]. As a result, parents are commonly affected by psychological and somatic problems that, in turn, negatively influence their child's care [18]. However, the etiology of sleep problems in children with LLCs and SPMI is not entirely clear [20,21]. To address this issue and to support an efficient diagnosis of sleep problems, reliable and valid measures are essential [4].

There are a number of sleep measures specifically developed for pediatric use. For instance, the "Sleep Disturbance Scale for Children" (SDSC; [22,23]), the "Children's Sleep Habits Questionnaire" (CSHQ; [14,24–27]) and the "Sleep Behavior Questionnaire" (SBQ; [28,29]) have been applied in numerous investigations [11]. However, these questionnaires were originally developed for use in healthy children and thus do not meet the special requirements of children with SPMI who commonly suffer from impaired language capability [21]. To address this problem, the "Sleep Questionnaire for Children with Severe Psychomotor Impairment" (Schlaffragebogen für Kinder mit Neurologischen und Anderen Komplexen Erkrankungen, SNAKE) was developed [21]. The SNAKE is a multidimensional and comprehensive proxy assessment that takes medical as well as psychosocial aspects of sleep problems in children with LLCs and SPMI into account. Its five scales are based on the ICSD-2 [5] and cover different sleep(-related) problems. Further, several items ask directly about sleep issues that may emerge from conditions linked to LLCs (for example medical care, need for repositioning, pain, epileptic seizures, breathing difficulties) and therefore are unique for the vulnerable population of severely disabled children and adolescents. Even though the SNAKE's reliability, its construct validity, and some aspects of criterion validity have been confirmed [21], the relationship between the scale's ratings and the caretakers' global assessment of the child's sleep quality has not yet been examined. The present paper addresses the question of how consistent the scores obtained in the SNAKE scales are with the caretaker's global rating. Concordance between the SNAKE scales and the global rating would be an additional confirmation of the questionnaire's validity and its practical benefit as a whole.

2. Materials and Methods

2.1. Dataset

Data were derived from a comprehensive dataset of $N = 226$ children and adolescents aged 1–25 years ($M = 10.39$) who had been diagnosed with LLCs and SPMI. Participants and their parents were originally recruited from one outpatient facility and three inpatient institutions within the scope of another study [21]. Ethical approval was obtained through the Ethics Committee of the Children's and Adolescent's Hospital Datteln, Germany (Approval code 2008/06/26/MB). Informed consent was obtained from all participants. Research ethics of this investigation comply fully with the Declaration of Helsinki and the German data protection law. A number of studies based on the same dataset have been published [18,21,30].

2.2. The Sleep Questionnaire for Children with Severe Psychomotor Impairment (SNAKE)

One challenge for the SNAKE is that the use of self-rating questionnaires in children with LLCs and SPMI is hindered by impaired cognitive and communicative abilities [21]. Hence, the SNAKE is based on proxy reporting by parents or other caregivers on behalf of their child with respect to the previous four weeks [21]. It consists of 54 items. Of these, 23 items belong to one of the following five scales:

- Disturbances going to sleep
- Disturbances remaining asleep
- Arousal and breathing disorders
- Daytime sleepiness
- Daytime behavior disorders

The remaining 31 items gather information on, for instance, sleep conditions, sleep duration, and efficacy, the core characteristics of the child and his or her family, and aspects of general sleep quality that do not feed into one of the SNAKE scales [21]. Core characteristics are the child's age, sex, weight, height, diagnosis or diagnoses, medication(s), the parents' marital status, where the child predominantly lives, the number of children in the household, the number of people in the household, and who filled out the questionnaire.

A confirmatory factor analysis conducted as part of the initial validation study showed a good fit. Test/retest reliability of the five factors ($r^{rt} > 0.7$) and internal consistencies (Cronbach's alpha > 0.7) are high [21]. The total score of a scale can be derived from the addition of its raw scores. For interpretation, a higher score on a particular scale corresponds with more problematic sleep or sleep-related behavior [31]. The SNAKE is available in English and German and can be requested free of charge as a download from the German Pediatric Pain Center and Pediatric Palliative Care Center [32].

2.3. Global Rating of Sleep Quality

The exact wording of the item asking for a global rating of the child's sleep is: "How would you rate your child's sleep quality overall?" The question can be rated by parents or other caregivers on a 5-point Likert scale (1 = very good, 2 = good, 3 = satisfactory, 4 = poor, and 5 = very poor). For some analyses the items were dichotomized from very good/good and satisfactory to (very) poor.

2.4. Statistical Analyses

Descriptive analyses were applied to describe the core characteristics of the included children and adolescents. The assumptions of normal distribution were checked through the Shapiro–Wilk test. As none of the examined variables were normally distributed (all $p < 0.05$), nonparametric tests were applied. Spearman–Rho correlations identified the relationships between the five SNAKE scales and the global rating, as well as between children's age and the sleep ratings. A correlation coefficient between 0.1 and 0.3 shows a weak association, whereas a coefficient between 0.3 and 0.5 reflects a medium association and a coefficient above 0.5 is indicative of a strong association. A Mann–Whitney U test was conducted and adjusted by Bonferroni correction to see if there were significant differences between the two dichotomized groups (global rating; very good/good–satisfactory to (very) poor) for the five SNAKE scales. The significance level was set at $p = 0.05$ (two-tailed). All analyses were conducted using SPSS (version 25, IBM, Chicago, IL, USA).

3. Results

3.1. Sample Characteristics

Of the $N = 226$ children and adolescents, $n = 14$ had to be excluded ($n = 12$ core parameters incomplete/more than 50% missing; $n = 2$ SNAKE incomplete/more than 50% missing). The final sample consisted of $n = 212$ children and adolescents ($n = 99$, 46.7% female; $n = 113$, 53.3% male) aged between 1 and 25 years ($M = 10.4$; SD = 5.5). Cerebral palsy ($n = 54$, 26.3%), global developmental retardation ($n = 35$, 17.1%), different rare syndromes ($n = 28$, 13.7%) and neurodegenerative diseases/metabolic disorders ($n = 21$, 10.2%) were the most common diagnoses in this sample.

The SNAKE was completed by the mother for $n = 187$ (88.2%) children and by the father for $n = 14$ (6.6%) children (mother and father together: $n = 5$, others: $n = 6$).

Referring to the global sleep rating, $n = 42$ (19.8%) children were rated as having very good, $n = 67$ (31.6%) good, $n = 70$ (33%) satisfactory, $n = 26$ (12.3%) poor, and $n = 7$ (3.3%) very poor sleep during the past four weeks. Children were nearly equally allocated to the two dichotomized groups that reflected the child's general sleep quality (very good/good: $n = 109$, 51.4%; satisfactory to (very) poor: $n = 103$, 48.6%).

3.2. Relationship between the Global Rating of a Child's Sleep and the SNAKE Scales

Table 1 demonstrates the Spearman–Rho correlations between the SNAKE scales and the global sleep rating (all $p < 0.01$). It is clear that each of the five scales correlates positively and significantly with the global rating. The association with the global rating is strong for disturbances in terms of going to sleep and disturbances with respect to remaining asleep, medium for arousal and breathing disorders as well as daytime behavior disorders, and weak for daytime sleepiness.

Table 1. Correlations between five Sleep Questionnaire for Children with Severe Psychomotor Impairment (SNAKE) scales and the global rating of a child's sleep.

Measure	1	2	3	4	5
1. Disturbances going to sleep	-	-	-	-	-
2. Disturbances remaining asleep	0.57 **	-	-	-	-
3. Arousal and breathing disorders	0.34 **	0.45 **	-	-	-
4. Daytime sleepiness	0.10	0.36 **	0.37 **	-	-
5. Daytime behavior disorders	0.45 **	0.50 **	0.30 **	0.14 *	-
6. Global sleep rating	0.61 **	0.73 **	0.41 **	0.23 **	0.44 **

* $p < 0.05$, ** $p < 0.01$.

Mann–Whitney U testing revealed that children who were classified as having a satisfactory to (very) poor sleep during the past four weeks scored significantly higher in all five SNAKE scales as compared to children who were classified as having a very good/good sleep during the abovementioned time frame (Figure 1). This result was also confirmed after Bonferroni correction.

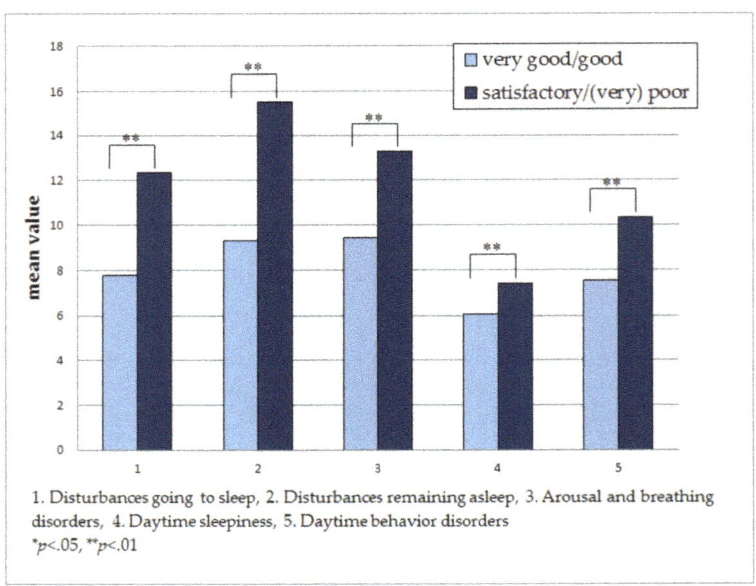

Figure 1. Differences between global sleep quality in the two subgroups for all five scales of the Sleep Questionnaire for Children with Severe Psychomotor Impairment (SNAKE).

3.3. Relationship between Age and Sleep Ratings

Because of the broad age range of children and adolescents that were included in analyses, we further tested if there were any relationships between children's age and the reported sleep problems. "Disturbances going to sleep" ($r = -0.14$, $p < 0.05$), "Daytime sleepiness" ($r = -0.18$, $p < 0.01$) and "Daytime behavior disorders" ($r = -0.23$, $p < 0.01$) correlated negatively and significantly with children's age, i.e., the younger the child, the stronger the sleep disturbance. The remaining two SNAKE scales ("Disturbances remaining asleep" and "Arousal and breathing disorders") and the global rating of a child's sleep did not correlate with children's age (all $p > 0.05$).

4. Discussion

Results show that the two examined sources of information, the global rating of a child's sleep, which directly measures the parents' assessment of their child's sleep quality, and the five SNAKE scales, which indirectly measure the child's sleep behavior, are consistent. The highest concordance with the global rating was achieved for disturbances going to sleep and disturbances remaining asleep.

Analyses reveal positive correlations between all five scales and the global rating. Even though this result must not be interpreted as evidence of causality, it is an important clue that both sources of information tend towards the same direction. This assumption is also supported by the fact that in comparison with children who slept very well or well during the past four weeks, children who were identified as having slept only satisfactorily, poorly or very poorly during that period concurrently obtained significantly higher values for each of the five SNAKE scales and therefore suffered from more sleep problems than children in the other group. This result emphasizes, once more, that the scales seem to be appropriate for mapping sleep(-related) problems in the vulnerable group of children with LLCs and SPMI [21]. Interestingly, the differences between the mean values of the two groups (very good/good; satisfactory to (very) poor) differed between the five scales: They were the largest for scale 2 (disturbances remaining asleep) and the smallest for scale 4 (daytime sleepiness). Thus, some specific aspects of sleep problems in children with LLCs and SPMI seem to distinguish between children with good and poor sleep more strongly than others. Nonetheless, as our questioning and the analyses we conducted do not allow any conclusions to be drawn about the causality of the relationship, we cannot clearly interpret this finding and instead defer to future studies. Three of the five SNAKE scales, but not the global rating of a child's sleep, correlate negatively with children's age. That result indicates that severely disabled children's specific sleep problems decline with children's increasing age; this has also been shown in prior studies [13]. Another explanation could be that parents monitor their child's sleep more intensively when he or she is younger and therefore can make a more precise report on specific sleep problems than parents of older children. Nevertheless, we did not find a relationship between a child's sleep problems in general and the child's age. There are also studies that did not find or do not assume such a decline of sleep problems with increasing age [10,19]. It must be considered that the actual age of children and adolescents with LLCs and SPMI commonly differs from their developmental age, which might be a reason for our inconclusive result. Therefore, investigations are needed to better understand the impact of children's age or developmental age on sleep problems.

In nearly 90% of the cases included in this study, mothers completed the questionnaire. As the mother is often the primary caretaker of their ill child [18,19,33], it can be expected that in general their statements are reliable because of the expertise they have regarding their child's general condition and their child's sleep. Nevertheless, it must be noted that our data are highly subjective and should therefore be underpinned with objective measures such as polysomnography or actigraphy in future research efforts.

In the current sample, children and adolescents of different ages and with different diagnoses are represented. It can therefore be concluded that our results are valid for a broad range of severely disabled children. Nevertheless, we did not consider special characteristics that go along with the children's diagnoses (e.g., need for repositioning, use of ventilation); this additional information would be helpful to refine our findings. Furthermore, we did not compare our results for different groups of diagnoses. Within the framework of this study, this must not be seen as a deficiency because our aim was to make a general statement on the SNAKE's methodological quality. Notwithstanding, the comparison of sleep characteristics of children with different life-limiting diagnoses would be an interesting approach for future studies in general. The global sleep rating of the children and adolescents included in this study was mainly in the "very good", "good", or "satisfactory" range. This result is different from studies that describe a high range of sleep problems in severely disabled children [4]. A reason for that could be that the LLC cohort includes a very heterogeneous group of children and adolescents with various illnesses, comorbidities, and personal characteristics [34]. Therefore, a direct comparison between prevalence rates of different studies on that heterogeneous population is only feasible to a limited extent [35].

A clear limitation of the SNAKE is its lack of cutoff values [21], which makes it impossible to state whether the values the included children reached for the five SNAKE scales are clinically meaningful or not. The implementation of cutoff values is urgently needed to strengthen the usefulness of the SNAKE in clinical contexts.

In summary, the five scales of the SNAKE that indirectly assess different aspects of sleep(-related) problems seem to correspond with the parent's direct judgment on their child's sleep quality. Therefore, our results are additional proof that the SNAKE is a valid questionnaire for assessing sleep problems in severely disabled children. Furthermore, it underscores that in contrast with other pediatric sleep questionnaires [22–24], the SNAKE meets the challenges of children with LLCs and SPMI. Future research should primarily address the development of cutoff values for the SNAKE and the inclusion of objective measures. These efforts would advance knowledge regarding sleep problems in this vulnerable population.

Author Contributions: L.A.S., B.Z. and J.W. made substantial contributions to the conception of the work; L.A.S. performed the statistical analysis and drafted the paper; B.Z., M.B. and J.W. added to the interpretation of data and revised the paper critically for important intellectual content; all authors gave their final approval of the version to be published.

Conflicts of Interest: The authors declare no conflict of interest.

References

1. Fraser, L.K.; Miller, M.; Hain, R.; Norman, P.; Aldridge, J.; McKinney, P.A.; Parslow, R.C. Rising national prevalence of life-limiting conditions in children in england. *Pediatrics* **2012**, *129*, e923–e929. [CrossRef] [PubMed]
2. Fraser, L.K.; Lidstone, V.; Miller, M.; Aldridge, J.; Norman, P.; McKinney, P.A.; Parslow, R.C. Patterns of diagnoses among children and young adults with life-limiting conditions: A secondary analysis of a national dataset. *Palliat. Med.* **2014**, *28*, 513–520. [CrossRef] [PubMed]
3. Garske, D.; Schmidt, P.; Hasan, C.; Wager, J.; Zernikow, B. Palliativversorgung auf der pädiatrischen palliativstation "lichtblicke"—Eine retrospektive studie. *Palliativmedizin* **2016**, *17*, 302–307. [CrossRef]
4. Tietze, A.L.; Blankenburg, M.; Hechler, T.; Michel, E.; Koh, M.; Schluter, B.; Zernikow, B. Sleep disturbances in children with multiple disabilities. *Sleep Med. Rev.* **2012**, *16*, 117–127. [CrossRef] [PubMed]
5. American Academy of Sleep Medicine. *International Classification of Sleep Disorders: Diagnostic and Coding Manual*, 2nd ed.; American Academy of Sleep Medicine: Westchester, IL, USA, 2005.
6. Stores, G. Children's sleep disorders: Modern approaches, developmental effects, and children at special risk. *Dev. Med. Child Neurol.* **1999**, *41*, 568–573. [CrossRef] [PubMed]
7. Atmawidjaja, R.W.; Wong, S.W.; Yang, W.W.; Ong, L.C. Sleep disturbances in malaysian children with cerebral palsy. *Dev. Med. Child Neurol.* **2014**, *56*, 681–685. [CrossRef] [PubMed]
8. Annaz, D.; Hill, C.M.; Ashworth, A.; Holley, S.; Karmiloff-Smith, A. Characterisation of sleep problems in children with Williams syndrome. *Res. Dev. Disabil.* **2011**, *32*, 164–169. [CrossRef] [PubMed]
9. Vandeleur, M.; Walter, L.M.; Armstrong, D.S.; Robinson, P.; Nixon, G.M.; Horne, R.S. How well do children with cystic fibrosis sleep? An actigraphic and questionnaire-based study. *J. Pediatr.* **2017**, *182*, 170–176. [PubMed]
10. Newman, C.J.; O'Regan, M.; Hensey, O. Sleep disorders in children with cerebral palsy. *Dev. Med. Child Neurol.* **2006**, *48*, 564–568. [CrossRef] [PubMed]
11. Bloetzer, C.; Jeannet, P.Y.; Lynch, B.; Newman, C.J. Sleep disorders in boys with Duchenne muscular dystrophy. *Acta Paediatr.* **2012**, *101*, 1265–1269. [CrossRef] [PubMed]

12. Pera, M.C.; Romeo, D.M.; Graziano, A.; Palermo, C.; Messina, S.; Baranello, G.; Coratti, G.; Massaro, M.; Sivo, S.; Arnoldi, M.T.; et al. Sleep disorders in spinal muscular atrophy. *Sleep Med.* **2017**, *30*, 160–163. [CrossRef] [PubMed]
13. Ingram, D.G.; Churchill, S.S. Sleep problems in children with agenesis of the corpus callosum. *Pediatr. Neurol.* **2017**, *67*, 85–90. [CrossRef] [PubMed]
14. Larson, A.M.; Ryther, R.C.; Jennesson, M.; Geffrey, A.L.; Bruno, P.L.; Anagnos, C.J.; Shoeb, A.H.; Thibert, R.L.; Thiele, E.A. Impact of pediatric epilepsy on sleep patterns and behaviors in children and parents. *Epilepsia* **2012**, *53*, 1162–1169. [CrossRef] [PubMed]
15. Romeo, D.M.; Brogna, C.; Musto, E.; Baranello, G.; Pagliano, E.; Casalino, T.; Ricci, D.; Mallardi, M.; Sivo, S.; Cota, F.; et al. Sleep disturbances in preschool age children with cerebral palsy: A questionnaire study. *Sleep Med.* **2014**, *15*, 1089–1093. [CrossRef] [PubMed]
16. Wirrell, E.; Blackman, M.; Barlow, K.; Mah, J.; Hamiwka, L. Sleep disturbances in children with epilepsy compared with their nearest-aged siblings. *Dev. Med. Child Neurol.* **2005**, *47*, 754–759. [CrossRef] [PubMed]
17. Ramgopal, S.; Shah, A.; Zarowski, M.; Vendrame, M.; Gregas, M.; Alexopoulos, A.V.; Loddenkemper, T.; Kothare, S.V. Diurnal and sleep/wake patterns of epileptic spasms in different age groups. *Epilepsia* **2012**, *53*, 1170–1177. [CrossRef] [PubMed]
18. Tietze, A.L.; Zernikow, B.; Michel, E.; Blankenburg, M. Sleep disturbances in children, adolescents, and young adults with severe psychomotor impairment: Impact on parental quality of life and sleep. *Dev. Med. Child Neurol.* **2014**, *56*, 1187–1193. [CrossRef] [PubMed]
19. Morelius, E.; Hemmingsson, H. Parents of children with physical disabilities—Perceived health in parents related to the child's sleep problems and need for attention at night. *Child Care Health Dev.* **2014**, *40*, 412–418. [CrossRef] [PubMed]
20. Adlington, K.; Liu, A.J.; Nanan, R. Sleep disturbances in the disabled child—A case report and literature review. *Aust. Fam. Physician* **2006**, *35*, 711–715. [PubMed]
21. Blankenburg, M.; Tietze, A.L.; Hechler, T.; Hirschfeld, G.; Michel, E.; Koh, M.; Zernikow, B. Snake: The development and validation of a questionnaire on sleep disturbances in children with severe psychomotor impairment. *Sleep Med.* **2013**, *14*, 339–351. [CrossRef] [PubMed]
22. Bruni, O.; Ottaviano, S.; Guidetti, V.; Romoli, M.; Innocenzi, M.; Cortesi, F.; Giannotti, F. The sleep disturbance scale for children (SDSC). Construction and validation of an instrument to evaluate sleep disturbances in childhood and adolescence. *J. Sleep Res.* **1996**, *5*, 251–261. [CrossRef] [PubMed]
23. Cohen, R.; Halevy, A.; Shuper, A. Children's sleep disturbance scale in differentiating neurological disorders. *Pediatr. Neurol.* **2013**, *49*, 465–468. [CrossRef] [PubMed]
24. Owens, J.A.; Spirito, A.; McGuinn, M. The children's sleep habits questionnaire (CSHQ): Psychometric properties of a survey instrument for school-aged children. *Sleep* **2000**, *23*, 1043–1051. [CrossRef] [PubMed]
25. Churchill, S.S.; Kieckhefer, G.M.; Bjornson, K.F.; Herting, J.R. Relationship between sleep disturbance and functional outcomes in daily life habits of children with down syndrome. *Sleep* **2015**, *38*, 61–71. [CrossRef] [PubMed]
26. Breau, L.M.; Camfield, C.S. Pain disrupts sleep in children and youth with intellectual and developmental disabilities. *Res. Dev. Disabil.* **2011**, *32*, 2829–2840. [CrossRef] [PubMed]
27. Wayte, S.; McCaughey, E.; Holley, S.; Annaz, D.; Hill, C.M. Sleep problems in children with cerebral palsy and their relationship with maternal sleep and depression. *Acta Paediatr.* **2012**, *101*, 618–623. [CrossRef] [PubMed]
28. Cortesi, F.; Giannotti, F.; Ottaviano, S. Sleep problems and daytime behavior in childhood idiopathic epilepsy. *Epilepsia* **1999**, *40*, 1557–1565. [CrossRef] [PubMed]
29. Byars, A.W.; Byars, K.C.; Johnson, C.S.; DeGrauw, T.J.; Fastenau, P.S.; Perkins, S.; Austin, J.K.; Dunn, D.W. The relationship between sleep problems and neuropsychological functioning in children with first recognized seizures. *Epilepsy Behav.* **2008**, *13*, 607–613. [CrossRef] [PubMed]
30. Tietze, A.L.; Zernikow, B.; Otto, M.; Hirschfeld, G.; Michel, E.; Koh, M.; Blankenburg, M. The development and psychometric assessment of a questionnaire to assess sleep and daily troubles in parents of children and young adults with severe psychomotor impairment. *Sleep Med.* **2014**, *15*, 219–227. [CrossRef] [PubMed]

31. Otto, M.T.; Tietze, A.-L.; Zernikow, B.; Wager, J. *Sleep Questionnaire for Children with Severe Psychomotor Impairments—Manual*; The German Paediatric Pain Centre and Paediatric Palliative Care Centre, Children's and Adolescents' Clinic Datteln: Datteln, Germany; University of Witten/Herdecke: Witten, Germany, 2014.
32. Sleep Questionnaire for Children with Severe Psychomotor Impairments Version 1.0. German Paediatric Pain Centre and Paediatric Palliative Care Centre. Available online: http://www.deutsches-kinderschmerzzentrum.de/fileadmin/media/PDF-Dateien/englisch/Snake_engl_23_06_15.pdf (accessed on 31 January 2018).
33. Raina, P.; O'Donnell, M.; Rosenbaum, P.; Brehaut, J.; Walter, S.D.; Russell, D.; Swinton, M.; Zhu, B.; Wood, E. The health and well-being of caregivers of children with cerebral palsy. *Pediatrics* **2005**, *115*, e626–e636. [CrossRef] [PubMed]
34. Zernikow, B. *Palliativversorgung von Kindern, Jugendlichen und Jungen Erwachsenen*; Springer: Heidelberg, Germany, 2013; Volume 2.
35. Zernikow, B.; Gertz, B.; Hasan, C. Pädiatrische Palliativversorgung—Herausfordernd Anders. *Bundesgesundheitsblatt* **2017**, *60*, 76–81. [CrossRef] [PubMed]

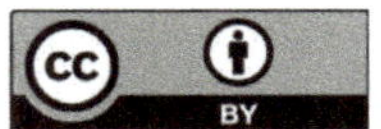

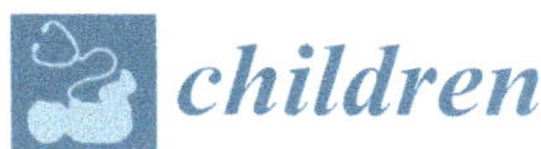
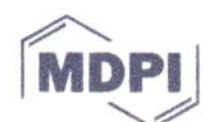

Article

A Review of Apps for Calming, Relaxation, and Mindfulness Interventions for Pediatric Palliative Care Patients

Taelyr Weekly [1], Nicole Walker [2], Jill Beck [2], Sean Akers [2] and Meaghann Weaver [2,*]

[1] Department of Cardiology, University of Nebraska Medical Center, South 42nd Street and Emile Street, Omaha, NE 68198, USA; tjmiller@unmc.edu

[2] Children's Hospital and Medical Center 8200 Dodge Street, Omaha, NE 68114, USA; niwalker@childrensomaha.org (N.W.); jibeck@childrensomaha.org (J.B.); sakers@childrensomaha.org (S.A.)

* Correspondence: meweaver@childrensomaha.org; Tel.: +402-955-5432

Received: 9 November 2017; Accepted: 18 January 2018; Published: 26 January 2018

Abstract: Patients and families increasingly use mobile apps as a relaxation and distraction intervention for children with complex, chronic medical conditions in the waiting room setting or during inpatient hospitalizations; and yet, there is limited data on app quality assessment or review of these apps for level of engagement, functionality, aesthetics, or applicability for palliative pediatric patients. The pediatric palliative care study team searched smartphone application platforms for apps relevant to calming, relaxation, and mindfulness for pediatric and adolescent patients. Apps were reviewed using a systematic data extraction tool. Validated Mobile Application Rating Scale (MARS) scores were determined by two blinded reviewers. Apps were then characterized by infant, child, adolescent, and adult caregiver group categories. Reviewer discussion resulted in consensus. Sixteen of the 22 apps identified were included in the final analysis. The apps operated on either iOS or Android platforms. All were available in English with four available in Spanish. Apps featured a relaxation approach (12/16), soothing images (8/16), and breathing techniques (8/16). Mood and sleep patterns were the main symptoms targeted by apps. Provision of mobile apps resource summary has the potential to foster pediatric palliative care providers' knowledge of app functionality and applicability as part of ongoing patient care.

Keywords: technology; mobile applications; meditation; multimedia; children; palliative; relaxation; stress

---

1. Introduction

Technology represents an entertainment presence for culture; this anecdotally is recognized in the increased presence of audiovisual material use as a distraction technique by parents in waiting rooms and hospital rooms. Approximately three-quarters (77%) of Americans now own a smartphone and half own a tablet computer [1]. Smartphones are near universal among younger adults, with >90% of adolescent and young adults owning a smartphone [1]. With the widespread ownership and access to technology, our pediatric palliative care team wondered whether we may consider leveraging current technology use to include apps for calming, relaxation, and mindfulness rather than strictly gaming apps.

In considering the role of technology in a pediatric clinical setting, our study team considered the roles of both relaxation and distraction (Table 1). Our study team differentiated between relaxation and distraction in terms of the level of participant engagement/activity required. A relaxation app was one that involved active entrance into a focused state of calm such as participatory mindfulness, engaged visualization, or body scan. A distraction app was defined by the study team as one that included a passive receptivity to sound/visual diversion or recreation. Both relaxation and distraction apps each shared an endpoint of a lifting of tension, soothing of anxiety, and restoration to a sense of peace. The vibrant imaginations and full engagement of pediatric patients means that even a distraction app can foster a tranced-equilibrium of deep relaxation.

Electronic interventions such as mindfulness apps and relaxation-based apps have been noted for their positive effect on the general health and psychological well-being of patients with chronic, complex medical conditions [2–4]. Technology distraction is noted to be accepted by pediatric patients [5,6] with improvement in pain management and cooperation.

Table 1. Role of technology in a pediatric medical setting.

App Role	Relevant Clinical Scenario	Examples of App Technique
Relaxation—Actively fosters entering a state of calm; focusing mind; releasing tension	8-year-old hospitalized oncology patient struggling with insomnia limited to hospital setting 12-year-old female with sickle cell disease reporting increased "all over" body pain during month of parents' divorce	Mindfulness Yoga/body movement Meditation, hypnosis, or visualization Body scan
Distraction—Passively offers a diversion or recreation for stress reduction and anxiety alleviation	8-year-old male frightened of needles in lab for blood draw 12-year-old female feeling nervous in busy waiting room while waiting to see doctor for scheduled chemotherapy	Games Soothing images Calming audio

Nervous or anxious feelings are noted as a significant symptom for children in medical settings [5]. The aim of our study was to investigate what apps for relaxation and distraction exist for pediatric palliative patients and to describe the features, qualities, and intended audience.

2. Materials and Methods

2.1. Eliciting Pediatric Relaxation Apps

Smartphone application platform stores, Blackberry World App (Blackberry, Waterloo, ON, Canada), App Store iOS (Apple Inc., Cupertino, CA, USA), and Google Play (Google, Mountain View, CA, USA), were searched between May and July 2017 using keywords: child, pediatric, adolescent, palliative, mindfulness, relaxation, and calm. An announcement was posted on a national Child Life e-mail list to gather additional relaxation application recommendations.

2.2. Procedure for Reviewing the Relaxation Apps

Three reviewers (MW, NW, AW) independently performed eligibility assessments of apps utilizing a pre-determined eligibility checklist. Inclusion criteria included pediatric-specific apps, free apps, and privacy-protecting apps. Exclusion criteria included apps which were not pediatric-specific, apps with a cost, and any app with "open discussion" format of interaction electronically (to protect children from exposure to unknown co-app users). These independent reviewers reached consensus for exclusion/inclusion decision with >88% inter-rater agreement. Five apps were discussed to reach inclusion/exclusion consensus.

The team developed a data extraction sheet in Microsoft Excel (Microsoft, Albuquerque, NM, USA), which underwent a pilot test on three randomly selected apps. Items on the extraction sheet included app name, cost, platform availability, brief summary of the app as posted by the app store, listing of app features, targeted age group, and consumer rating. Each app was reviewed for specific mention of symptom profiles such as stress, anxiety, bullying, trauma, sleep disorders, and depression. Each app was further reviewed for specific mention of relaxation approaches such as stress management, symptom tracking, body scanning, calming audio, diary or journaling, meditation, mood tracking, hypnosis, cognitive behavioral therapy, crisis management, yoga or body movements, brainwave frequencies, spirituality/religious support, breathing techniques, or heart rate and breathing tracking. The data extraction sheet included items for study team members to indicate their perspective on the positive and concerning features of each app, age appropriateness, and level of app interaction (specifically whether the app could be used for children with fine motor skill limitations). Reviewers provided descriptions of app relevance to pediatric palliative care.

Reviewers utilized the Mobile Application Rating Scale (MARS) classification score to measure app aesthetics, engagement, functionality, and overall quality [7]. The MARS is a validated, objective, and reliable tool for assessing the quality of mobile health apps [7]. The 23-item MARS questionnaire results in a mean score from 1–5 specific to engagement, functionality, aesthetics, and information domains. Higher mean score per domain represents higher quality.

A team of six reviewers (MW, AW, SA, JB, NW, TM) from disciplines of palliative care, psychology, child life (child development specialist), and nursing systematically reviewed apps in full with two reviewers downloading and using each app program a minimum of one session per reviewer. These two study team members independently completed the data extraction per app and each reviewer entered the data into an Excel extraction template designed by two study team members (MW and AW) to enable consistent data formatting for team analysis. A minimum of one additional study team member also downloaded each app, utilized the app for a full session, and checked data extraction to recognize differences of opinion and recirculate these findings back to primary and secondary reviewers for agreement.

2.3. Data Analysis

Data analysis followed a pre-determined quantification of extracted items and content analysis. This approach facilitated the recognition of patterns, variations, and relationships from extracted data. The two reviewers' MARS scores were averaged per engagement, functionality, aesthetics, and information domains.

3. Results

A total of 22 apps were identified with two then excluded on full application review as they were not pediatric-specific, three excluded due to cost, and one excluded due to "open discussion" format of electronic interaction. Two nonduplicative applications were added from the listserv project announcement. This resulted in 16 total apps for inclusion.

Apps used either the iOS (Apple Inc.) or Android (Google) operating systems with 15/16 (94%) available on both platforms. All of the apps included were available in English, with four of the apps available in Spanish. All of the included apps were available for free. Nine of the apps were identified as potentially relevant for the infant group, 14 for the elementary group, 16 for the adolescent group, and 15 for the adult caregiver category. The study team analyzed the apps for level of required interaction to determine each app's feasibility for children with limited fine motor coordination, of which eight of the 16 (50%) apps could be started and then required no further user-initiated action.

Symptoms specifically targeted by the apps included: stress (50%), sleep disorders (38%), anxiety (38%), general mental health (25%), and depression (19%). There were two apps that did not fit any of the specifically mentioned symptoms (Fluid app [8] and Kindoma Drawtime app [9]).

A majority of the apps, 12/16 (75%), featured a relaxation approach and 11/16 (69%) used a stress management technique. A total of 8/16 (50%) featured soothing images and 8/16 (50%) included a guided breathing technique. Apps targeted specific coping mechanisms such as: calming music (44%), calming words (44%), mindfulness approach (38%), meditation (38%), yoga (31%), body scan (25%), symptom tracking (19%), mood tracking (19%), cognitive behavioral therapy (13%), games (13%), and brainwave frequencies (6%).

MARS domain scores are available in Table 2.

Table 2. App listing and characteristics.

App Name	Description	Language Available	MARS Engagement	MARS Functionality	MARS Aesthetics	MARS Information	Suggested Age Group	App Approach
Breathe, Think, Do with Sesame [10]	Teaches breathing techniques while offering fun interactive games.	English/Spanish	High 4.6	High 4.7	High 4.7	High 4	Infant, Preschool	Game simulation for breathing exercises
Breathe2Relax [11]	Animated video with demonstration of breathing technique. Customizable breathing app.	English	High 3.8	High 4.8	High 4	High 4.6	Elementary and above	Breathing exercises
Smiling Mind [12]	Guided meditations separated by age group.	English	Medium 3	High 4	High 3.7	High 3.4	Elementary and above	Meditation
Calm [13]	App for mindfulness, meditation, breathing, and improved sleep.	English	High 4.4	High 4.8	High 5	High 3.5	Elementary and above	Meditation and breathing exercises
MyCalmBeat [14]	Breath training to slow breaths to six breaths per minute.	English	High 3.6	High 4.8	High 5	High 4	Elementary and above	Breathing exercises
Nature Sounds [15]	This app offers different relaxing sounds. You can make playlists and save your favorites.	English/Spanish	Medium 3	High 5	High 4.7	High 4.4	Elementary and above	Relaxing audio sounds
Headspace [16]	Teaches a new meditation technique each day.	English	High 4	High 4	High 4	High 3.8	Elementary and above	Meditation
Mindshift [17]	Anxiety specific. Coping with and facing anxiety.	English	High 4.8	High 5	High 4.3	High 4.5	Adolescent and above	Meditation, yoga, and cognitive therapy
Kindoma Drawtime [9]	Video chat for young children and their loved ones to draw together.	English	High 4.2	High 4.3	High 4.7	High 4	All	Real time video chat; relational and creative
Kindoma Storytime [18]	Video chat plus books for young children and their loved ones to read together.	English	High 4.4	High 4.3	High 4.7	High 4	All	Real time video chat; relational
Nature Sounds [19]	Relaxation, using audio sounds, nature images for background.	English	Medium 2.6	High 4	Medium 2.6	Medium 2.3	All	Relaxing audio sounds
Art of Glow [20]	Create kinetic colorful art e.g., fireworks, colors glow.	English	Medium 2.8	High 3.5	Medium 3	Medium 3	All	Relaxing visual images
Nature Sounds Relax and Sleep [21]	Nature sounds to promote relaxation and sleep.	English	Medium 2.8	High 4	Medium 2.3	Medium 2.6	All	Relaxing audio sounds
Relax Melodies [22]	Offers 52 sounds and melodies that can be combined by user preference. Has timer and alarm. Also offers five-day meditation programs.	English/Spanish	High 3.6	High 4.8	High 4.7	High 3.7	All	Relaxing audio sounds
Fluid [8]	Touch screen into liquid surface—makes drops/waves.	English	Medium 3	High 4	Medium 3.3	Medium 2.4	All	Relaxing visual images
Koi Pond Lite [23]	Nature scene, water, fish, flowers—can customize.	English/Spanish	Medium 3	High 4	High 3.6	Medium 2.4	All	Relaxing visual images

MARS: Validated Mobile Application Rating Scale.

4. Discussion

Increased availability and acceptance of mobile technology offers interesting, creative, and vibrant exposure to various relaxation techniques. However, this requires provider knowledge of what apps exist and what activity options are available. The study team utilized a novel systematic approach to investigate apps by assigning two blinded reviewers per app and by utilizing a validated app quality rating tool (MARS). This approach to app review was entertaining and educational for reviewers but was also challenging due to the seemingly subjective nature of app approval (interestingly, inter-rater agreement was high at 88%). This study offers the foundational information needed to inform providers of available applications which can serve as the base for increased use of technology for calming, relaxation, and mindfulness.

While our study team prioritizes the role for human interaction in calming techniques and strategies, the reality is that many of our patients currently already use "gaming" as a form of distraction. As a care team, we have collectively opted to still prioritize and emphasize relational relaxation techniques as our primary relaxation intervention. For those families who are already incorporating technology for distraction, we pursued app review to emphasize the relaxation component of technology use rather than just the distraction component. Our study team is now working on creating a handout of calming, relaxation, and mindfulness app resources for patients and families and loading tablets with symptom-specific apps for children and families to "try out" with a knowledgeable care provider while in the medical setting. The goal of "trying out" is to foster relational and interaction component to use that could be continued in a home setting with parent-child interaction. This study purposed to research relaxation apps targeted to pediatric age groups to create a reference guide for families. When families are utilizing technology with children, the format of technology would ideally be not just individual gaming activities but purposeful, relational relaxation using technology tools [24].

The apps which most compelled our study team were those with creative, relational use of calming technology for children include Kindoma [9,18], which allows parents to actively color/draw with their child even from a distance, or apps which allow a parent to read a bedtime story to a child from a distance. Calm [13] and Mindshift [17] apps allowed for a speaker version which would allow a parent and child to breathe together for a partnered relaxation approach. Fluid allows more than one finger or hand to pull colors on the screen at one time, allowing a parent and child to co-design calming patterns.

Although the app search was focused on pediatric age ranges, the calming kinetics of nature imagery, soothing music, and guided meditations have potential to appeal to both pediatric patients and their parental caregivers. Further research will explore the effectiveness of these apps in clinical practice. Next steps for engagement include pilot studies grounded in participatory approach to measure not only the self-reported experience of pediatric palliative care patients and their family members through qualitative inquiry and patient reported outcomes but also meaningful concurrent biometric outcomes such as measured physiologic changes with app use. Most exciting would be the eventual development of a pediatric palliative care app for calming, relaxation, and mindfulness designed with children and families receiving palliative care based on a combined culmination of favorite app features and patient-specific feedback on app quality.

5. Conclusions

The provision of a mobile apps resource summary has the potential to foster pediatric palliative care providers' knowledge of app functionality and applicability as part of ongoing patient care.

Acknowledgments: The study team wishes to thank the Hand in Hand Pediatric Palliative care team.

Author Contributions: M.W. and T.W. worked on study design. All authors participated in data extraction and app review. M.W. and T.W. co-wrote the manuscript with all authors approving final edition.

Conflicts of Interest: The authors declare no conflict of interest.

References

1. Record Shares of Americans Now Own Smartphones, Have Home Broadband. Available online: http://www.pewresearch.org/fact-tank/2017/01/12/evolution-of-technology/# (accessed on 18 August 2017).
2. Mikolasek, M.; Berg, J.; Witt, C.M.; Barth, J. Effectiveness of mindfulness- and relaxation-based eHealth interventions for patients with medical conditions: A systematic review and synthesis. *Int. J. Behav. Med.* **2017**. [CrossRef] [PubMed]
3. Munster-Segev, M.; Fuerst, O.; Kaplan, S.A.; Cahn, A. Incorporation of a stress reducing mobile app in the vare of patients with type 2 diabetes: A prospective study. *JMIR mHealth uHealth* **2017**, *5*, e75. [CrossRef] [PubMed]
4. Guided education and training via smartphones in subthreshold post-traumatic stress disorder. *Cyberpsychol. Behav. Soc. Netw.* **2017**, *20*, 470–478. [CrossRef]
5. Bagnasco, A.; Pezzi, E.; Rosa, F.; Fornonil, L.; Sasso, L. Distraction techniques in children during venipuncture: An Italian experience. *J. Prev. Med. Hyg.* **2012**, *53*, 44–48. [CrossRef] [PubMed]
6. Törnqvist, E.; Månsson, Å.; Hallström, I. Children having magnetic resonance imaging. *J. Child Health Care* **2015**, *19*, 359–369. [CrossRef] [PubMed]
7. Stoyanov, S.R.; Hides, L.; Kavanagh, D.J.; Zelenko, O.; Tjondronegoro, D.; Mani, M. Mobile app rating scale: A new tool for assessing the quality of health mobile apps. *JMIR mHealth uHealth* **2015**, *3*. [CrossRef] [PubMed]
8. *Fluid*, version 3.0; David Samuel: Hong Kong, China, 2015.
9. *Kindoma Drawtime*, version 2.7; Kindoma Inc.: Palo Alto, CA, USA, 2017.
10. *Breathe, Think, Do with Sesame*, version 1.5.7; Sesame Workshop: New York, NY, USA, 2016.
11. *Breath2Relax*, version 2.9; National Center for Telehealth & Technology: Joint Base Lewis-McChord, WA, USA, 2016.
12. *Smiling Mind*, version 3.2.6; Smiling Mind: Carlton, Australia, 2018.
13. *Calm*, version 3.12.1; Calm: San Francisco, CA, USA, 2018.
14. *MyCalmBeat*, version 2.4; MyBrainSolutions: San Francisco, CA, USA, 2015.
15. *Nature Sounds*, version 3.0.2; Relaxio: Petrzalka, Slovakia, 2017.
16. *Headspace*, version 3.2.5; Headspace, Inc.: Santa Monica, CA, USA, 2018.
17. *Mindshift*, version 1.2.3; Anxiety Disorders Association of British Columbia: Vancouver, BC, Canada, 2017.
18. *Kindoma Storytime*, version 4.7.0; Kindoma Inc.: Palo Alto, CA, USA, 2017.
19. *Nature Sounds*, version 3.3; Dream_Studio: Dąbrówka, Poland, 2018.
20. *Art of Glow*, version 1.0.8; Natenai Ariyatrakoo, 2015.
21. *Nature Sounds Relax and Sleep*, version 2.10; Zodinplex: Lipniki, Poland, 2016.
22. *Relax Melodies*, version 6.7.4; Ipnos Software: St-Bruno, QC, Canada, 2018.
23. *Koi Pond Lite*, version 1.1.1; 3Planesoft: Vologda, Russia, 2013.
24. Culbert, T. Prespectives on Technology-Assisted Relaxation Approaches to Support Mind-Body Skills Practice in Children and Teens: Clinical Experience and Commentary. *Children* **2017**, *4*, 20. [CrossRef] [PubMed]

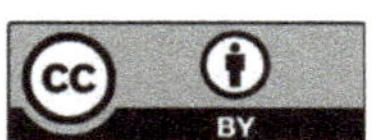

MDPI
St. Alban-Anlage 66
4052 Basel
Switzerland
Tel. +41 61 683 77 34
Fax +41 61 302 89 18
www.mdpi.com

Children Editorial Office
E-mail: children@mdpi.com
www.mdpi.com/journal/children

www.ingramcontent.com/pod-product-compliance
Lightning Source LLC
Chambersburg PA
CBHW051728210326
41597CB00032B/5643
* 9 7 8 3 0 3 8 9 7 3 5 0 8 *